OPTIMISING FEMALE ATHLETIC PERFORMANCE

Optimising Female Athletic Performance presents a comprehensive overview of the wide range of factors that underpin female athletic performance based on the most up-to-date research. This book draws from the disciplines of anatomy, physiology, psychology, and sociology to develop an integrated approach and illustrates how female athletes can be safely prepared for training and performance in a way that benefits their health and optimises their performance. The book covers the specific challenges active females encounter as they move through their lives from childhood, puberty, adolescence, adulthood, potentially motherhood, and on to the menopausal stage.

As well as presenting the key knowledge and research around female athletic performance, each chapter includes real-world examples in the form of case studies and athletes' experiences. Each chapter concludes with a summary offering key points and takeaway messages for coaches and practicing athletes, as well as end-of-chapter quizzes to allow students to assess their own learning and knowledge.

Optimising Female Athletic Performance is key reading for undergraduate students studying sports science and sports coaching degrees who aspire to a career working with female athletes in a range of contexts and environments. Content has been presented in a way that is easily accessible to students and to facilitate the practical application of knowledge by practitioners in a range of sport and exercise settings. It is also useful to active females to understand their own performance and enhance their experience of sport and fitness.

Jess Pinchbeck, PhD is a Senior Lecturer in Sport and Fitness at The Open University, UK and has over 18 years of teaching experience in both further and higher education, she is deeply committed to promoting and empowering women and girls to engage in positive sports experiences.

Candice Lingam-Willgoss, PhD has worked for 22 years in higher education across a range of sport science disciplines, her research interests focus closely on improving our understanding of females' experiences in sport, specifically how females navigate their journey through sport.

Simon Rea is a Senior Lecturer in Sport and Fitness at The Open University, UK and has spent over 20 years teaching in higher education and has worked in several sports science-related roles and written extensively about many disciplines in sports science. He is committed to producing resources to help male coaches and personal trainers understand the female experience of sport and fitness.

OPTIMISING FEMALE ATHLETIC PERFORMANCE

Jess Pinchbeck, Candice Lingam-Willgoss and Simon Rea

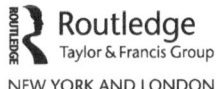
Routledge
Taylor & Francis Group

NEW YORK AND LONDON

Designed cover image: Getty images

First published 2025
by Routledge
605 Third Avenue, New York, NY 10158

and by Routledge
4 Park Square, Milton Park, Abingdon, Oxon OX14 4RN

Routledge is an imprint of the Taylor & Francis Group, an informa business

Library of Congress Cataloging-in-Publication Data
A catalog record for this title has been requested

ISBN: 978-1-032-36070-6 (hbk)
ISBN: 978-1-032-36069-0 (pbk)
ISBN: 978-1-003-33011-0 (ebk)

DOI: 10.4324/9781003330110

Typeset in Sabon
by Taylor & Francis Books

CONTENTS

FIGURES

TABLES

BOXES

1

INTRODUCTION

Jess Pinchbeck, Candice Lingam-Willgoss and Simon Rea

Introduction

This book provides a comprehensive overview of the broad range of factors that underpin female athletic performance. The crucial term used in this book is 'female athletic performance' which encompasses the performance and participation of women and girls involved in physical activity. This includes those who exercise to improve health and fitness, as well as those involved in recreational and competitive sport, spanning all the way to elite athletes operating at the pinnacle of their respective sports. Optimising female athletic performance can be achieved through the application of empirical evidence from a range of disciplines to ensure that female athletes are working with their unique physiologies in safe, supportive environments. This book emphasises a holistic approach to female athletic performance and draws attention to the complex interactions between the physiological, psychological, and sociological factors that impact on female athletes.

From our own research into the field of female athletic performance we have concluded that there is an increasing demand for greater knowledge and understanding of the multidimensional influences on the performance of female athletes. This necessitates the integration of high-quality research to inform and advance this area of study. Throughout their lives females will go through significant lifecycle changes. These changes commence during childhood as they move through puberty, into their adolescent years, onto adulthood and potentially motherhood. Following that, they move into their menopausal and post-menopausal stages. Each stage of the lifecycle brings with it specific physical, psychological, and social challenges that can affect women's performance, their attitudes towards physical activity and the amount of time that they can invest in it. While there is existing research in this area more knowledge is required to

DOI: 10.4324/9781003330110-1

construct a comprehensive understanding of female athletes and assess the specific support they may need at different stages of their athletic development.

One area where more research is required is around the anatomical and physiological differences between male and female athletes, with particular attention paid to the menstrual cycle, breast health and pelvic floor function in relation to sports performance. Furthermore, it is imperative that research evidence in this area is accessible to a range of different audiences. This accessibility can help athletes and coaches better understand the menstrual cycle and how it can impact on athletic performance, potentially contribute to injury risk, be affected by hormonal contraception, and suffer disruption from low energy availability. Yet, collectively as academics from three different disciplines we advocate the significance of the person as well as the athlete, extending beyond the anatomical and physiological differences to further encompass sociological and psychological areas of study.

This book draws upon our own research, for example, Jess's thesis explored sociocultural factors that influence female sports participation, whereas Candice's thesis examined the transitional experiences of elite female athletes. Jess's work is grounded in sociology and emphasised the extent to which childhood experiences of sport may shape adult participation and the complexities of this connection. Jess's research highlighted the social processes that influence the behaviours, tastes, and judgements of women at different life stages. Candice's area of expertise lies within the discipline of psychology and focuses on the stages around pregnancy and the transition into motherhood. Candice's research exposed the lack of knowledge by key stakeholders around how to support the pregnant athlete, in terms of how to support training during pregnancy as well as the return to sport from a physical, psychological, and sociological perspective. Furthermore, this research highlighted how many sports environments remain heavily gendered with women poorly supported. Simon has produced a range of resources in the area of female athletic performance in conjunction with *The Well HQ* to support active females but also to support the work of coaches and trainers. In particular, he has written a free online course for The Open University and created several educational animations around key issues affecting female athletes.

In addition to our academic and professional roles we also have applied experience of working with female athletes. Simon has a wealth of practical experience having worked with females of all ages as a personal trainer. Jess is a Level 2 netball coach working with 11–16-year-olds and Candice is a Level 2 triathlon coach who specialised in coaching youth athletes including elite performers. Also, as mothers of teenage daughters, and as active women, Candice and Jess also hold a personal interest and have their own experiences of what it means to be an active female.

Rationale for the book

Over the past few decades there has been a significant increase in female participation in sport and exercise. Women's sport has become increasingly professionalised with football, rugby union, netball and cricket now being played by full time, professional athletes in the UK and many other countries. With this professionalisation, there has been a parallel increase in demand for expertise to support female athletic performance. Sports coaches, fitness trainers and strength and conditioning coaches require specific knowledge to enable them to work effectively with female athletes to achieve optimal performance and to protect their health.

While there is a need to support female athletes better, women's sport has been failed spectacularly by research and science that for many years has focused on researching male athletes with the assumption that findings must also apply to females. Thus, up until recently, females have predominantly used male-centric training methods and techniques, and worn clothing and footwear designed for male athletes. Data shows that sport science research has focused predominantly on using male participants with only around 6 per cent of sports science research focusing exclusively on female athletes (Cowley et al., 2021). To address these issues there is a developing body of knowledge around female sporting performance with research being published in journals and the pub-lication of seminal academic texts such as *The Exercising Female* (Forsyth and Roberts, 2019) and books aimed at a wider audience such as *The Female Body Bible* (Ross et al., 2023) that are seeking to educate female athletes and those who support them.

The rationale for writing this book was to complement the existing texts in this area and create an accessible, evidence-based resource that applies the aca-demic study of female athletes to practical settings. Its purpose is twofold: first to assist undergraduate students studying sport-related degrees who aspire to work with female athletes in a variety of roles and settings. This text will sup-port them to develop their understanding and comprehension of the area by offering information and recommendations to optimise performance. Second, the text aims to extend its impact through the accessible content to allow it to provide a valuable resource for a broader audience including female athletes, those working in coaching roles, as well as the wider groups who may have an interest in female athletic performance. The use of case studies and real-life examples show how the content of each chapter can be applied by both female athletes and those working with them to optimise performance. As women's sport continues to rise in prominence, at both recreational and elite level, this book serves as a valuable teaching resource that contributes towards the exist-ing gap in women's sport literature.

Introduction to content

To achieve the aims of this book, we have selected topics that we, as academics, coaches, and researchers ourselves, consider have most relevance to female athletes and coaches to enable them to optimise performance. We begin in Chapter 2 by drawing attention to the gender gaps in sport and sports science research that may contribute to some of the challenges female athletes face in sporting environments. In Chapter 3 research on the impact of the menstrual cycle on training and performance is examined, assessing how coaches and athletes can work with a female's biology rather than working against it. Chapter 4 investigates the topic of hormonal contraception as it is often used by female athletes to mitigate the impact of the menstrual cycle, and an assessment of research evidence informs the discussion as to whether this is a good strategy to adopt.

The impact of the menstrual cycle remains a key theme throughout the book as it can influence virtually every aspect of a female's health. Chapter 5 covers the link between low energy availability, caused by an inadequate diet, and the loss, or disruption, to the menstrual cycle that can have serious consequences for a female's health. Chapters 6 to 8 consider some specific anatomical concerns for female athletes; first, in Chapter 6 the role of breast support and its impact on health and performance outcomes is explored, concluding with recommendations on how this can be managed by the female athlete and their coach. Chapter 7 investigates the pelvic floor, assessing how a healthy pelvic floor should perform, and looking at the two main types of pelvic floor dysfunction women experience. In Chapter 8 the theme of musculoskeletal concerns is continued by reviewing the research evidence around whether there are specific injuries that female athletes are more prone to experience, with a focus on anterior cruciate ligament (ACL) injuries and concussions. In each chapter, the authors use scientific evidence to review the topic and apply this to real world scenarios alongside their recommendations for practice.

In Chapters 9 to 13 we move on to consider a broader range of psychological and social influences across the various life stages of the female athlete and the specific challenges they can create. This starts in Chapter 9 which focuses on the adolescent athlete and the challenges faced as girls move through puberty into the teenage years. The impact on participation in sport and sports performance is discussed along with practical recommendations for coaches, parents, and the athlete themselves.

The timing of a female's athletic career may coincide with peak fertility, and many athletes navigate pregnancy and the post-natal period alongside participation and performance. Chapter 10 examines hormonal changes that occur during pregnancy creating significant musculoskeletal, cardiovascular, and psychological transformations in the female and these offer both opportunities and challenges to the female when training or competing. Understanding the impact of these changes is vital to training safely and effectively during the three trimesters of pregnancy as well as the post-natal stage and the considerations that need to be taken into account when returning to training.

Following on from pregnancy Chapter 11 moves into an exploration of motherhood drawing upon literature as well as primary research by Jess and

Candice to inform the debate. Motherhood is a key transition in a woman's life and can have a significant impact on both participation in sport and athletic performance. This chapter focuses on the psycho-social factors that women combining motherhood with athletic performance may face, both at recreational and elite level. Chapter 12 explores sociological research, drawing on the literature and Jess's own research into the role of the family and how the family environment can shape a girl's participation in and attitude to sport that may carry on to their adulthood. Family is often integral to athletic performance, as both physical and emotional support are vital to develop an environment where the female athlete can succeed.

In Chapter 13 the focus shifts to the later stage of a female's lifecycle when they may still be competing in masters/seniors events or exercising recreationally. As the female passes through her 40s into her 50s she is likely to experience physical and emotional changes in response to a reduction in the hormones that drove her menstrual cycle. Again, this stage can have its own challenges as women may experience menopausal symptoms that can affect daily life. Finally in Chapter 14 aspects of the coach-athlete relationship are explored to assess whether there are differences in how coaches, male and female, should approach coaching female athletes. There is a particular focus on how females may prefer to communicate and the coaching styles they may respond to best. Understanding these subtle variations is vital for coaches when creating a positive coaching environment, and also for the female athlete so they know when they are part of a coaching environment that can optimise their performance.

Our manifesto: the past, present, and future of women's sport

This book is our own manifesto demonstrating our passion towards closing the gender gap in sports participation and optimising female sports performance. Based on our individual experiences of researching in this area it is evident that significant gaps exist within the female sports science literature and that existing research is often lacking in quality or the breadth and depth of studies to accurately draw conclusions. As women's sport continues to grow, and to enable female performances to consistently improve, it is our aim to educate, through a variety of means, female athletes themselves as well as those coaching girls and women in sport to create an environment where females can thrive. To achieve this we feel that research, teaching, and practice in female sport needs to be based upon the following three principles:

1   Quality sport and exercise science research with female participants.

   Ensuring that sport and exercise science research is equally inclusive of female athletes and female sport with specific studies focusing on female anatomical and physiological features such as menstruation, breast health, pregnancy, and musculo-skeletal injuries, and the application to training and performance.

2 Research on female participation and performance needs to be multidisciplinary.

Research into female sports participation and performance should include research from multiple disciplines to adopt a holistic and bio-psycho-social approach to female sports performance and participation. A multi-disciplinary approach offers a greater solution to address the wider issues within female sport participation and performance such as family support, adolescence, pregnancy, motherhood, and the menopause.

3 Dissemination of research to key stakeholders in female sport and exercise.

Research from all sport science disciplines should be disseminated using appropriate resources to all stakeholders to educate both athletes themselves and those working with female athletes to possess the appropriate knowledge and understanding to create a positive training environment and to optimise performance. This includes educating the coach educators and encouraging coach-athlete dialogue using language and vocabulary pertaining to the female body. In this way everyone will feel comfortable discussing these natural processes and any 'taboo' elements can be eliminated.

We sincerely hope that the content of this book will go some way to supporting these principles and making sporting environments equally fulfilling for male and female athletes.

Note on terminology

The content in this book relates to athletes who identify as cisgender women and girls. When we use the terms 'sports woman' and 'female athletes' we are referring to those people who have female genitals, have gone through puberty as a female, and have, or had, a menstrual cycle.

References

Cowley, E.S., Olenick, A.A., McNulty, K.L. and Ross, E.Z. (2021) '"Invisible sportswomen": the sex data gap in sport and exercise science research', *Women in Sport and Physical Activity Journal*, 29(2), 146–151. Available at: https://journals.humankinetics.com/ view/ journals/wspaj/29/2/article-p146.xml (Accessed: 16 May 2023).

Reuters (2023) 'Women's World Cup final draws record TV figures in Spain, England'. Available at: www.reuters.com/sports/soccer/womens-world-cup-final-draws-record-tv-figures-spain-england-2023-08-21 (Accessed: 22 August 2023).

Ross, E.Z., Moffat, B. and Smith, B. (2023) *The Female Body Bible*. London: Penguin.

Seary, K. (2023) 'Female Athlete Health Report'. Available at: *The Female Athlete Health Report 2023 – Kyniska Advocacy* (Accessed: 22 August 2023).

Sport England (2022) *Active Lives Survey* 21–22. Available at: www.sportengland.org/research-and-data/data/active-lives/active-lives-data-tables#november-2021-22-22323 (Accessed: 29 August 2023).

Statista (2023) *Number of women who participated in sport and physical activity at least twice in the last 28 days in England from 2016 to 2021.* Available at: https://www.statista.com/statistics/1024168/female-sport-physical-activity-participation-england/ (Accessed: 22 August 2023).

2

THE RESEARCH GENDER GAP AND ITS IMPACT ON FEMALE HEALTH AND ATHLETIC PERFORMANCE

Candice Lingam-Willgoss

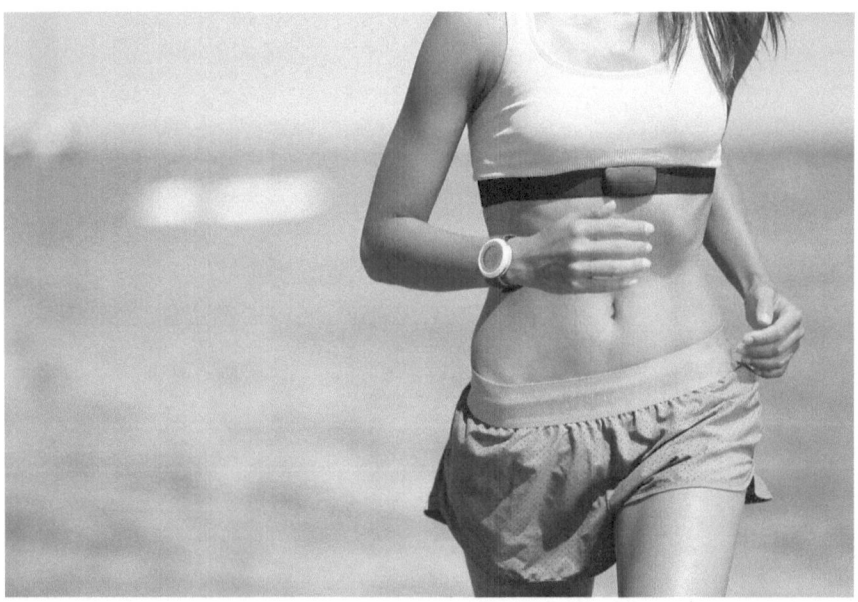

Introduction

The prevalence and representation of women in elite sport has increased significantly in recent years, with representation at the Tokyo 2020 Olympic Games seeing near parity in terms of events and medals available to females, with female competitors representing 48 per cent of athletes (Smith et al., 2022). While these tangible improvements in participation and performance are evident, they still fail

DOI: 10.4324/9781003330110-2

to be replicated within sport science and sports medicine research where there remains a significant research gender gap. These gaps present a challenge when looking to develop an evidence-informed approach to practice. Evidence developed with male athletes cannot simply be applied to female athletes, owing to the numerous biological differences between the sexes. Within this chapter the aim is to explore in depth why these research gaps exist and the implication this has on both recreational and elite female athletes in terms of health and performance. Through examining the disservice that limited gender specific research has on female athletes this chapter will start to look at the benefits of adopting a female-centric approach to planning training and recovery schedules that are tailored for female athletes.

While progress has been made, challenges remain regarding both equality in society and also within sport, with sport remaining a heavily gendered area that can position women as the outsiders (Fink, 2008). As touched on, in recent years the growth in female participation in sport has led to more focus and interest in female athletes (Castanier et al., 2021), and as a result there has been a significant rise in both the professionalism and the profile of elite female sports and athletes (Fink, 2015). However, even with increased airtime and coverage for female sports there remains a disparity between male and female sports in terms of opportunity and exposure, which is also reflected in the sports performance literature (Emmonds et al., 2019). Even though biological gender has been shown to be a determining factor in athletic performance, for example in terms of aerobic capacity, weight and muscle mass (Perez-Gomez et al., 2008), research conducted using male participants is still being used to explain female performance.

Yet, things are starting to change and with the evolution of professionalism within women's sport, which has afforded women the opportunity to be full-time athletes, a growing body of research is emerging within sport science and sport medicine. This research seeks to understand more of the gendered experiences of female athletes. For example, Brown et al.'s (2021) research focused on the experience and perception of menstruation on training and sport performance: 17 elite female athletes from a range of different sports were interviewed, with results suggesting that all athletes had needed to manage the stages of their cycle appropriately, owing to a range of factors, for example, mood disturbance and reduced motivation to train. Notably, even those athletes who did not experience discernible changes did report this time to be a potential distraction during times of competition.

A further implication of Brown's study was that it identified a lack of openness in discussing issues unique to the female athlete such as the menstrual cycle. This topic is discussed in more depth in Chapter 3 but it does highlight one key area that requires more female specific research to be conducted. This suggests there is a real need to develop more positive conversations in order to facilitate open and honest understanding between athlete and coach, especially when the coach is male (de Haan and Norman, 2020). The importance of this is even more significant when we consider how there tend to be more men in positions of power (e.g. coaching) within sport (Norman, 2018).

While female specific research has become more established in recent years, most research is comparative in design as it examines gender differences rather than solely exploring the female journey (e.g. de Subijana et al., 2020). Statistics show that female only research is rare with just 6 per cent of publications using female only participants compared with 31 per cent using male subjects (Cowley et al., 2021).

Why is research using female participants important?

The female experience within sport has several unique factors that have the potential to impact on all aspects of performance and health. Furthermore, it is important to recognise that as well as the biological differences between the sexes there are a range of psychological and social factors that require more research. These factors are illustrated in Figure 2.1 which also highlights key areas covered within this book. Through gaining a deeper understanding of the female athletic experience from a bio-psycho-social perspective, all those involved in sport, from athlete to coach, to parent or partner, can ultimately provide better support to the athlete.

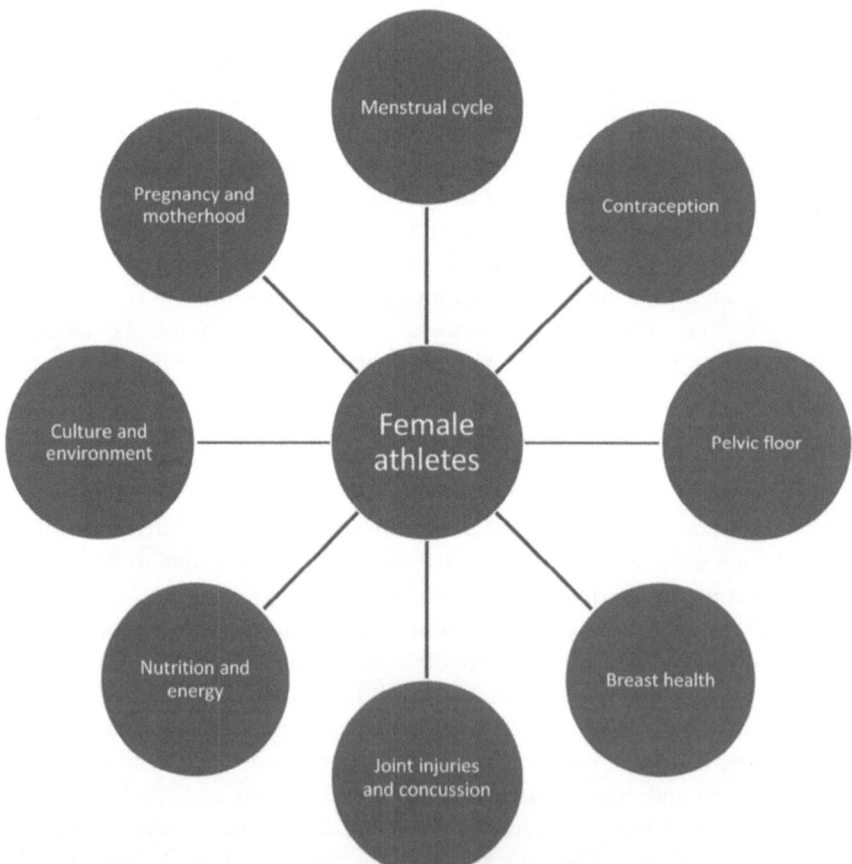

FIGURE 2.1 Factors to consider when working with female athletes
Source: Adapted from Rea, 2022.

Before we start to look at the gender research gap in more depth, Box 2.1 introduces Rebecca, an elite snowboarder, who was involved in a sport where there is very little understanding or consideration of female athletes.

BOX 2.1 REBECCA (SNOWBOARDER)

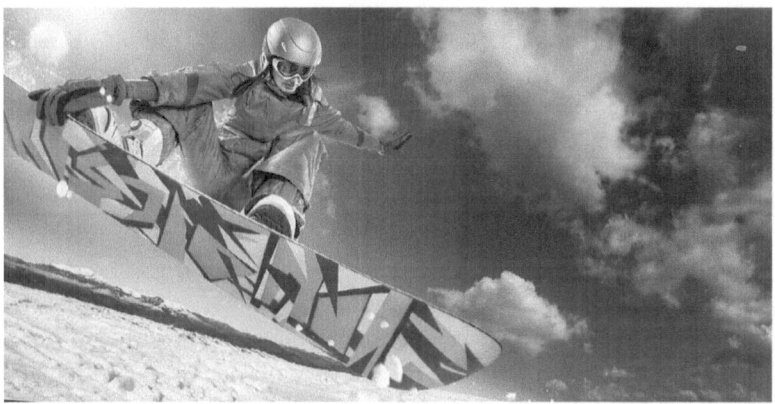

Rebecca is a 45-year-old snowboard coach. As a child growing up in a family of snow sport athletes Rebecca started snowboarding at the age of five, owing largely to her desire to be like her older brothers. Being the youngest sibling, she typically used second hand kit handed down from her brothers.

At the age of 14 she joined a club where all the coaches were men and she was the only girl in the team. The coaches were very experienced and great at coaching, but as a young girl Rebecca often felt isolated and a bit of an outsider. Training was also undertaken with everyone together and when Rebecca reached 16 and started to engage with strength and conditioning work she found herself being compared to the boys, this often felt quite demoralising and she did consider giving up as she just wasn't hitting the same numbers as them.

At the age of 22 she was selected for Team GB and started to receive lottery funding and while there remained disparity, in terms of specific support such as the structure of training sessions and management of injury, Rebecca was very successful gaining World Cup podiums and an Olympic medal. This saw her elevated to a fully funded athlete, however, the lack of support she received as a women became even more magnified when she fell pregnant and also upon her post-natal return to sport. During her pregnancy her coaches were unsure about what training she could do and what was safe and it took a lot of her own research to work out a plan that allowed her to still train. This failure to accommodate the needs of the pregnant athlete was also seen when she had to eventually stop training to have her son, which saw her lose all of her funding (something largely connected to those 'in charge' not believing she would return as they didn't think it feasible). When Rebecca did return it was not because she wanted to or felt ready to but she felt forced to return to competition when her son was only eight weeks old to ensure she could gain back her ranking and in turn her funding. Rebecca acknowledged that it wasn't necessarily the fault of her coaches but more a lack of knowledge and information about how to train females and a failure to develop policies that were specific to returning mothers.

When Rebecca retired from elite sport aged 32 she decided to enter into coaching fuelled by her desire to share her experience and provide better support for young female athletes.

Rebecca's experiences in snowboarding are likely to be similar to those of athletes who are involved in sports with heavily gendered environments. These environments typically see men in the positions of power in terms of policy making and coaching which often results in the practices that have worked for male athletes being applied to women. Rebecca's story raises a key point that there is a need for more female specific research to understand the experiences of women in different sporting contexts that can be used to inform practice.

What are the challenges of using female only research participants?

While it is apparent there is a need for more multidisciplinary research investigating female athletes the fact remains that there is not sufficient research being carried out to reflect the level of female participation in sport. Furthermore, research that is conducted with female participants has often been of low quality and poorly designed (McNulty et al., 2020). Researching women can be more challenging, owing to the complexities of the female reproductive and biological system which can see research take more time and cost more money (Mujika and Taipale, 2022). These factors have meant that researchers have tended to steer away from basing research on women (Emmonds et al., 2019). Without research of this kind, it becomes impossible to develop an evidence-based practice approach to any aspect of female sports performance. These issues were exemplified by Rebecca our Snowboarder who recognised how the lack of knowledge within her sport meant she didn't get the right support, particularly during her pregnancy.

Researching women involves controlling more variables, but those very variables highlight the importance of understanding women as a discrete group. Emmonds et al. (2019) examined the challenges of undertaking research in female sport highlighting several of the complexities that female athletes may present. From the highly specific issues around menstruation, such as the impact of fluctuations in hormones at different stages of the menstrual cycle which have been found to have an impact on injury risk, as well as the more overarching performance implications that may occur at different stages of the cycle, to the difference in the biomechanics of men and women. These complexities indicate that female athletes will require different approaches to training, nutrition and recovery to their male counterparts, and these strategies may have further nuances at particular stages of their menstrual cycle.

Mujika and Taipale (2019) further support the work of Emmonds et al. (2019) through their reflections on research with male and female participants. They reflected how at the start of their research journey people steered away from researching women because they were more complicated, owing to the hormonal fluctuations that could impact physiological research. However, conversely they reported that while this research may require more detailed planning, when research is conducted with women the participants are fully invested to learn more about their own physiology and performance and in their words will 'go the extra mile' to support the research.

This investment by female participants in the research can also be a reaction to social norms that have seen women in the subordinate role and often lacking a voice or appearing marginalised (LaVoi, 2016). Involvement in research, particularly qualitative studies using in-depth interviews or focus groups can give women voice to their ideas and thoughts. Although it is important to note as Reinharz and Chase (2003) discuss elite women (such as athletes) are generally more comfortable being heard. This marginalisation of women further relates to other sociocultural norms dictated by society. Sport remains a predominantly patriarchal environment with both sports science and medical provision being limited for female athletes, as well as there often being a lack of funding and poor access to expert staff. These are all considerations when embarking on research as proposals may not have support, not be prioritised, or appear to lack value (Elliott-Sale et al., 2021).

Another potential reason for the lack of research on women could link to there being fewer female researchers, with evidence suggesting that women are more likely to research women (Stanley and Wise, 2002). Martinez-Rosales et al. (2021) examined the lack of representation of women within sports science both in terms of publications and editorial leadership. Through analysis of the sex of both first and second authors and identification of the sex of the editorial board they concluded that only 24.8 per cent of research had women as first author with only 19.7 per cent of board positions being held by women. Their findings emphasise how women are hugely underrepresented in terms of authoring and within editorial positions within sport science which is likely to contribute to the lack of female specific research.

Researching female athletes: what needs to be considered?

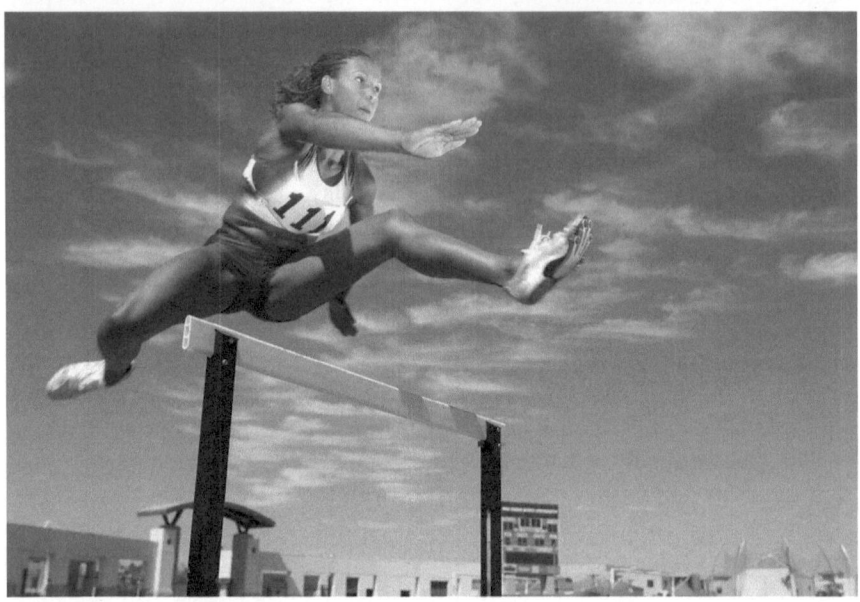

As Emmonds et al. (2019) discuss there are significant difficulties when it comes to applying evidence developed with male subjects to females largely down to the biological differences between the sexes. Pointing to a need to develop research that is specific to female athletes. While there has been a growth in the research area surrounding female athletes there are still somewhat dated stereotypes at play that can have an impact on research with women. It is important to contextualise these to understand why there remains a lack of female centric research within sport.

There are several implications when it comes to applying research conducted on men to women, for example what is considered safe for men may not be safe for women. Or there may be training protocols that could be tailored to be more beneficial to women if undertaken differently. Those working with athletes, for example coaches, need to understand these female specific issues as well as those related to female psychology and trends in female injury (Pitchers and Elliot-Sale, 2019).

Lingam-Willgoss (2023) highlights the implication of this lack of research in her study looking at the experience of elite female athletes on their return to sport after childbirth. Through a case study analysis of five elite female athletes from running and winter sports the study uncovered how those from a winter sports background, which was also heavily gendered, lacked the right evidence informed practical support during their career. One athlete recalled how the return from injury protocol (designed for men) was used to test her return to sport post-partum (only ten weeks after having her daughter). This had potentially very dangerous implications as two of the exercises were contraindicated (one being the single leg jump) during the postpartum period. This echoes some of Rebecca's experiences which also reflect a lack of knowledge about how to support female athletes during pregnancy and post-partum periods. This example highlights how a lack of specific research on the returning mother within some sports could have a significant long term health implication.

In contrast to these negative experiences are those of Moore et al. (2022) who examined the fuelling needs of female athletes, specifically around carbohydrate and protein, with a focus on the implications around the menstrual cycle. Findings supported an individualised approach that allows personal symptoms around menstruation to be factored in along with sport specific demands and competitive goals. While not suggesting anything radical this study emphasised the need for personalisation, something that is lacking in research that is conducted on men and applied to women.

As touched on earlier, it is also important to recognise how it is not just biological and physiological differences between the sexes that can impact the athletic journey, but how psychological factors must also be taken into consideration. Ekengren et al. (2020) conducted a comparative study examining the experiences of elite handball players towards the end of their careers. Their findings highlighted the vast differences in gender specific themes from the athlete's early introduction to sport into retirement. Two psychological themes are illustrated below in Figure 2.3.

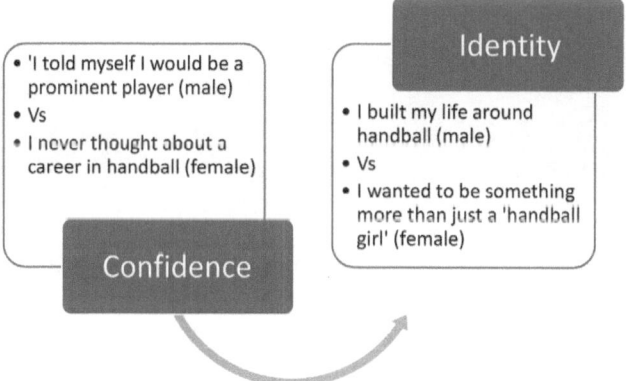

FIGURE 2.2 Two gender-specific themes describing career pathways of Swedish professional handball players
Source: Adapted from Ekengren et al. (2020)

Through looking at these two themes related to confidence and identity we can see how male and female athletes' approach and view sport in different ways. These findings draw parallels with the work of Tekavc (2017) who also identified confidence, in particular their ability to be an athlete, as a differentiating factor between male and female athletes. With confidence being such a fundamental factor for all elite athletes these subtle differences highlight how female centred research must not simply focus on the biological but include a psychological and social perspective as well.

Through developing research with female athletes at the forefront we will increase understanding of how best to support elite female athletes, including a better understanding of the physical capabilities of athletes, focusing on the specific demands of sports as well as developing sex specific recovery and injury rehabilitation strategies. These steps will allow progression of women's sport through allowing more tailored approaches to working with female athletes rather than rely on application from a male population.

What's gender got to do with it?

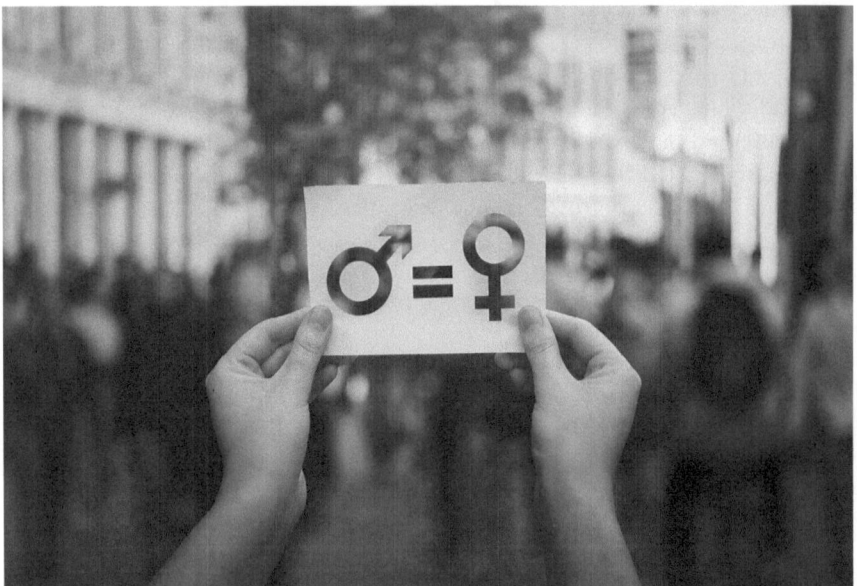

We have talked about the importance of differentiating between the sexes in terms of research. However, it is also important to recognise the influence that gender may have on the way that women act or behave and subsequently the impact on research within this area. Unlike sex, gender is widely accepted to be a social construct that allocates a set of suitable behaviours to the male or female sex, furthermore, these behaviours tend to conform to societal expectations of how men and women should act (Appleby and Foster, 2014). Taken a stage further, the concept of gender identity reflects how an individual understands themselves in terms of the cultural definitions of male and female (Wood and Eagly, 2015).

This point also suggests a need to examine the differences between men and women from more than just biological or psychological, but how a sociological perspective may also have a bearing, as men and women are likely to understand themselves within the constricts of their gender and the social norms. In the context of sport this also presents an interesting consideration as often the demands of sport may challenge the conventions of a given gender, for example women competing in combat sports (that requires typically male traits such as aggression) and in turn their experiences will be different to their male counterparts (Kavoura et al., 2015).

BOX 2.2 SPOTLIGHT ON: DEVELOPING OPENNESS – COMMUNICATION GAPS IN WOMEN'S SPORT

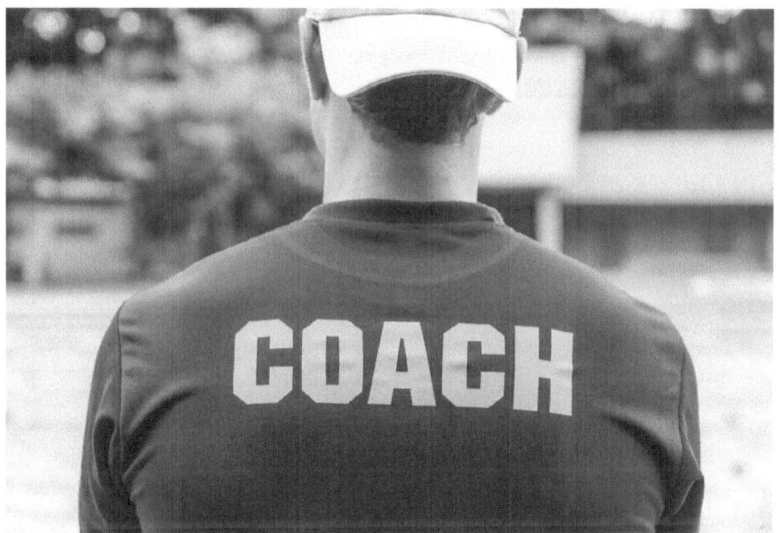

We have focused on the gaps that are apparent within the research domain related to female athletes. However, this also spotlights other gaps that need addressing if more parity between the sexes is to be achieved. A key aim of this book is to remove the stigma attached to many of the terms associated with women and their biology and create more open dialogues between those working in sport. As such a communication gap has to be acknowledged which sees many topics talked about in hushed tones or brushed aside as people don't want to talk about periods and breasts as they can make people feel uncomfortable.

This was something illustrated through Rebecca's experiences in sport as she felt uncomfortable talking about issues she experienced during puberty as all of her coaches were men. Rebecca felt embarrassment talking about anything connected to menstruation, something Ross et al. (2023) discuss in their book *The Female Body Bible*. Ross recounts how within her experiences of working within both the Olympic and Paralympic domain she heard a range of different euphemisms for periods as well other words related to sexual anatomy and reproduction. This is further exacerbated by the way parents teach their children euphemisms something Bobel (2020) recognises as the first stage of encouraging people to avoid the realities of the human body in order to avoid embarrassment and perpetuate the concept that menstruation is a taboo! This embarrassment is heightened when men and women interact – a problem when we consider that within sport this is perhaps the most common interaction with coaching remaining a predominantly male domain (UK Coaching, 2019).

The benefit of a female coach in terms of providing a more open space for athletes was discussed by Lorimer and Jowett (2009) who concluded that female coaches displayed more accurate levels of empathy than male coaches as well as being more accurate in their understanding of the athletes' feelings, subsequently fostering better quality and more open relationships. This links to Rebecca's motivation for wanting to work within her sport to provide a more open and supportive environment for female athletes.

It isn't just sport

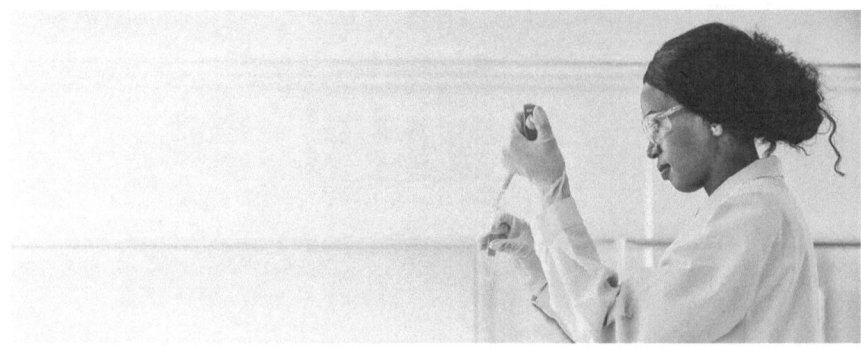

While the focus of this chapter has been on the gaps within sport-related research, an equally concerning gap is apparent within the medical literature. For example, Bohannon (2023) points out it wasn't until 1999 that researchers discovered sex differences in response to general anaesthetic with women waking faster than men! While females being left out of sport science research may have an impact on their ability to reach peak performance the gap within the medical research could result in serious health implications. In a similar way to sport based research, traditionally women have been excluded from medical research, owing to menstruation rendering female biology too variable as well as concerns over fertility implications (Merone et al., 2021). Like sport this has seen more research conducted on males and applied to females where they are considered to be similar to a 'small male'. It is worth noting that intersex, transgender and gender nonconformists are also victim to this trend (Wainer et al., 2020). Like sport, medicine remains a patriarchal institution and gender inequalities persist becoming particularly pronounced when looking at senior positions with women poorly represented in leadership and research resulting in the ongoing disproportionate ratio of male to female research (Jagsi et al., 2006). Furthermore, we see similar trends when female authorship is compared to male authorship of research, highlighting another area of under-representation (Sebo et al., 2020). The absence of research in both this domain and the sporting context diminishes the favourable health outcomes for females.

BOX 2.3 REAL-WORLD APPLICATIONS

As a female athlete, you should:

- Engage in conversations with fellow female athletes as they are likely to possess valuable information to share.
- Challenge coaches to create open environments that remove the stigma attached to certain topics around female health and performance.
- Refrain from comparing yourself to male athletes when training together as male and female athletes have many psychological and physiological differences.

As a coach, you should:

- Be aware that the majority of sport science/coaching research is conducted with male participants and therefore is not always applicable to female athletes and seek out alternative information sources.
- Consult with specialists in women's sport when working with female athletes who have specific concerns.
- Create an environment of openness and encourage open discussions about initially sensitive topics related to female health and performance.

Summary

This chapter has highlighted a gender-gap in terms of research within sport and medicine which can be attributed to a wide range of factors such as the complexity of the female menstrual cycle. The lack of females conducting research or within positions of authority both within academia and sporting environments has also perpetuated the highly androcentric nature of both sport and medicine. As a result this positioning of women as secondary and the assumption that research conducted on males can be applied to women persists.

The key messages to take away from this chapter are:

- The majority of research either compares male and female athletes or focuses on male athletes with only 6 per cent of research being conducted on women.

- Research exclusively focused on women has been avoided, owing to the perceived complexity arising from hormonal fluctuations that could potentially impact on physiological studies.
- Differences between male and female athletes are not purely biological, but also relate to their psychology as well as sociocultural norms.
- There remains a stigma attached to discussing female health, including menstruation, breast health and the menopause.
- The lack of women in positions of power within sporting environments has compounded the perpetuation of a singular point of view with men at the forefront and a lack of sensitivity towards female-related topics.

End-of-Chapter Quiz

Answers can be found after the References

1. What percentage of sports science research in 2020 was conducted on women only?

    a   61%
    b   35%
    c   6%
    d   11%

2. Which two of the following factors illustrate why female specific research is needed?

    a   Women can experience significant pelvic floor issues.
    b   Women's sports equipment is more expensive than men's.
    c   Women experience more joint injury and concussions.
    d   Women are less suited to playing sport than men.

3. Identify one reason why women are often excluded from research studies:

    a   There aren't enough elite female athletes.
    b   Hormonal fluctuations create too many variables.
    c   Research on men can be generalised to female athletes.
    d   There are no female researchers.

4. Which of the following psychological factors was recognised by Ekengren et al. (2020) as being different in men and women?

    a   Anxiety
    b   Confidence
    c   Motivation
    d   Concentration

5.   How can gender impact on research conducted?

    a   Women will interpret things in a different way to men.

    b   It has no impact.

    c   It is the same as the differences between sexes.

    d   It will stop women doing some sports.

References

Appleby K.M. and Foster, E. (2014). 'Gender and Sports Participation' in E.A. Roper (Ed.), *Gender relations in sport*. Springer Science & Business Media.

Bobel, C. (2020) *New blood: Third-wave feminism and the politics of menstruation.* Rutgers University Press.

Bohannon, C. (2023) *Eve: How the female body drove 200 million years of human evolution.* Hutchinson Heinemann.

Brown, N., Knight, C.J. and Forrest, L.J. (2021) Elite female athletes' experiences and perceptions of the menstrual cycle on training and sport performance. *Scandinavian Journal of Medicine & Science in Sports*, 31(1), 52–69.

Castanier, C., Bougault, V., Teulier, C., Jaffré, C., Schiano-Lomoriello, S., Vibarel-Rebot, N., Villemain, A., Rieth, N., Le-Scanff, C., Buisson, C. and Collomp, K. (2021) The Specificities of Elite Female Athletes: A Multidisciplinary Approach. *Life*, 11(7), 622.

Cowley, E.S., Olenick, A.A., McNulty, K.L. and Ross, E.Z. (2021) "Invisible sportswomen": the sex data gap in sport and exercise science research. *Women in Sport and Physical Activity Journal*, 29(2), 146–151.

de Haan, D. and Norman, L. (2020) Mind the gap: the presence of capital and power in the female athlete–male-coach relationship within elite rowing. *Sports Coaching Review*, 9(1), 95–118.

de Subijana, C.L., Galatti, L., Moreno, R. and Chamorro, J.L. (2020) Analysis of the athletic career and retirement depending on the type of sport: a comparison between individual and team sports. *International journal of environmental research and public health*, 17(24), 9265.

Ekengren, J., Stambulova, N., Johnson, U. and Carlsson, I.M. (2020) Exploring career experiences of Swedish professional handball players: Consolidating first-hand information into an empirical career model. *International Journal of Sport and Exercise Psychology*, 18(2), 156–175.

Elliott-Sale, K.J., Minahan, C.L., de Jonge, X.A., Ackerman, K.E., Sipilä, S., Constantini, N.W., Lebrun, C.M. and Hackney, A.C. (2021) Methodological considerations for studies in sport and exercise science with women as participants: a working guide for standards of practice for research on women. *Sports Medicine*, 51(5), 843–861.

Emmonds, S., Heyward, O. and Jones, B. (2019) The challenge of applying and undertaking research in female sport. *Sports medicine-open*, 5, 1–4.

Fink, J.S. (2008) Gender and sex diversity in sport organizations: Concluding comments. *Sex Roles*, 58, 146–147.

Fink, J.S. (2015) Female athletes, women's sport, and the sport media commercial complex: Have we really "come a long way, baby"? *Sport management review*, 18(3), 331–342.

Jagsi, R., Guancial, E.A., Worobey, C.C., Henault, L.E., Chang, Y., Starr, R., Tarbell, N.J. and Hylek, E.M. (2006) The "gender gap" in authorship of academic medical literature—a 35-year perspective. *New England Journal of Medicine*, 355(3), 281–287.

Kavoura, A., Ryba, T.V. and Chroni, S. (2015) Negotiating female judoka identities in Greece: A Foucauldian discourse analysis. *Psychology of Sport and Exercise*, 17, 88–98.

LaVoi, N.M. (2016) A framework to understand experiences of women coaches around the globe: The Ecological-Intersectional Model. In *Women in sports coaching*, pp. 13–34. Routledge.

Lingam-Willgoss, C. (2023) *Negotiating Identity: how elite athlete mothers navigate their journey through sport* (Doctoral dissertation, The Open University).

Lorimer, R. and Jowett, S. (2009) Empathic accuracy in coach–athlete dyads who participate in team and individual sports. *Psychology of Sport and Exercise*, 10(1), 152–158.

Martínez-Rosales, E., Hernández-Martínez, A., Sola-Rodríguez, S., Esteban-Cornejo, I. and Soriano-Maldonado, A. (2021) Representation of women in sport sciences research, publications, and editorial leadership positions: are we moving forward? *Journal of Science and Medicine in Sport*, 24(11), 1093–1097.

McNulty, K.L., Elliott-Sale, K.J., Dolan, E., Swinton, P.A., Ansdell, P., Goodall, S., Thomas, K. and Hicks, K.M. (2020) The effects of menstrual cycle phase in exercise performance in eumenorrheic women: a systematic review and meta-analysis. *Sports Medicine*, 50, 1813–1827.

Merone, L., Tsey, K., Russell, D. and Nagle, C. (2021). *Sex and gender gaps in medicine and the androcentric history of medical research*.

Moore, D.R., Sygo, J. and Morton, J.P. (2022) Fuelling the female athlete: Carbohydrate and protein recommendations. *European Journal of Sport Science*, 22(5), 684–696.

Mujika, I. and Taipale, R.S. (2019) Sport science on women, women in sport science. *International journal of sports physiology and performance*, 14(8), 1013–1014.

Norman, L. (2018) "It's sport, why does it matter?" Professional coaches' perceptions of equity training. *Sports Coaching Review*, 7(2), 190–211.

Perez-Gomez J., Rodriguez, G.V. and Ara, I. (2008) Role of muscle mass on sprint performance: gender differences? *European Journal of Applied Physiology*, 102, 685–694.

Pitchers, G. and Elliot-Sale, K. (2019) Considerations for coaches training female athletes. *Prof Strength Cond*, 55, 19–30.

Rea, S. (2022) Session 1: Mind the gap: gender differences in sport science research and its impact on female athletes. *Badged Open Course: Supporting female performance in sport and fitness*. Available at: Supporting female performance in sport and fitness: Session 8: Introduction − OpenLearn − Open University (Accessed: 12 September 2023).

Reinharz, S. and Chase, S.E. (2003) Interviewing women. *Inside interviewing: New lenses, new concerns*, pp. 73–90.

Ross, E., Moffat, B. and Smith, B. (2023) *The Female Body Bible*. London: Penguin.

Sebo, P., Maisonneuve, H. and Fournier, J.P. (2020). Gender gap in research: a bibliometric study of published articles in primary health care and general internal medicine. *Family Practice*, 37(3), 325–331.

Smith, E.S., McKay, A.K., Ackerman, K.E., Harris, R., Elliott-Sale, K.J., Stellingwerff, T. and Burke, L.M. (2022). Methodology review: a protocol to audit the representation of female athletes in sports science and sports medicine research. *International journal of sport nutrition and exercise metabolism*, 32(2), 114–127.

Stanley, L. and Wise, S. (2002) *Breaking out again: Feminist ontology and epistemology*. Routledge.

Tekavc, J. (2017) *Investigation into Gender Specific Transitions and Challenges Faced by Female Elite Athletes*. Brussels: Vubpress.

UK Coaching (2019) Coaching in the UK, 2019 Coach Survey. Available at https://www.ukcoaching.org/UKCoaching/media/coaching-images/Entity%20base/Downloadables/CPS_Coaches-_FINAL_2019.pdf / Accessed 12th February 2024

Wainer, Z., Carcel, C., Hickey, M., Schiebinger, L., Schmiede, A., McKenzie, B.*et al.* (2020) Sex and gender in health research: Updating policy to reflect evidence. *Med J Aust.*, 212(2), 57–62.

Wood, W. and Eagly, A.H. (2015) Two traditions of research on gender identity. *Sex Roles*, 73, 461–473.

Answers

1.   c
2.   a and c
3.   b
4.   b
5.   a

3

THE MENSTRUAL CYCLE AND FEMALE ATHLETIC PERFORMANCE

Simon Rea

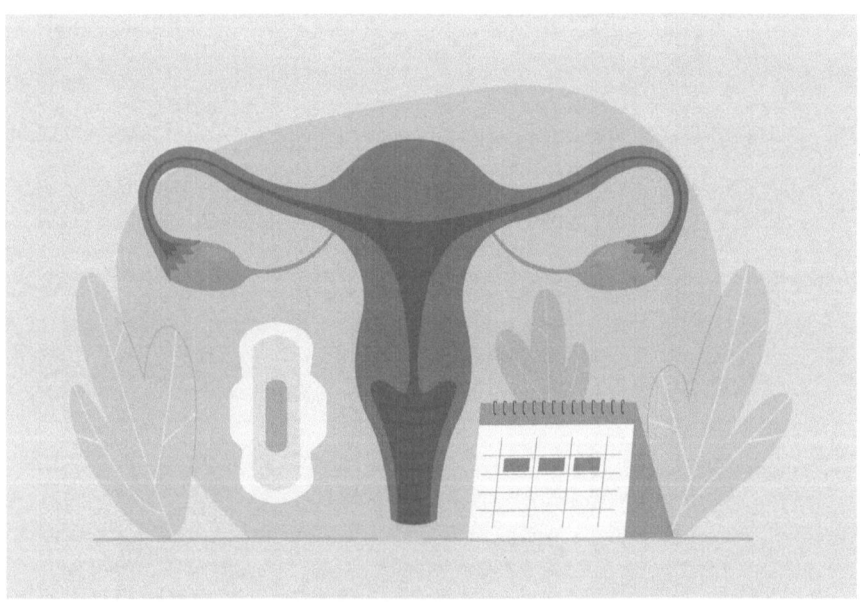

Introduction

The menstrual cycle is a recurring pattern of hormonal changes across a period of 28 days, although this can vary from 21 to 35 days between females and within individual cycles. It is an important process that prepares the body for a potential pregnancy and is driven by hormones. Having a regular period is viewed as a vital sign of whole body health in menstruating females with any variations to the cycle

DOI: 10.4324/9781003330110-3

being potentially dangerous (American College of Obstetricians and Gynaecologists, 2015). Disruptions, or irregularities, in the menstrual cycle (dysmenorrhoea) or the loss of the menstrual cycle (amenorrhoea) can have negative impacts on bone health, cognitive function, mood and fertility (Misra, 2015).

There remains a general lack of understanding around the menstrual cycle. In 2019 the Royal College of Obstetricians and Gynaecologists reported that women are 'woefully uneducated at every life stage' about what is happening in their bodies and how it relates to their physical and mental health. A study of 14,000 active women worldwide showed that 72 per cent had never had any education about exercise and the menstrual cycle and this rose to 82 per cent of participants in the study from the UK and Ireland (Strada, 2019).

Despite more discussion around the menstrual cycle in sporting environments and an openness about it from athletes it is often viewed, particularly by men, as a taboo subject that is difficult to approach. However, for the benefit of the health and performance of female athletes it is important that the menstrual cycle is treated as another performance variable to be considered by all coaches and trainers.

As discussed in Chapter 2, while female participation in sport has significantly risen, research into female athletic performance has not mirrored this increase in participation. Given the anatomical, physiological, and hormonal differences between men and women it is naïve, and even potentially dangerous, to attempt to apply research conducted on men to women. In order to advance women's sport it is vital to explore the effect of the menstrual cycle on performance in training and during competition.

Research around the menstrual cycle tends to focus on two areas: first, whether athletic performance is impacted by the phases of the menstrual cycle; second whether there are phases within the menstrual cycle where specific types of training will lead to greater gains than other phases. Both these research areas will be examined in this chapter but before we explore the menstrual cycle itself, read the case study, in Box 3.1, where you are introduced to Florence and her experiences of the menstrual cycle.

BOX 3.1 FLORENCE (FOOTBALLER)

Florence is a semi-professional footballer who trains with her team twice a week and typically plays in a competitive match once a week. She supplements her football training with two long runs and two strength and conditioning training sessions a week. She is highly motivated, and her goal is to play professionally in the Women's Super League.

Florence has always had a fairly regular menstrual cycle, although it does vary in its length which makes it difficult to predict when she will have her period. She does not usually notice any signs or symptoms that her period is about to start but when it does start she gets severe pain in her stomach. She also experiences heavy bleeding, muscle pain and cramps in her back and legs as well as abdominal bloating. She is often in so much discomfort that she finds she has to really push herself to go to training. Because she has such heavy periods she really worries about blood leaking out while she is training or playing during her period.

Florence's team has a male coach and although he talks openly about menstruation she does not feel comfortable talking to him about it. Despite often feeling poorly she tries to work through her period pain, although sometimes she has to stop training and claims she has an injury or is ill. She is afraid to give the real reason in case she is dropped from the team. She does find that gentle exercise can ease some of her symptoms once she gets started but she really struggles during high intensity sessions. When her period has passed Florence starts to feel energised and motivated in training to do more and more. She notices that she often performs best in the two weeks after her period has finished.

Her teammates have advised her that tracking her cycle using an app may be beneficial to her as that way she will be able to anticipate what is coming up and prepare for it. Florence does start to do this and after a couple of months she sees patterns in her cycle and is able to identify how she will feel physically and emotionally at different stages. She feels more in control and can prepare for when her period will start and ensure she has plans in place for this.

Florence's experiences and concerns may be fairly typical of female athletes, and we will revisit her experiences as we progress through this chapter.

The hormones of the menstrual cycle

The menstrual cycle is controlled by hormones, in particular progesterone and oestrogen (estrogen in the US). Hormones are described as 'chemical messengers' as they travel in the bloodstream and send messages to specific sites in the body to perform certain functions (Hill, 2019). However, oestrogen and progesterone are just two of the many hormones involved in the cycle that starts in the brain when the hypothalamus gland sends signals to the pituitary gland to release two hormones – follicle stimulating hormone (FSH) and luteinising hormone (LH). Box 3.2 summarises the roles of four hormones that are central to the menstrual cycle.

BOX 3.2 THE HORMONES OF THE MENSTRUAL CYCLE

Follicle stimulating hormone (FSH) – FSH stimulates follicles in the ovaries to grow until a dominant follicle is chosen, and this follicle will start to produce oestrogen. Then, along with luteinising hormone, FSH will help the selected follicle to release an egg (ovulation).

Luteinising hormone (LH) – LH provides the power behind ovulation as it combines with FSH in the days before ovulation to stimulate the chosen follicle to produce more oestrogen and allow ovulation to occur.

Oestrogen – oestrogen is produced by the dominant follicle that has been chosen to release an egg. This follicle will then form the corpus luteum that continues to produce oestrogen and also progesterone for the length of the menstrual cycle. Oestrogen's role is to thicken the lining of the uterus allowing a fertilised egg to embed itself in the wall of the uterus.

Progesterone – progesterone will maintain the lining of the uterus and prevent it from overgrowing.

Source: Adapted from Hill (2019)

The phases of the menstrual cycle

As shown in Figure 3.1 the menstrual cycle is divided into two phases across a 'textbook' 28-day cycle, although it is reported that only around 12 per cent of women actually have a 28-day cycle (Hill, 2019). The first 14 days of the cycle are called the follicular phase and this lasts from the start of the period until ovulation. The second 14 days of the cycle are called the luteal phase and it runs from ovulation to end of the cycle before menstruation starts.

The first significant events of the menstrual cycle actually happen in the final days of the previous cycle. Figure 3.1 shows that in Days 26–28 of the cycle both oestrogen and progesterone fall to low levels. This fall in hormones triggers the release of prostaglandins that cause the blood vessels of the endometrium (lining of the uterus) to contract and reduce blood supply. This deprives the endometrium of oxygen, so it dies and is discarded by the uterus, via the vagina, as part of the period. It is also the release of prostaglandins that are responsible for producing stomach cramps, and along with the low levels of oestrogen and progesterone, cause other pre-menstrual symptoms (Hill, 2019).

The menstrual cycle starts on Day 1 with the period, or menstrual bleeding that lasts for 5–6 days. During this time oestrogen and progesterone levels are

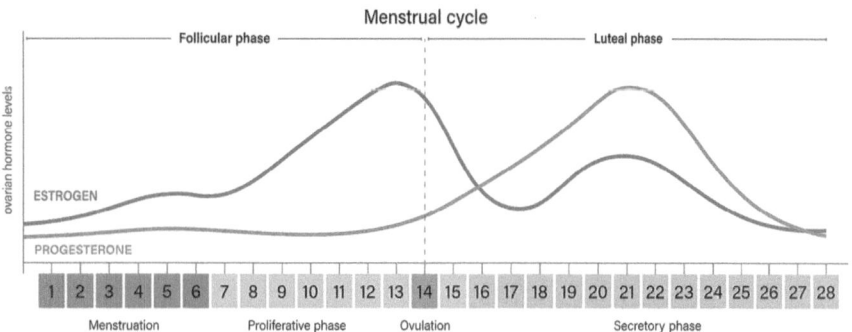

FIGURE 3.1 The phases of the menstrual cycle
Source: Shutterstock

relatively low but after Day 5 oestrogen starts to rise and peaks around Day 12, just before ovulation that occurs around Days 13–15. Oestrogen can make females feel energised and motivated, although it can differ between individuals. This may be because oestrogen promotes the production of serotonin that is regarded as a 'feel good' hormone. Research has shown that in active women the motivation to train is highest around ovulation which coincides with oestrogen's peak (Crewther and Cook, 2018), and confidence and competitiveness can increase as well (Buser, 2012).

Ovulation signals the end of the follicular phase (proliferative phase) and a reduction in oestrogen levels leading into the start of the luteal phase (secretory phase). The luteal phase is characterised by an increase in progesterone up to around Day 21. Progesterone is the pro-gestation hormone that will support a pregnancy when required, and it creates a different environment by promoting calmness, good mood, and sleep (Ross et al., 2023). Progesterone soothes the nervous system and acts as a natural anti-anxiety medication (Joffe et al., 2020). The luteal phase is also characterised by a slight increase in basal metabolic rate and an accompanying increase in temperature of around half a degree (Ross et al., 2023). This rise in body temperature can cause an increase in sweat rate, especially during exercise (Lee et al., 2014).

These changes in the hormonal environment across the menstrual cycle offer opportunities to design training programmes that match the effects of these hormones on the female athlete, and we will investigate these in a later section. These hormone shifts also explain why training schedules designed for males may not suit female athletes.

Towards the end of the cycle (Days 26–28) oestrogen and progesterone levels drop significantly unless the egg has been fertilised. This fall causes a 'hormone hangover' where women may experience a withdrawal from the effects of the hormones and experience some of the reported 150 symptoms of premenstrual syndrome (PMS), some of which are shown in Figure 3.2.

The menstrual cycle and athletic performance

As mentioned previously, the primary functions of oestrogen and progesterone are to support reproduction. However, fluctuations in these two hormones across the menstrual cycle have a complex range of effects on the cardiovascular, respiratory, metabolic, and muscular systems (McNulty et al., 2020). All of these systems play important roles in athletic performance. The BBC Elite British Sportswomen's survey (Lofthouse, 2020) showed that 60 per cent of sportswomen believed that their athletic performance had been affected by their period. This included missing training or competitions. In 2022 British sprinter, Dina Asher-Smith, blamed her cycle for the cramp in her calf when she pulled up in the final of the European Championships 100 m. However, as is common with many human experiences, the menstrual cycle affects all females differently. In Box 3.3 we can see two athletes with radically differing experiences of training and competing during their period.

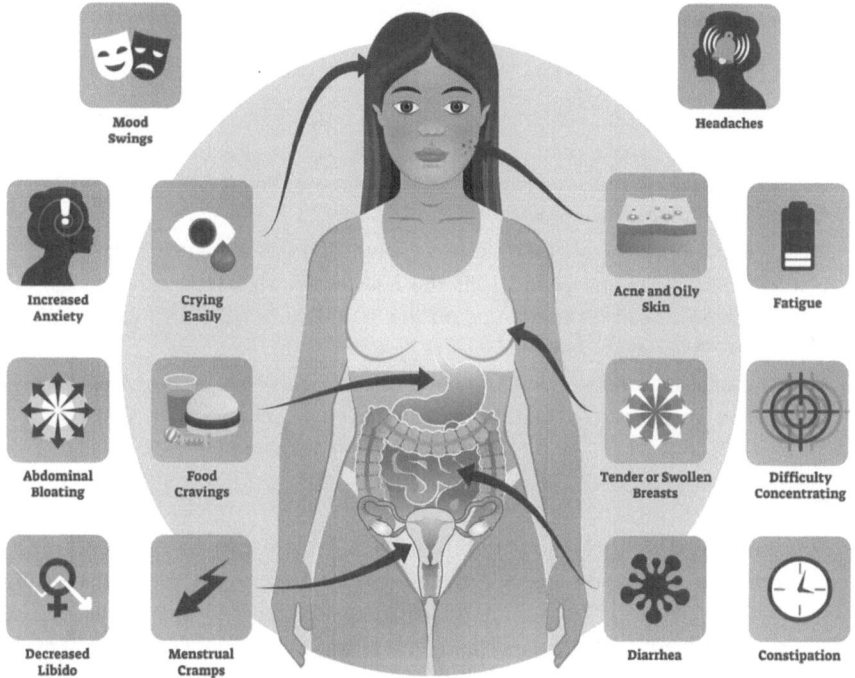

FIGURE 3.2 Some of the reported 150 symptoms of premenstrual syndrome
Source: Shutterstock

BOX 3.3 WHAT DO THE ATHLETES SAY?

Jazmin Sawyers (European Indoor Long Jump Champion 2023)

I have always said my period has FOMO, the fear of missing out, because for every major final it turns up. I had an experience at the Olympics where I thought I wasn't going to be able to compete because the pain that I had with my period was so bad.

I was taking medication that was supposed to delay it, and it had worked all year. But three hours before I'm supposed to be competing in the Olympics I am writhing around on the floor in pain.

It's something that I really needed to get a handle on because it was affecting my competition, and if I couldn't walk I definitely couldn't do the long jump. On that day, I ended up pumping myself full of as many pain-killers as I could handle, and I just got out there and managed.

I think the reason that I didn't get this dealt with earlier is that I felt like I couldn't have that conversation with my coaches.

Andrea Spendolini-Siriex (two time European and two-time Commonwealth Diving Champion)

I'm very lucky and very blessed to have a coach who understands me and who doesn't make me feel like I can't talk to him about it (the menstrual cycle) because it does affect the training session, and it does affect if I can go on the 10-metre board.

Quite honestly when I'm on my period I do feel extremely strong, and when I am on my period I lift the heaviest in S&C (strength and con-ditioning). I can do more reps on the 10 metre board, and I can do the harder dives more easily.

I actually won the Commonwealth Games when I was at the peak of my period, and when I was bleeding the most I won a Commonwealth gold medal.

(Adapted from Team GB, 2023)

This illustrates clearly how different each female can be, and the differ-ences between the experiences of their menstrual cycle. As we can see some females, like Andrea Spendolini-Siriex, experience few symptoms during their period, some females experience moderate symptoms and some females experience debilitating symptoms, as shown by Florence in the case study and Jazmin Sawyers in Box 3.3.

These differences can leave us asking, why are there pronounced variations between females' experiences, and also between the individual cycles of each female? The answer is due to the differing effects of hormones. There are hormone receptor sites on cells across the whole body that affect how organs such as the brain, gut, blood vessels and muscles function. As levels of oes-trogen and progesterone fluctuate the changes in the amounts of oestrogen and progesterone available to the cells of the body can alter producing physical and emotional symptoms. Each female will have variations in the levels of their hormones and importantly their sensitivity to the effects of these hor-mones. These variations in explain why females experience their cycle differ-ently and encounter different symptoms.

In Chapter 2 we explained how research using females was made more challenging, owing to their cycles. The example in Box 3.3 of two athletes having opposing experiences of their period illustrates one of the complexities into researching females and producing definitive results that can be accurately applied to all female athletes.

What does the research say?

First, it must be said that this is an area where research is still in its infancy and the research is often contradictory. One significant study is a metanalysis by McNulty et al. (2020) that combined the results of 51 studies into the impact of the menstrual cycle on athletic performance. It concluded that exercise performance in women was not significantly affected by any phase of the menstrual cycle, apart from minor amounts during the early follicular phase (Days 1–5). This metanalysis showed that the impact of fluctuations in hormones did not affect the physiological capacity of women to perform in terms of performance markers, such as strength, power, and aerobic endurance. However, they did conclude that in 2020 there was very little good quality research conducted on how the menstrual cycle impacts on performance.

More recent research has shown that oestrogen and progesterone do have important implications for how females respond to exercise (Gault and Smith, 2023). As oestrogen is an anabolic hormone, that promotes the development of muscle and storage of energy, it can increase the body's ability to recover quickly from high intensity exercise and increase the body's muscle building capacity (Chidi-Ogbulu and Baar, 2018). These responses can be beneficial during the training period. Progesterone can increase body temperature (by around half a degree) and increase the resting heart rate with a potentially detrimental effect on performance. Progesterone levels rise during the second half of the cycle (luteal phase) and studies have shown that when testing for endurance, muscle fatigue and VO_2max, that athletes performed better in the follicular phase (Days 6–12) than those in the luteal phase (Days 16–28) (Julian et al., 2017; Graja et al., 2020).

Research into the effects of the menstrual cycle on anaerobic performance are inconclusive, although some studies have linked the follicular phase to increased muscular strength, while others have attributed this effect to increased energy levels and motivation during this stage (Gault and Smith, 2023).

Jazmin Sawyers's experiences, as shown in Box 3.3, illustrate the contradiction that while the menstrual cycle has no significant impact on the markers of athletic performance, the ability to access these markers can be compromised by the symptoms of the menstrual cycle, such as pain and stomach upsets. This supports the experiences of athletes from the BBC Survey (Lofthouse, 2020) that found the majority experienced symptoms that impacted performance.

Adapting training to match the phases of the menstrual cycle

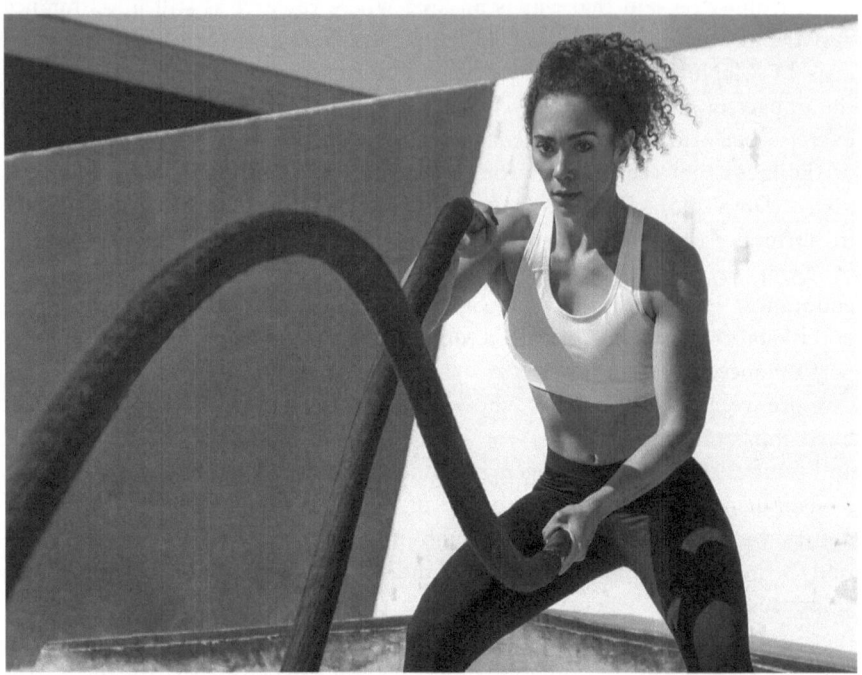

The hormones oestrogen and progesterone have been shown to have differing impacts on mood and energy level. As oestrogen can increases motivation and energy it is logical that the time in the cycle when oestrogen is peaking, between Days 7 and 14, may be an ideal time to train hard. In contrast, progesterone is associated with feelings of calmness and slowing down, so it may be a good time to schedule in recovery.

In addition to this, these hormones also promote other processes within the body. Oestrogen is an anabolic hormone associated with the development of muscle and storage of energy, while progesterone has a catabolic effect in that it breaks down body's structures, including muscle (Rocha-Rodrigues et al., 2021). The follicular stage, where oestrogen levels are high, may present opportunities for coaches and athletes to exploit by increasing volume and intensity of training. While every woman will respond differently to these hormones, learning how to 'train around the menstrual cycle' may be beneficial for some female athletes.

This approach is also based on changes in metabolism across the menstrual cycle as during the follicular phase, particularly the days after the period, the body is better able to metabolise carbohydrates for energy, meaning more glucose can be supplied to muscles (Eckerson, 2019). High intensity exercise is dependent on a fast supply of glucose to the muscles and thus this stage can be a good time to perform high intensity aerobic training and strength training (Ross et al., 2023).

Sung et al. (2014) showed that concentrating strength and resistance training in the first half of the cycle achieved greater gains in strength and muscular development compared to performing strength training evenly across the cycle. This method of stacking strength training in the follicular stage and performing it less frequently in the luteal phase was shown to increase strength by up to 40 per cent, compared to a 27 per cent increase when the pattern was flipped (Sung et al., 2014). Sims (2016) advocates this approach, and recommends focusing on lower intensity, steady state training during the luteal phase to allow the body to recover. However, in contrast Elliott-Sales (2022) urges caution with this approach as there is a lack of conclusive scientific evidence to back up this approach and promotes an individualised approach taking account of variations between female athletes and within their own cycles.

In 2023 a significant meta-analysis and systematic review on the impact of phases of the menstrual cycle concluded that there was very little evidence to support a focus on strength in the follicular stage (Colenso-Semple et al., 2023). The authors analysed studies that investigated the relationship between the development of strength, hypertrophy and exercise performance and the phases of the menstrual cycle. Their conclusion was that the findings were inconsistent and there was insufficient evidence to make any association. The researchers did acknowledge that there were significant differences in the magnitude of responses to hypertrophy training between individuals, but these are common to men and women. Owing to this commonality it is less likely that there will be significant differences in the effect of resistance training within each person during their cycle, even though the levels of oestrogen and progesterone fluctuate across a menstrual cycle (Jeukendrup, 2023).

A major problem is that across the studies in the meta-analysis there was a pattern of poor and inconsistent methodological practices making it difficult to come to exact conclusions (Colenso-Semple et al., 2023). While in the future front loading resistance training may prove to be effective, and should not be ruled out completely, in the absence of high quality evidence it is premature to say that athletes and their coaches should make adaptations to training schedules to match the phases of the menstrual cycle.

Unfortunately, this is another example of a lack of high quality research working against female athletes, and until the number of research studies in this area increases there is limited weight of evidence to support female athletic performance and to inform training programme design and training scheduling.

Menstrual cycle phase and injury risk

In the run up to the 2023 World Cup there were at least eight international players who were ruled out of the tournament, owing to anterior cruciate ligament (ACL) injuries. Sports women are reported to be up to six times more likely to experience a non-contact ACL injury than their male counterparts (Parsons et al., 2021), and twice as likely as males to injure other joints in their body (Wolf et al., 2015). In women's football 88 per cent of ACL tears are non-contact injuries, and 66 per cent are associated with defensive pressing (Lucarno et al., 2021). ACL injuries are most likely to occur when there is a horizontal movement involving rapid deceleration of a limb, rapid changes of direction and single leg actions (Bailey and Ahearn, 2023). These are all characteristics of defensive actions, such as defensive pressing.

ACL injuries have been linked to performing in the late follicular phase of the menstrual cycle (Days 12–14) when oestrogen levels are at their peak. Oestrogen has the effect of increasing laxity of ligaments around joints (McDonald, 2018). This increased mobility around joints puts more pressure on the ACL to stabilise the joint and making it more prone to tears. Females also have a greater angle between the femur and the tibia at the knee (the Q-angle) when compared to men, and this may be a risk factor as well. However, the correlation between hormonal fluctuations, anatomical differences, and ACL injuries may offer too simplistic an explanation.

Increasing attention is being paid to the gendered environment that can work against females. Environmental elements such as often having to play on poorer quality pitches, having fewer quality coaches and less access to specific strength and conditioning programmes may also contribute to the increased probability of ACL injuries occurring in female footballers (Bailey and Ahearn, 2023). Ross (2023) points out that the mechanism for injury is complex and while hormones may be one risk factor we also need to consider factors such as fatigue or lack of sleep, previous injuries, conditions of the ground, previous training and conditioning, as well as the anxiety and stress that surround the perceived risk of injury at this stage of the menstrual cycle. Exploring the increased prevalence of ACL injuries in women's football is an example of the value of viewing women's sport from different scientific perspectives, so while physiology is important, sociocultural, and psychological perspectives on participation and performance can also contribute vital information.

Another risk factor for female footballers relates to the football boots they are wearing. Traditionally females have either worn men's boots or female versions of male boots that have been made in smaller sizes. However, the female foot is anatomically different as females have smaller feet, a wider forefoot in relation to the length of their foot, higher arches, a greater ankle circumference and narrower heels (Krauss et al., 2010). Therefore, it is not appropriate to use boots made for men. Finally, we are starting to see footwear designed specifically for female athletes, such as football boots designed by Ida Sports.

Once again there are problems with a lack of quality research in this area. There have been several studies into the causes of ACL injuries, but they usually involve self-recall to establish what stage the athlete was in their menstrual cycle, and self-recall can be a less reliable method of research. Also as the length of menstrual cycle can vary in the individual it is difficult to accurately assess whether a single hormone was present in high levels (Pitchers and Elliott-

Sale, 2019). Once again this highlights the need for further research in the domain of female sports performance and another example of where women are being let down by a lack of empirical evidence and exploration.

What can female athletes do to support their performance across the phases of the menstrual cycle?

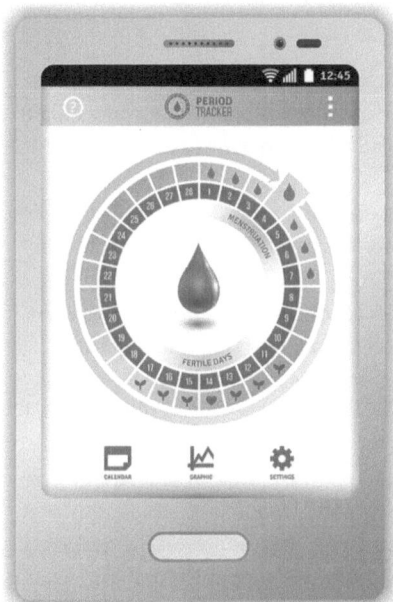 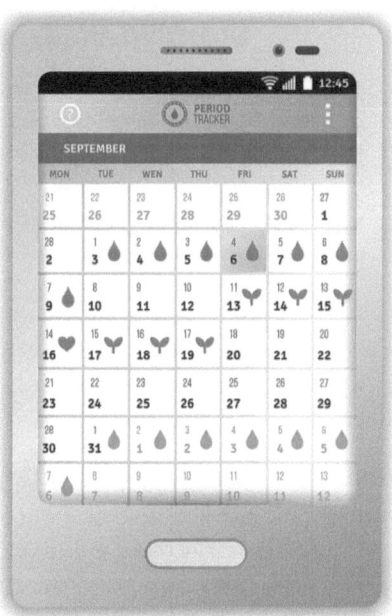

Women can start to take some control, improve their body literacy and gain a deeper understanding of how their body functions by tracking their menstrual cycle. Tracking the menstrual cycle helps women to increase awareness of what their own cycle feels like, and it can form an important element of self-care for women (Hill, 2019). This can be done by using a calendar, diary, or a period tracking app. There are apps that an athlete can share with their coach, if they have given permission to share their data. Cycle tracking has many advantages as it can help females to understand when their hormones may make them feel more motivated and energetic, and when their symptoms can become more challenging. This is important because if a woman can anticipate how they may be going to feel at any stage in their cycle then they can be proactive and start to make plans for any changes. In the case study of Florence in Box 3.1 she was advised to start tracking her cycles as it would help her to prepare for any potential problems that may arise.

Being prepared for each stage of the cycle is referred to as 'menstrual resilience' by Ross et al. (2023), as they see resilience as being able to respond to what may happen by changing your approach or doing something differently. Menstrual resilience will help females know what they need, when they need it so they can have the best experience of their cycle. There may be a drawback to tracking periods as it could influence how an individual thinks they should be feeling. For example, at a certain point in their cycle they may have previously felt lethargic so expecting to do so again at that point may actually bring on feelings of lethargy.

BOX 3.4 SPOTLIGHT ON: PERIOD CLOTHING AND UNDERWEAR

In 2022 Puma and Modibodi conducted research into why teenage girls were leaving sport in such large numbers. They discovered dropout rate was as high as 50 per cent and their research showed the following statistics:

- 1 in 2 teenagers skipped sport because of their period.
- 3 in 5 teenagers skipped sport, owing to fear of leaking blood, or revealing their period.
- 3 in 4 teenagers experienced anxiety or lack of concentration when participating in sport and physical exercise while on their period, owing to fear of leakage.
- 75% of teenagers never discussed their period with their coach.

(Baker, 2022)

Modibodi and Nixi Body are among companies who now manufacture underwear designed to absorb blood from a period and enable the athlete to carry on without fear of leakage or visible blood stains. The underwear is designed with an ultra-thin absorbent lining that is around 3 mm thick that can hold between 10–25 ml of blood, equivalent to between two and four tampons' worth of blood. Sports have taken measures to support sportswomen on their period as shown by the next three examples.

In November 2022 Wimbledon announced that their policy of wearing all white clothing would be relaxed from 2023. As a result players could wear dark coloured underwear if they wanted, providing they are no longer than the length of their skirt. As a result in the first round of Wimbledon 2023 Elena Rybakina, the defending champion, and her opponent, Shelby Rogers of the US, both wore black undershorts. British tennis player Heather Watson said that she was relieved at this decision as in 2022 she had used the contraceptive pill to avoid having her period during the event. Other players explained how they were so anxious that they developed signals with their support team to let them know if they noticed that they were bleeding.

Before the 2023 Football World Cup it was announced that the England team would no longer wear white shorts with their home strip and that both home and away strips would incorporate blue shorts. They joined Australia and New Zealand in having specially designed kits that featured a leak protection liner in their shorts. Domestically, Bristol City now wear red shorts as part of their kit and join

Manchester City, Stoke, Swansea and West Bromwich Albion by playing in dark coloured shorts. Other sports have been slower to implement changes, such as England's cricketers still playing in all white kits during Test matches.

Period swimwear that is designed with five layers to absorb and seal in menstrual blood is also available from manufacturers such as Ruby Love. This is an answer to a serious problem as it is not possible to wear sanitary pads in swimming pools and some women do not feel safe or comfortable using tampons while swimming.

As shown by the example of Heather Watson in Box 3.4 some athletes do turn to hormonal contraceptives to limit menstrual symptoms or manage the timing of their period. Research shows that 70 per cent of female athletes use hormonal contraception at some point in their career (Martin et al., 2018) but not all athletes want to take additional medication and in Chapter 4 you will explore the use of hormonal contraception among female athletes.

Period pain is partly caused by prostaglandins which are chemicals released around the first day of the period that can cause inflammation leading to stomach pain and upset. Non-steroidal anti-inflammatory drugs (NSAIDs), such as ibuprofen and aspirin, can be effective as painkillers to treat these symptoms of a period. They were used by Florence in the case study and helped to enable Jasmin Sawyers to compete in long jump at the Olympics as shown in Box 3.3. Using heat treatments, such as a hot water bottle or heat pad, can also help to alleviate stomach cramps and pain.

Increasingly nutrition is being seen as having an important role to play in managing menstrual symptoms. In particular the following four strategies can be trialled to see if they reduce symptoms:

- Consuming fruit and vegetables may help reduce menstrual cramps and pain (Fernández-Martínez et al., 2018). In particular the intake of foods rich in magnesium and zinc are beneficial in regulating prostaglandins responsible for inflammation (Parazzini et al., 2017).
- Eating fish and seafoods that provide rich sources of omega 3, such as salmon, tuna, chia seeds and walnuts, can reduce inflammation and thus period pain (Rahbar et al., 2012).
- Drinking 6–8 glasses of water to maintain hydration as menstrual blood loss can contribute to dehydration and may cause headaches.
- Taking the spice turmeric, which has an active ingredient, curcumin, that acts as an anti-inflammatory and mimics NSAIDs like ibuprofen can help reduce inflammation and period pain (Hesami et al., 2021).

In addition to the four strategies above some women find that exercise can relieve some symptoms through the production of hormones that act as natural painkillers and enhance mood. Exercising can be challenging when menstrual symptoms are significant but even low intensity exercise such as walking may be beneficial.

BOX 3.5 REAL-WORLD APPLICATION

As a female athlete, you should:

1. Educate yourself about the physiology of the menstrual cycle and under-stand why you may have variations in energy levels, mood, or psycholo-gical state during different phases.
2. Use an app or diary to track your cycle and increase your awareness of what your own menstrual cycle feels like through its different phases, and so you can predict when your period may start.
3. Understand the different effects that oestrogen and progesterone have on training and recovery and adapt your schedule if you find it beneficial to train harder or rest more during the different phases of your menstrual cycle.
4. Be prepared for the start of your period and ensure that you have every-thing in place to support you through these days. This includes making sure you have the right clothing and sanitary wear.
5. Experiment with changes in diet and pain-relieving medication to assess whether they may be beneficial when you have to compete or train during your period.
6. Be comfortable opening conversations about your menstrual cycle with people around you who will benefit from knowing what is happening with your cycle, for example, your partner, coach, and fellow athletes.

As a coach, you should:

1. Understand the different phases of the menstrual cycle and any potential impact they can have on a female athlete's mood, motivation, or other psychological factors.
2. Consider any physiological changes that may occur and how they might impact on performance in competition and training.
3. Appreciate that every female will experience their cycle differently and take time to understand how individual athletes may be impacted.
4. Develop a coaching environment where you are able to have honest and open conversations with female athletes about their menstrual cycle.

Summary

The impact of the menstrual cycle on female athletic performance is a complex area that is not currently being effectively supported by sufficient amounts of high-quality research. As a result, we are not fully clear on the relationship between athletic performance and the phases of the menstrual cycle. In addition to this the individual female experience is a significant factor to consider when establishing this relationship, owing to the inter-individual differences in the severity of menstrual symptoms and the differing amounts of hormones released throughout the cycle. As there are no guidelines currently around exercise and the menstrual cycle it is dependent upon female athletes and their coaches to develop their own individualised approach.

The key messages to take away from this chapter are:

1.   The menstrual cycle lasts for around 28 days and is divided in two phases – the follicular phase between the start of the period and ovulation when oestrogen predominates, and the luteal phase between ovulation and the end of the cycle when progesterone predominates.
2.   Although each female will experience the menstrual cycle differently oestrogen usually promotes high energy and motivation levels, while progesterone can promote calmness and good mood.
3.   There is some evidence to suggest that strength training and high intensity aerobic training may produce greater adaptations if concentrated in the follicular phase, with low intensity aerobic training and periods of recovery more prevalent in the luteal phase.
4.   Research currently shows that athletic performance is relatively unaffected by the phases of the menstrual cycle; however, the ability to attain peak athletic performance may be compromised by symptoms of the menstrual period in the early days of the cycle.
5.   Owing to its effect on joint stability, research shows a slight potential increase in the risk of joint injury around the point where oestrogen levels peak.
6.   Female athletes can increase their body literacy and develop menstrual resilience by tracking their menstrual cycle using an app or diary.

End-of-Chapter Quiz

Answers can be found after the References

1.   Identify which of the following statements about the menstrual cycle is false:

a   A textbook menstrual cycle lasts around 28 days in length.
b   A women's menstrual cycle may vary in length between cycles.
c   The menstrual cycle starts when the ovaries are stimulated to release oestrogen.
d   Amenorrhoea refers to the loss of periods when the cycle is disrupted.

2.   Identify which of the following statements about the hormones of the menstrual cycle is true:

a   At the end of the menstrual cycle oestrogen will be high and progesterone will be low.
b   At the end of the menstrual cycle oestrogen will be low and progesterone will be high.

c At the end of the menstrual cycle oestrogen and progesterone will both be low.

d At the end of the menstrual cycle oestrogen and progesterone will both be high.

3. Identify what impact the menstrual cycle may have on athletic performance:

a The menstrual cycle will have a minor effect on a female's endurance and strength.

b The menstrual cycle will impact significantly on training performance and recovery time.

c The menstrual cycle can impact positively on a female's aerobic capacity.

d The menstrual cycle can impact negatively on flexibility and skill levels.

4. Oestrogen is identified as an anabolic hormone, meaning that it can promote:

a rest and relaxation

b muscle development

c joint flexibility

d higher heart rates

5. Identify which two interventions may help female athletes best prepare for physical and emotional symptoms associated with different phases of the menstrual cycle:

a Booking days off when they know they will experience bad symptoms.

b Building rest periods and recovery days into their training schedule.

c Opening up conversations with their coach and people in their support network.

d Adjusting nutrition to meet the needs of different phases of their cycle.

e Tracking their menstrual cycle to predict when they may experience symptoms.

References

American College of Obstetricians and Gynaecologists (2019) Menstruation in Girls and Adolescents: Using the Menstrual Cycle as a Vital Sign. Available at: www.acog.org/clinical/clinical-guidance/committee-opinion/articles/2015/12/menstruation-in-girls-and-adolescents-using-the-menstrual-cycle-as-a-vital-sign (Accessed 18 September 2023).

Bailey, M. and Ahearn, N. (2023) How to tackle the increased rate of ACL injuries in women's football. Available at: www.boa.ac.uk/resource/how-to-tackle-the-increased-rate-of-acl-injuries-in-women-s-football.html#:~:text=Biologically%20female%20athletes%20have%203,as%20a%20significant%20challenge4 (Accessed 4 October 2023).

Baker, M. (2022) PUMA and Modibodi® commissioned a global survey to investigate why 1 in 2 girls are leaving sport. Available at: *PUMA and Modibodi® commissioned a global survey to investigate why 1 i – Modibodi US* (Accessed 4 October 2023).

Buser, T. (2012) 'The impact of menstrual cycle and hormonal contraceptives on competitiveness', *Journal of Economic Behavior and Organization*, 83(1), 1–10.

Chidi-Ogbulu, N. and Baar, K. (2019) 'Effect of estrogen on musculoskeletal performance and injury risk', *Frontiers in Physiology*, 9(1834). doi:10.3389/fphys.2018.01834.

Colenso Semple, L.M., D'Souza, A.C., Elliott-Sale, K.J. and Phillips, S. (2023) 'Current evidence shows no influence of women's menstrual cycle phase on acute strength performance or adaptations to resistance exercise training', *Frontiers in Sports and Active Living*, 5, 1054542. doi:10.3389/fspor.2023.1054542.

Crewther, B.T. and Cook, C.J. (2018) 'A longitudinal analysis of salivary testosterone concentrations and competitiveness in elite and non-elite women athletes', *Physiology and Behaviour*, 188, 157–161.

Eckerson, J.M. (2019) Energy and nutritional needs of the exercising female. In J. Forsyth and C.M. Roberts (Eds), *The Exercising Female: Science and its Application*. Oxford: Routledge.

Elliott-Sales, K.J. (2022) 'Cycle Races', *The Economist*, 444(9306), 72.

Elsesser, K. (2023) Wimbledon Allows Dark Shorts To Ease Period Leakage Worries. Available at: www.forbes.com/sites/kimelsesser/2023/07/05/wimbledon-allows-dark-shorts-to-ease-period-leakage-worries (Accessed 4 October 2023).

Fernández-Martínez, E., Onieva-Zafra, M.D. and Parra-Fernández, M.L. (2018) 'Lifestyle and prevalence of dysmenorrhea among Spanish female university students', *PLoS One*, 13(8). doi:10.1371/journal.pone.0201894.

Gault, M. and Smith, K. (2023) 'The menstrual cycle: a look back on the understanding and its impact on athletic performance', *American College of Sports Medicine*, 27(5), 6–10.

Graja, A., Kacem, M., Hammouda, O., Borji, R., Bouzid, M.A., Souissi, N. and Rebai, H. (2020) 'Physical, biomechanical, and neuromuscular responses to repeated sprint exercise in eumenorrheic female handball players: effect of menstrual cycle phases', *Journal of Strength and Conditioning Research*, 38(8), 2268–2276.

Hesami, S., Kavianpour, M., Nooshabadi, M.R., Yousefi, M., Lalooha, F. and Haghighian, H.K. (2021) 'Randomised double blind, placebo-controlled clinical trial studying the effects of turmeric in combination with mefanic acid in patients with primary dysmenorrhea', *Journal of Gynecology Obstetrics and Human Reproduction*, 50(5), 101840.

Hill, M. (2019) *Period Power*. London: Bloomsbury.

Jeukendrup, A. (2023) Strength training based on menstrual cycle phase. Available at: *No evidence to adapt training to the phase of the menstrual cycle* (mysportscience.com) (Accessed 9 October 2023).

Joffe, H., de Wit, A., Coborn, J., Crawford, S., Freeman, M., Wiley, A., Athappilly, G., Kim, S., Sullivan, K.A., Cohen, L.S. and Hall, J.E. (2020) 'Impact of estradiol variability and progesterone on mood in perimenopausal women with depressive symptoms', *Journal of Endocrinology and Metabolism*, 105(3), 642–650.

Julian, R., Hecksteden, A., Fullager, H.H. and Meyer, T. (2017) 'The effects of the menstrual cycle phase on physical performance in female soccer players', *Plos One*, 12(3).

Krauss, I., Valiant, G., Horstmann, T. and Grau, S. (2010) 'Comparisons of female foot morphology and last design in athletic footwear – are men's lasts appropriate for women?' *Research in Sports Medicine*, 18(2), 140–156.

Lee, H., Petrofsky, J., Shah, N., Awali, A., Shah, K, Alotaibi, M. and Yim, J.E. (2014) 'Higher sweating rate and skin blood flow during the luteal phase of the menstrual cycle', *Tohuku Journal of Experimental Medicine*, 234(2),11–22.

Lofthouse, A. (2020) BBC Elite British Sportswomen's survey. Available at: https://www.bbc.co.uk/sport/53705777 (Accessed 2 October 2023).

Lucarno, S, Zago, M., Buckthorpe, M., Grassi, A., Tosarelli, F., Smith, R., Della Villa, F. (2021) 'Systematic Video Analysis of Anterior Cruciate Ligament Injuries in Professional Female Soccer Players', *American Journal of Sports Medicine*, 49(7), 1794–1802. doi:10.1177/03635465211008169.

Martin, D., Sale, C., Cooper, C. and Elliott-Sale, K.J. (2018) 'Period prevalence and perceived side effects of hormonal contraceptive use and the menstrual cycle in elite athletes', *International Journal of Sports Physiology and Performance*, 13(7), 926–932.

McDonald, I. (2018) *The Women's Book Volume 1: A Guide to Nutrition, Fat Loss and Muscle Gain.* Austin, TX: Lyle McDonald.

McNulty, K.L., Elliott-Sale, K.J., Dolan, E., Swinton, P.A., Ansdell, P., Goodall, S., Thomas, K. and Hicks, K.M. (2020) 'The effects of menstrual cycle phase in exercise performance in eumenorrheic women: a systematic review and meta-analysis', *Sports Medicine*, 50, 1813–1827.

NHS (2023) Pre-menstrual syndrome (PMS). Available at: *PMS (premenstrual syndrome) – NHS* (www.nhs.uk) (Accessed 2 October 2023).

Parazzini, F., Di Martino, M. and Pellegrino, P. (2017) 'Magnesium in the gynecological practice: a literature review', *Magnesium Research*, 30(1), 1–7.

Pitchers, G. and Elliott-Sale, K.J. (2019) 'Considerations for coaches training female athletes', *Training Female Athletes*, 55, 19–30.

Rahbar, N., Asgharzadeh, N. and Ghorbani, R. (2012) 'Effect of omega-3 fatty acids on intensity of primary dysmenorrhea', *International Journal of Gynaecology and Obstetrics*, 117(1), 45–47.

Rocha-Rodrigues, S., Sousa, M., Reis, P.L., Leao, C., Cardaso-Marinho, B., Massada, M. and Afonso, J. (2021) 'Bidirectional Interactions between the Menstrual Cycle, Exercise Training, and Macronutrient Intake in Women: A Review', *Nutrients*, 13(2), 438. doi:10.3390/nu13020438.

Ross, E. in BBC Sports Desk (Host) (2023, 8 March) Women's Sport Matters – We're not all the same. Period. (Audio Podcast). *BBC*. Available at: www.bbc.co.uk/sounds/play/p0f7b8jn (Accessed 4 October 2023).

Ross, E., Moffat, B. and Smith, B. (2023) *The Female Body Bible.* London: Bantam.

Sims, S. (2016) *Roar.* USA: Rodale.

Sung, E., Han, A., Hinricks, T., Vorgerd, M., Manchado, C. and Platen, P. (2014) 'Effects of follicular versus luteal phase-based strength training in young women', *Springer Plus*, 3, 668.

Team GB (2023) Sporty AF (And Female) Our Cycles - The Menstrual Cycle in Sport Episode 2, uploaded 20 September 2023. Available at: www.youtube.com/watch?v=yYJteJZCUuA (Accessed 2 October 2023).

Answers

1. c
2. c
3. a
4. b
5. c and e

4

HORMONAL CONTRACEPTION AND ATHLETIC PERFORMANCE

Jess Pinchbeck

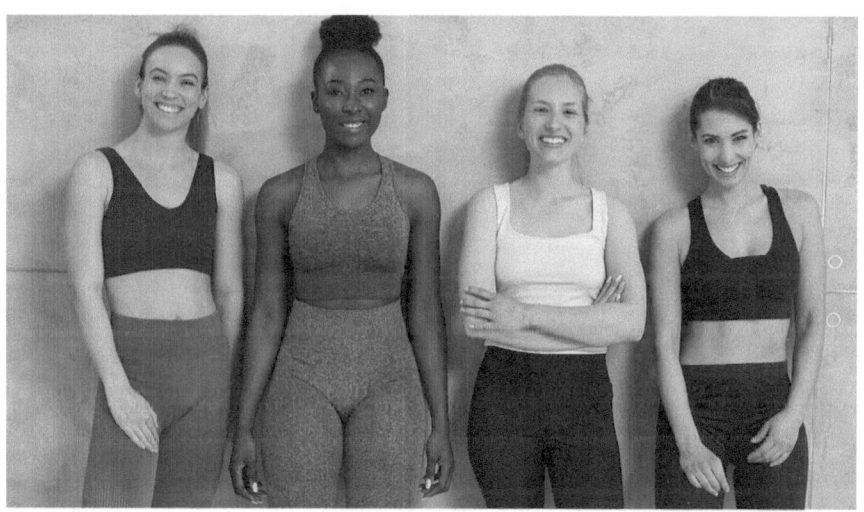

Introduction

The consideration of physiological factors related to menstruation are often neglected when planning training schedules for active females as is the use of hormonal contraception. Yet, contraception is a crucial consideration for many athletes as their peak fertility can often coincide with the time in their career when they are striving for optimal performance (Bø et al., 2018). There are a variety of contraceptive methods that women can use to prevent pregnancy the selection of which is an extremely personal choice. Contraception can include non-hormonal methods, such as condoms and the diaphragm, as well as a range of hormonal contraceptives such as the oral

DOI: 10.4324/9781003330110-4

contraceptive pill, intrauterine system (IUS) (known as the coil), implants, patches, and the injection. This chapter focuses on the use of hormonal contraception. The reason for this is that hormonal contraception has an impact on normal hormonal fluctuations during the menstrual cycle which causes physiological changes. Therefore, it is important that female athletes and those working with them have a knowledge and understanding of the uses and implications of hormonal contraception and factor this into a female athlete's training and nutrition plan.

As discussed in Chapter 3 the menstrual cycle involves several endogenous hormones (naturally occurring within the body), two of which are oestrogen and progesterone. All forms of hormonal contraception involve the introduction of exogenous (external synthetic or artificial) forms of oestrogen and/or progesterone into the body (Pitchers and Elliot-Sale, 2019). Each type of hormonal contraception will contain slightly different amounts of synthetic hormones and therefore may have slightly different effects on the body. This chapter will explore the different types of hormonal contraception available, how they work, and the impact that each type has on the hormones of the menstrual cycle. It will examine the prevalence of hormonal contraception used by athletes and active women and the reasons behind their use. The effect that hormonal contraception may have on training and performance is explored alongside the debate regarding the benefits of a natural menstrual cycle against those gained from a synthetic cycle as produced by hormonal contraception. The use of hormonal contraception can also mask any menstrual problems that an athlete is experiencing, such as irregularity or absence of natural periods, which also needs considering when working with female athletes.

But first read the case study, in Box 4.1, where you are introduced to Safa who is encountering typical issues connected with periods and hormonal contraception.

BOX 4.1 SAFA (COUNTY CRICKETER)

Safa is a 25-year-old county level cricketer and has been taking the contraceptive pill since she was aged 17. The main reason Safa started taking the pill was to allow her to control her periods in relation to cricket to ensure that a bleed never coincided with a county championship game. These matches are 50-over games and are divided into the first inning lasting 3 hours and 20 minutes, followed by a break of around 40 minutes, and then the second inning which also lasts 3 hours 20 minutes, with neither inning exceeding 50 overs. This means that Safa can be on the field for over 3 hours without a break wearing white cricket trousers. When Safa was 17, she had a heavy bleed during the game and leaked through her whites, she was mortified and felt so embarrassed, hence her resorting to oral contraception to prevent this happening again. Although the rules state that players can ask for a break Safa didn't feel confident enough to draw attention to herself and ask for a break plus, at age 17, she didn't always know how heavy her flow was until it was too late. Safa's natural cycle was quite irregular, and she often experienced quite bad menstrual cramping and so ultimately being on her period on competition days just wasn't an option. Prior to taking the pill Safa tried wearing a tampon as well as a sanitary towel but sometimes that wasn't enough protection. Also, the toilets at many of the facilities are not always equipped for women and lack suitable sanitation disposal.

The contraceptive pill has worked well for Safa and she tends to take about three packets of combined pills back-to-back without a break to prevent her from having a breakthrough bleed. When she does decide to allow a bleed she manipulates when she starts and stops the packet to plan for competition. This means that Safa hasn't had a natural period for 8 years. However, in the last few months she has started experiencing low mood and depression as well as getting headaches which are beginning to interfere with her training. These seem to subside during the time when she does take a 7-day break between packs and so she wonders whether this may be associated with taking the same pill now for 8 years. She doesn't feel confident talking to her male coach about it and so booked in to see her GP who has advised her to come off the pill to ascertain what is happening naturally. Safa has reluctantly agreed but is worried about the impact of this and the practicality of no longer being able to manage her cycle. This in itself is causing her worry and anxiety.

What the case study illustrates is why some athletes may choose to use hormonal contraception for issues other than the prevention of pregnancy. It also highlights the benefits of such an approach as well as the potential impact of taking hormonal contraception on women's health and also sports performance. Safa's situation also shows the lack of knowledge and education that many girls and women have regarding hormonal contraception and the difficulties that women often feel discussing this with a coach. For example, Armour et al. (2020) found that over three-quarters of athletes and coaches in their study did not amend training, owing to the menstrual cycle, and 76 per cent of athletes did not discuss menstruation with their coaches.

Safa's case study will be referred to throughout this chapter, and some of her experiences can be linked to issues reported in the research. But first hormonal contraception is considered in more detail including the potential health and performance-related implications for athletes.

How do oral hormonal contraceptives work?

The most common type of hormonal contraception is the oral contraception pill. There are two main types of contraceptive pill: the combined contraceptive pill and progestogen only pill. The next sections look at these in more detail.

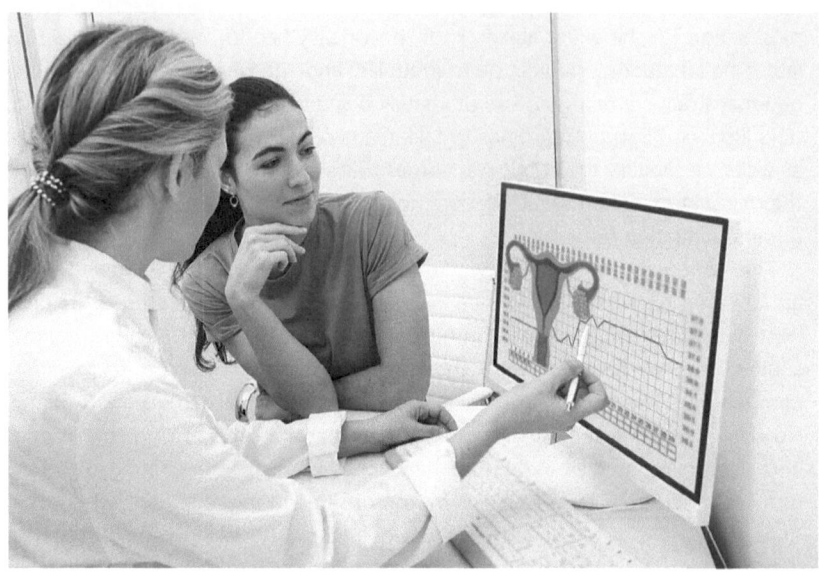

Combined contraceptive pill

The combined contraceptive pill is the most common type of hormonal contraception and is typically just called 'the pill' (NHS, 2023a). Within the UK they are also the most frequently used hormonal contraceptive by elite sportswomen (Martin et al., 2018). The combined pill contains artificial versions of oestrogen and progesterone, and it works by keeping these hormones at a consistent level replicating the second half of the menstrual cycle. This means that ovulation is prevented, and no egg is released. There are lots of different brands of combined pills but the (NHS, 2023a) states there are three main types:

- Monophasic 21-day pills – these are the most common type. Each pill contains the same amount of hormones and 1 pill is taken for 21 days, followed by a 7 day break of no pills before the cycle starts again. During the pill free week, a bleed is likely to occur, although this is like a period it is a withdrawal bleed and not a natural period. Sometimes it is possible to reduce the break to 4 days, or even take the packs continuously back-to-back without a break such as Safa has done.
- Phasic 21-day pills – you take these for 21 days and then have a 7-day break, however, there are 2 or 3 different coloured sections with each pack each containing different levels of hormones. The pills have to be taken in the correct order.
- Every day (ED) pills – these packs contain 28 tablets, 21 of which are active pills and contain hormones, and 7 that are placebo tablets containing no hormones. Each pill is taken in the correct order for 28 days and then the next pack is taken straight away. During the 7 days taking the placebo tablets a bleed is likely to occur.

Progestogen-only pill

The progestogen-only pill typically prevents pregnancy by preventing sperm reaching the egg through increasing the thickness of the mucus in the cervix, however, the desogestrel progestogen only pill can also stop ovulation (NHS, 2023e). Each pack contains 28 pills and 1 pill is taken daily with no break between packs, however, there are two different types of progestogen only pill each of which has different time requirements for taking the pills:

- 3-hour progestogen only pill – these are the older traditional forms of progestogen-only pills (commonly referred to as the mini pill) and they must be taken within the same 3-hour time slot every day to be effective
- 12-hour progestogen only pill – these are the new generation pills (desogestrel progestogen only pill), and they have a 12-hour window to take the pill which can be less restrictive and easier to manage if athletes have an unpredictable schedule or lots of travel.

Around half of women do not experience any bleeding using this form of contraception, or for those that do bleed it is typically much lighter breakthrough bleeding, because the uterus lining is being kept thin all the time. However, these are not the only choices that women have.

What other types of hormonal contraceptives are there?

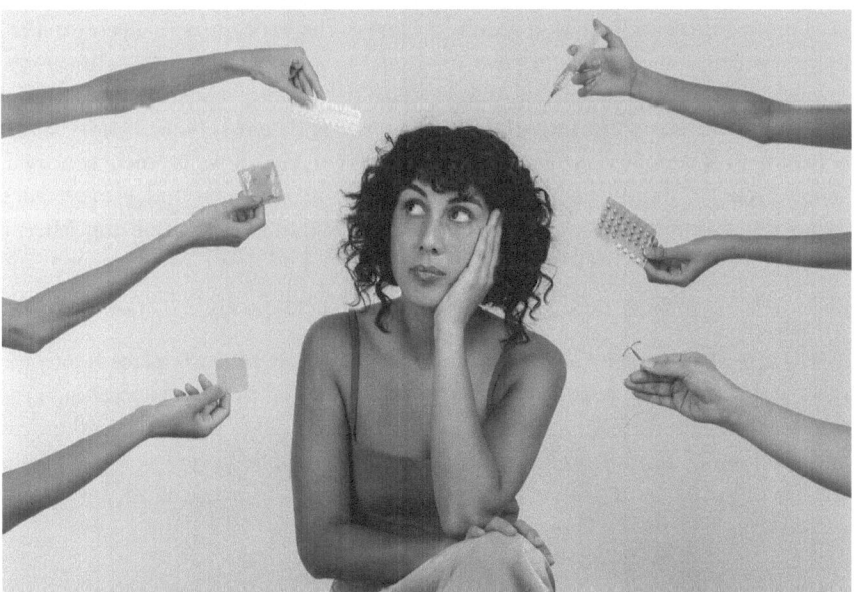

In addition to the oral contraceptive pill there are Long-Acting Reversible Contraceptives (LARCs). These include the implant, an injection, and they can include a hormonal coil. LARCs deliver the synthetic dose of hormones that stay in your system for various lengths of time depending on the approach you use.

The contraceptive implant is a small plastic rod which is inserted into the upper arm just underneath the skin. It works by releasing synthetic progestogen into the bloodstream to prevent the release of an egg, increasing the thickness of the mucus in the cervix to prevent sperm from getting through and thinning the lining of the womb. The implant can last up to three years, however, once it is removed fertility resumes. A common side effect of the implant is that periods stop completely (NHS, 2023b). The contraceptive injection is similar to the implant in that it works by releasing synthetic progestogen into the bloodstream to protect against pregnancy and this can last 8–13 weeks depending upon the type of injection. However, the main difference is that once the injection wears off it can take up to a year for fertility to return to normal (NHS, 2023c).

There are two types of coils, which is a small plastic device that is implanted into the uterus, but only one of these uses hormones. One type of coil is an intrauterine device also called the coil or 'copper coil' (IUD) as it releases copper into the uterus, not synthetic hormones. The presence of copper in the contraceptive alters the cervical mucus, preventing sperm to reach and survive near the egg. The second is an intrauterine system (IUS), which releases progestogen to prevent pregnancy. This type of contraception is slightly different in that it doesn't supress the reproductive cycle of hormones because it delivers a low dose of the hormone very locally at the uterus. This keeps the uterus lining thin to avoid pregnancy rather than delivering the hormone into the bloodstream and across your whole body. Some may experience the loss of ovulation but for most women the menstrual cycle, ovulation and the cyclical release of oestrogen and progesterone can occur (NHS, 2023d). Therefore, when using an IUS such as the Mirena coil, women still experience the natural highs and lows of oestrogen and progesterone however periods can become lighter and may even stop completely.

There is also the shorter acting contraceptive patch which is placed onto the skin, and it works by releasing synthetic oestrogen and progestogen through the skin into the bloodstream to prevent ovulation, thickening of the cervical mucus and thinning of the womb lining. A new patch is applied every week for three weeks, followed by a patch free week where a withdrawal bleed may occur before repeating the cycle again.

Why might athletes use hormonal contraception?

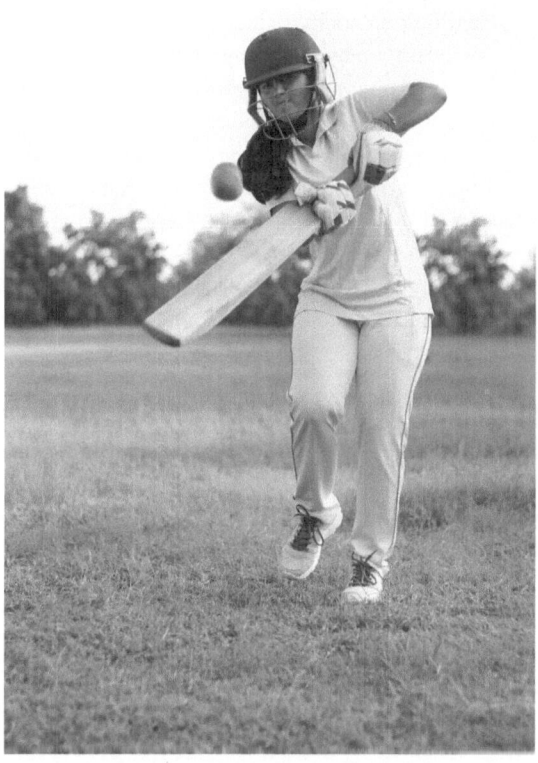

The prevalence of hormonal contraceptive use is higher in elite athletes than in the general UK population (Martin et al., 2018). Athletes will use hormonal contraception to prevent pregnancy, however, it can also be used for non-traditional means such as for menstrual management, just as Safa has done. This can be beneficial for athletes to be able to ensure their cycle is regulated so they can predict when they will bleed as well as managing some of the more unpleasant symptoms of the menstrual cycle, such as heavy bleeding, bloating, headaches, and severe period pain, known as dysmenorrhoea, all of which can impact athletic performance. As well as the management of physical symptoms associated with menstruation there are also the practicalities of managing the timing and frequency of bleeding, owing to women's sport often still following rules or structures that were initially implemented for the male game, such as those experienced by Safa. For example, wearing white uniform, length of competitions that last for hours without scheduled breaks, and even the lack of female sanitation facilities at certain sports grounds.

The actions taken by Safa are common among female athletes and Schaumberg et al. (2018) reported that 74 per cent of active women deliberately managed their use of oral contraceptives to prevent their withdrawal bleed, and 29 per cent did so at least four times within a year. The study concluded that this common strategy of manipulating menstruation potentially reduces hormone-related barriers to exercise participation and consequently may positively impact female participation and performance. Hormonal contraception can therefore be an effective tool for female athletes to be able to manage their menstruation around important competitions, yet it is not a straightforward process and individual circumstances should be considered. For example, Brown, Knight and Forrest (2021) found that while some participants enjoyed the convenience of using hormonal contraceptives to prevent bleeding others encountered negative symptoms such as headaches, with some athletes unaware of the negative symptoms until they ceased taking the contraceptive pill. Box 4.2 shows some individual athlete experiences of using hormonal contraception.

BOX 4.2 WHAT DO THE ATHLETES SAY?

Do as much research as you can before you decide which form of contraception is right for you. A lot of women only start thinking about their hormones when they start trying to get pregnant – I wish I'd had a better understanding much earlier.

Jess Ennis-Hill, former GB heptathlete, (cited in Hedges, 2023)

I have skipped my period using the pill because I did not want to bleed through clothing.

Heather Watson, British tennis player (cited in Watson, 2023)

They told me they had to take me off that pill because the headaches I was having highly increase your chances of having a stroke [...] The advice from the private doctor was to take a supplementary pill once a day, or stop heading the ball. I thought: 'I'm a defender, I can't not head a ball'.

Rachel Newborough, footballer, (cited in Lofthouse, 2023)

I learned a lot and feel proud to have gone from a young teenager with very irregular and painful periods, being put on the pill to "fix the problem" coming off the pill and now understanding, helping my body to be regular, managing and be healthy.

Hannah Miley, swimmer (cited in British Swimming, 2023)

I tried a Mirena coil but I really hated it. It had this odd suppressive effect on my mood [...] I am someone who has high highs and low lows, but this somehow just made me feel almost dead inside. I just didn't enjoy how it felt at all and eventually had it removed.

Isabella Burke, bobsleigher, (cited in Lofthouse, 2023)

The athlete's stories show that hormonal contraception and the body's response can be a very individual experience. In the BBC (2020) Elite British Sportswomen's survey, which received 537 responses, 59.8 per cent of athletes said their performance was affected by their period or they had missed training/ competition because of their period. In addition, 28.2 per cent of elite athletes said they took the contraceptive pill specifically to control the impact their period had on their performance, yet 39.9 per cent did not feel comfortable discussing their period with their coaches. A study by O'Donnell, White and Dobbin (2023) explored menstruation in netballers and reported that some players used hormonal contraception for various reasons such as to control their heavy bleeding, reduce pain and even control their acne. Participants cited menstruation as "an extra thing that makes me feel uncomfortable" and that the use of hormonal contraceptives "controls this really well", "was a nice side effect" and was "definitely handy because if you've got a game on your first day then it's not a good feeling". However, other participants in the study expressed concerns around long-term contraceptive use and previous disruption of the menstrual cycle, such as amenorrhoea, which is always a concern when female athletes are undertaking a high volume of training.

BOX 4.3 SPOTLIGHT ON: AMENORRHOEA AND HORMONAL CONTRACEPTION

Amenorrhoea is the loss of periods and as shown in Chapter 5 is one of the warning signs of RED-S. Worryingly the absence of a menstrual cycle has to some extent been normalised and even celebrated within female sport and hormonal contraceptives are often used to treat amenorrhoea, owing to disruption of the menstrual cycle.

A study by Cheng et al. (2021) reported that the use of hormonal contraception was prevalent within female collegiate athletes, and 24 per cent cited irregularities with their menstrual cycle as the main reason for their use. However, recent thinking warns against this approach as oral contraceptives induce an "imposter period" which is not the equivalent of a healthy menstrual cycle that comprises fluctuating hormones (Elliott-Sale and Hicks, 2018). Rather than acting as a cure taking oral contraceptives instead masks the underlying cause of the menstrual dysfunction, as the withdrawal bleed can lead athletes to falsely believe that their natural menstrual cycle has returned (Ross, Moffat and Smith, 2023). It is important for those working with athletes experiencing amenorrhoea to understand what is causing irregular or absent periods and work with healthcare professionals on restoring a healthy cycle, before considering the use of hormonal contraceptives.

The pros and cons of hormonal contraception

The highs and lows of oestrogen and progesterone and their contrasting effects were discussed in Chapter 3. Specifically, how oestrogen can make women feel energised and motivated while progesterone can promote feelings of calm and relaxation. Taking hormonal contraception results in these natural feelings being lost or less prevalent.

Using hormonal contraception can be effective for menstruation management, however, it is also important that athletes are fully informed about the choices they are making, including gaining an understanding of some of the potential implications on performance, physically and psychologically, and being aware of any unwelcome side effects such as unwanted weight gain and low mood. Different hormonal contraception will suit different athletes and the use of hormonal contraception is not a one size fits all approach. Women often try several different methods of contraception to find the method that works best for them. It is advisable for athletes to keep a diary when starting hormonal contraception to monitor any emotional or physical changes that they encounter and whether these changes have an impact on their training and performance.

There are inevitably practical benefits for athletes using hormonal contraception, mainly the prevention of bleeding or menstrual symptoms at key times in the performance calendar but there can also be drawbacks. Martin et al. (2018) reported 19 negative and 23 positive categories of side effects in hormonal contraceptive users as shown in Figure 4.1.

The study did show, however, that the side effects varied by the type of hormonal contraception used. For example, 17.8 per cent of participants using combined hormonal contraception reported less negative side effects compared with 39.1 per cent of those using progestin-only contraception (progestin is the synthetic form of progesterone) and the implant reported a higher incidence of negative effects compared to other forms of hormonal contraception (Martin et al., 2018). Despite the negative side effects documented approximately 30 per cent of sportswomen used progesterone-only contraceptives, owing to the perception that they bring about amenorrhoea, which can be seen as normal and even desirable in some sports.

The prevalence of hormonal contraceptive use and reported side effects of the menstrual cycle and hormonal contraceptive use in powerlifters and rugby players was investigated by Nolan, Elliot-Sale and Egan (2023). Findings revealed that 51.1 per cent of athletes were using hormonal contraception. Of those players not using hormonal contraceptives 83.5 per cent experienced side effects of the menstrual cycle including cramping (42.4 per cent), headache (24.5 per cent), and fatigue (24.5 per cent). In contrast only 40 per cent of those using hormonal contraceptives reported side effects, including mood changes (17.9 per cent), stomach pain (8.3 per cent), and headaches (6.9 per cent). This shows that the symptoms experienced by both those using hormonal contraception and those on a natural cycle are extensive and vary between individuals. Such side effects are likely to impact on athletic performance although future investigation in this area is needed to fully explore such effects.

Positive Effects	Negative Effects
Ability to predict/change cycle date	Weight gain
Regular period	Mood changes/swings
Cessation/less frequent periods	Irregular periods
Improved mood	Poor skin
Reduced bleeding/lighter periods	Headaches/migraines
Improved skin	Altered cycle length
Reduced period pain	Breast issues (bigger/sore)
Reduced cramps (unspecified)	Constant/irregular bleeding
Reduced pain (unspecified)	Spotting
Reduced headaches/migraine	Tiredness/fatigue/lethargy
Increased iron	Effect on training/performance
Less ill/sick	Nausea/sickness/vomiting
Resumption of cycle from amenorrhea	Water retention
Reduced stomach cramps	Abnormal liver function
Couldn't forget to take	Bloating
Effect on training/performance	Hormone imbalance
Reduced bloating	Increased appetite
Improved bone density	Stomach pain
Less faint	Unspecified pain
Reduced fluctuations in water retention	
Reduced fluctuations in weight	
Reduced PCOS side effects	
Helps PMT	

FIGURE 4.1 Positive and negative effects of hormonal contraception
Source: Adapted from Martin et al. (2018)

Hormonal contraceptives and athletic performance

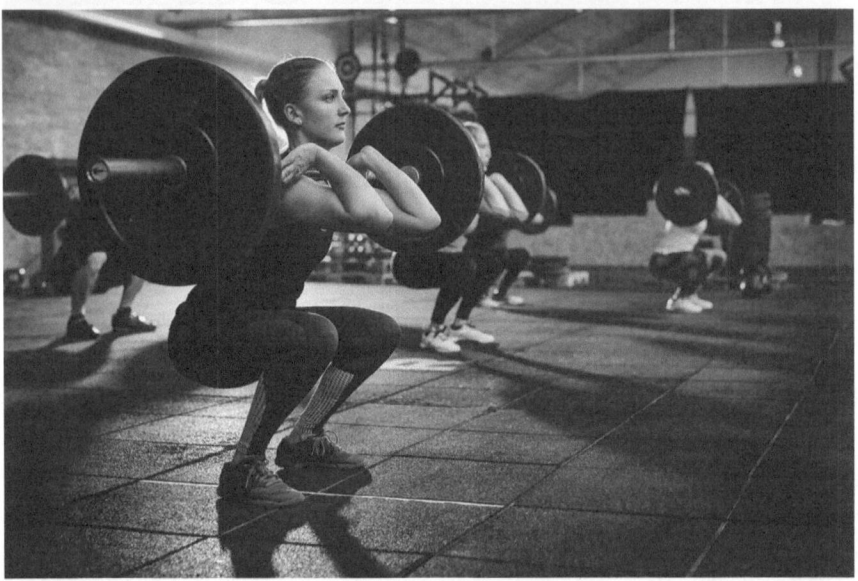

The relationship between hormonal contraceptive use and athletic performance is not completely clear and while some studies suggest that hormonal contraception can influence factors such as aerobic capacity, muscular strength and body composition further research is needed. For example, research has reported that females using oral contraceptives are potentially exposed to a higher risk of muscle damage during sport, owing to the changes in the concentrations of ovarian hormone exposure (Elliott-Sale, cited in Roberts and Forsyth, 2018). Furthermore, a study of 53 elite Olympic athletes by Larsen et al. (2020) found that those athletes who were taking an oral contraceptive compared to those that were on a natural cycle had higher concentrations of CRP (C-reactive protein) which is an indicator of inflammation and tissue damage and has also been linked to an increased risk of developing cardiovascular disease. Oral contraceptive use has also been reported by Riechman and Lee (2022) to impair the development of lean muscle mass in young women following a resistance exercise training programme, owing to the impact that hormones have on the processes of muscle development in the body. However, although an analysis of 42 studies showed that oral contraception users might have a slightly poorer exercise performance compared to those with a natural menstrual cycle the difference was so trivial that generalised guidance on the use of hormonal contraception and athletic performance would not be appropriate (Elliott-Sale et al., 2020).

Similar to that highlighted in Chapter 1 research with women has shown contradictory evidence or is poorly designed. Literature documenting oral contraceptive use and the effects on resistance training shows conflicting findings, with studies typically restricted by low numbers of participants and poor methodology, but overall research does suggest that the response to resistance training may be impacted by female hormones (Thompson et al., 2020). There are many different factors that make it difficult to fully understand the impact of oral contraceptives on female athletic performance, and one of the key issues is the number of variations in the type of hormonal contraception containing different doses of synthetic oestrogen and progesterone (Martin et al., 2018). Hirschberg (2022) similarly acknowledged that type, dose, and mode of administration of the hormonal contraceptives must be accounted for when interpreting the impact on physical performance and the risk of injury. The same article concluded that the interpretation of findings regarding the use of oral contraception on athletic performance are 'conflicting and non-conclusive' expounded somewhat by their methodological limitations. Although this is still an emerging area of research Box 4.4 provides some general considerations around hormonal contraception for coaches and athletes.

BOX 4.4 REAL-WORLD APPLICATION

As a female athlete, you should:

1. Consider the reasons why you want to use hormonal contraception and whether this is the right choice for you.
2. Fully research the different types of hormonal contraception, the way they work, the physiology, and potential side effects to make an informed choice.
3. If you do start to use hormonal contraception keep a note and monitor any changes that you notice on your health, mood, and performance.
4. Talk to your coach about your choice of hormonal contraception or menstrual issues that you are experiencing.
5. Remember that most forms of hormonal contraception stop the natural menstrual cycle and that a withdrawal bleed is not a true period and therefore not an indicator of health.

As a coach, you should:

1. Talk to your athletes about their periods and whether they are using hormonal contraception, either to prevent pregnancy or for some form of menstrual management.
2. Understand the potential impact of hormonal contraception on health and performance and discuss these with your athlete, however, always refer your athlete to a healthcare professional for medical advice.
3. When planning a training programme and nutritional plan always consider the individual.
4. Encourage your athlete to track their menstrual cycle and if using hormonal contraception to monitor any changes or side effects.
5. Be aware that if an athlete is using hormonal contraception then they will typically not be experiencing a natural cycle and the hormone fluctuations associated with the menstrual cycle.

Hormonal contraceptives provide reliable contraception and allow athletes to have better control over their menstrual cycles, which can be beneficial for negotiating training and competition schedules. They can also help regulate hormonal fluctuations, reduce menstrual symptoms, and prevent conditions like iron deficiency anaemia. However, the use of hormonal contraceptives may also have potential side effects, such as changes in mood, weight, or performance. It is important that athletes are fully aware of the potential benefits and drawbacks to make an informed decision and find the most suitable contraceptive option that balances their reproductive health needs alongside their athletic performance goals.

Summary

The messages to take away from this chapter are:

- There are several different types of hormonal contraception including the combined pill, progestogen only pill, the intrauterine system (IUS), hormone patches, implants and injections.
- Hormonal contraception works by introducing synthetic versions of the hormones oestrogen and/or progesterone into the body.
- The synthetic hormones in hormonal contraceptives typically work by tricking the brain into thinking that the body is always in the second half of the menstrual cycle and thus ovulation does not occur.
- Hormonal contraceptives may be taken by athletes for menstrual management to control symptoms such as menstrual bleeding, stomach cramps, headaches and bloating.
- There are positive and negative effects of using hormonal contraceptives and also of the natural menstrual cycle and these will vary from individual to individual.
- Hormonal contraception may have an impact on athletic performance however there are many complexities and contradictions within the findings and further research is needed.

End-of-Chapter Quiz

Answers can be found after the References

1. What is the most common type of hormonal contraception used in the UK?

    a   The coil
    b   The combined Pill
    c   The mini-pill
    d   The hormonal patch

2. Why might athletes choose to use hormonal contraception other than for the prevention of pregnancy?

a To lose weight
b To reduce the likelihood of illness
c To control menstrual symptoms
d To become stronger

3. Why is using the pill not suitable for the treatment of amenorrhoea?

a Because it can mask the underlying health issues
b Because it can cause heavy bleeding
c Because it can disrupt sleep
d Because it can impact your appetite

4. What are the four main negative effects of using hormonal contraception cited in the study by Martin et al. (2018)?

a Acne, poor sleep, bloating and tiredness
b Headaches, stomach cramps, acne and achy muscles
c Weight loss, heavy periods, acne, and headaches
d Weight gain, mood changes/swings, irregular periods and poor skin

5. Identify which of the following statements about hormonal contraception is FALSE:

a Women often try several different methods of contraception to find the methods that works best for them
b The combined pill is the most suitable form of hormonal contraception for elite athletes
c The relationship between hormonal contraceptive use and athletic performance is not completely clear
d While some participants enjoy the convenience of using contraceptive to prevent bleeding, others encounter negative symptoms

References

Armour, M., Parry, K.A., Steel, K. and Smith, C.A. (2020) 'Australian female athlete perceptions of the challenges associated with training and competing when menstrual symptoms are present', *International Journal of Sports Science & Coaching*, 15(3), 316–323.

BBC (2020) *BBC Elite British Sportswomen's Survey results*. Available at: https://www.bbc.co.uk/sport/53593459 (Accessed: 6 October 2023).

Bø, K., Artal, R., Barakat, R., Brown, W.J., Davies, G.A., Dooley, M., Evenson, K.R., Haakstad, L.A., Kayser, B. and Kinnunen, T.I. (2018) 'Exercise and pregnancy in recreational and elite athletes: 2016/2017 evidence summary from the IOC expert group meeting, Lausanne. Part 5. Recommendations for health professionals and active women', *British Journal of Sports Medicine*, 52(17), 1080–1085.

British Swimming (2023) *Hannah helping push period conversation in sport*. Available at: https://www.britishswimming.org/news/general-swimming-news/hannah-helping-push-period-conversation-sport/ (Accessed: 6 October 2023).

Brown, N., Knight, C.J. and Forrest, L.J. (2021) 'Elite female athletes' experiences and perceptions of the menstrual cycle on training and sport performance', *Scandinavian Journal of Medicine & Science in Sports*, 31(1), 52–69.

Cheng, J., Santiago, K.A., Abutalib, Z., Temme, K.E., Hulme, A., Goolsby, M.A., Esopenko, C.L. and Casey, E.K. (2021) 'Menstrual irregularity, hormonal contraceptive use, and bone stress injuries in collegiate female athletes in the United States', *PM&R*, 13 (11), 1207–1215.

Elliott-Sale, K. J. and Hicks, K. M. (2018) 'Hormonal-based contraception and the exercising female', in J. Forsyth and C. Roberts (ed.) The Exercising Female: Science and its Application. Oxon: Routledge, 30–43.

Elliott-Sale, K.J., McNulty, K.L., Ansdell, P., Goodall, S., Hicks, K.M., Thomas, K., Swinton, P.A. and Dolan, E. (2020) 'The effects of oral contraceptives on exercise performance in women: a systematic review and meta-analysis', *Sports Medicine*, 50 (10), 1785–1812.

Hedges, F. (2023) *Jessica Ennis-Hill: I want to help more women understand their bodies.* Available at: https://www.harpersbazaar.com/uk/beauty/mind-body/a44483505/jessica-ennis-hill-jennis-hormone-health-app/ (Accessed: 18 October 2023).

Hirschberg, A.L. (2022) 'Challenging aspects of research on the influence of the menstrual cycle and oral contraceptives on physical performance', *Sports Medicine*, 52(7), 1453–1456.

Larsen, B., Cox, A., Colbey, C., Drew, M., McGuire, H., Fazekas de St Groth, B., Hughes, D., Vlahovich, N., Waddington, G. and Burke, L. (2020) 'Inflammation and oral contraceptive use in female athletes before the Rio Olympic Games', *Frontiers in Physiology*, 11, 497.

Lofthouse, A. (2023) *BBC Women's Sport Survey: Periods, the pill and the effect on female athletes.* Available at: https://www.bbc.co.uk/sport/53705777 (Accessed: 6 October 2023).

Martin, D., Sale, C., Cooper, S.B. and Elliott-Sale, K.J. (2018) 'Period prevalence and perceived side effects of hormonal contraceptive use and the menstrual cycle in elite athletes', *International Journal of Sports Physiology and Performance*, 13(7), 926–932.

NHS (2023a) *Combined Pill.* Available at: https://www.nhs.uk/conditions/contraception/combined-contraceptive-pill/ (Accessed: 6 October 2023).

NHS (2023b) *Contraceptive implant.* Available at: https://www.nhs.uk/conditions/contraception/contraceptive-implant/ (Accessed: 6 October 2023).

NHS (2023c) *The contraceptive injection.* Available at: https://www.nhs.uk/conditions/contraception/contraceptive-injection/ (Accessed: 18 October 2023).

NHS (2023d) *Intrauterine system (IUS).* Available at: https://www.nhs.uk/conditions/contraception/ius-intrauterine-system/ (Accessed: 19 October 2023).

NHS (2023e) *The progestogen-only pill.* Available at: https://www.nhs.uk/conditions/contraception/the-pill-progestogen-only/ (Accessed: 6 October 2023).

Nolan, D., Elliott-Sale, K.J. and Egan, B. (2023) 'Prevalence of hormonal contraceptive use and reported side effects of the menstrual cycle and hormonal contraceptive use in powerlifting and rugby', *The Physician and Sportsmedicine*, 51(3), 217–222.

O'Donnell, J., White, C. and Dobbin, N. (2023) 'Perspectives on relative energy deficiency in sport (RED-S): A qualitative case study of athletes, coaches and medical professionals from a super league netball club', *PloS one*, 18(5), e0285040.

Pitchers, G. and Elliot-Sale, K. (2019) 'Considerations for coaches training female athletes', *Professional Strength and Conditioning*, 55, 19–30.

Riechman, S.E. and Lee, C.W. (2022) 'Oral contraceptive use impairs muscle gains in young women', *Journal of Strength and Conditioning Research*, 36(11), 3074–3080.

Roberts, C.-M. and Forsyth, J. (2018) 'Consensus statement: The inaugural women in sport & exercise conference: Blood, sweat and fears', *Women in Sport and Physical Activity Journal*, 26(2), 1–10.

Ross, E.Z., Moffat, B. and Smith, B. (2023) *The Female Body Bible*. London: Penguin.

Schaumberg, M.A., Emmerton, L.M., Jenkins, D.G., Burton, N.W., de Jonge, X.A.J. and Skinner, T.L. (2018) 'Use of oral contraceptives to manipulate menstruation in young, physically active women', *International Journal of Sports Physiology and Performance*, 13(1), 82–87.

Thompson, B., Almarjawi, A., Sculley, D. and Janse de Jonge, X. (2020) 'The effect of the menstrual cycle and oral contraceptives on acute responses and chronic adaptations to resistance training: a systematic review of the literature', *Sports Medicine*, 50, 171–185.

Watson, H. (2023) 'Let's start talking openly about periods and call time on this taboo.' *Telegraph*. Available at: https://www.telegraph.co.uk/tennis/2023/06/15/lets-start-talking-openly-about-periods-call-time-taboo/ (Accessed: 6 October 2023).

Answers

1.   b
2.   c
3.   a
4.   d
5.   b

5

RED-S SPELLS DANGER

The Impact of Low Energy Availability on Female Athletes

Simon Rea

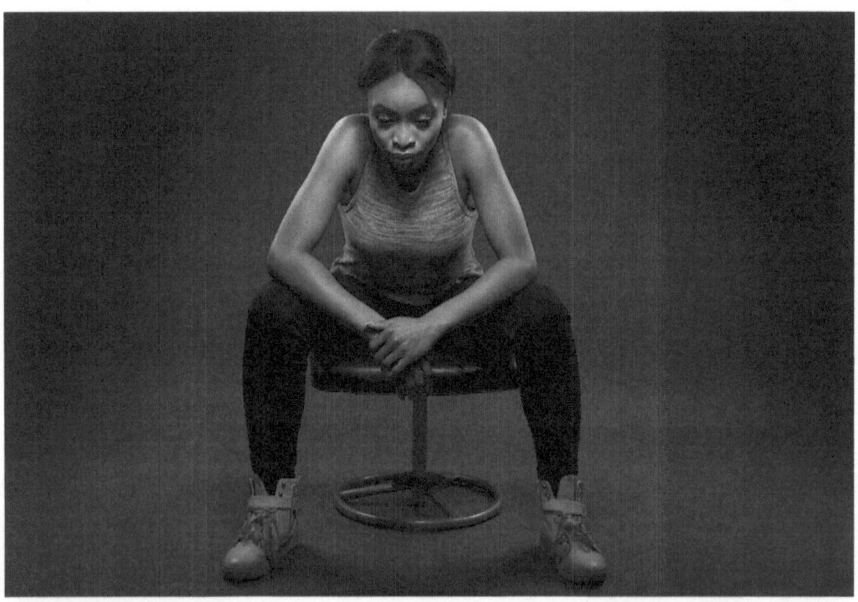

Introduction

Relative energy deficiency in sport, or RED-S, refers to the health and performance consequences of inadequate energy availability during sport and exercise (Mountjoy et al., 2014). Inadequate energy availability for training and competition over a prolonged period can impact on the maintenance of the body's optimal health. The relationship between low energy availability, disrupted menstrual function and bone health is referred to as the female

DOI: 10.4324/9781003330110-5

athlete triad. The term 'RED-S' was first used by the International Olympic Committee in 2014 to expand on the triad and include wider physiological, psychological and performance effects of low energy availability. 'RED-S' is a more inclusive term as it also recognised that the health and performance of male athletes, as well as athletes with a disability, can be negatively impacted by low energy availability.

Avoiding low energy availability is the single biggest challenge for female athletes due its impact on menstrual function and bone health (Pitchers and Elliott-Sale, 2019). But low energy availability (EA) impairs many other physiological processes in the body, including musculoskeletal health, gastrointestinal and cardiovascular function, growth, and development (Mountjoy et al., 2018).

In this chapter we will examine low energy availability and RED-S in detail and identify ten potential health and ten potential performance-related effects of RED-S. We will assess some of the causes of RED-S, and the warning signs that may indicate an athlete may be experiencing low energy availability before the condition becomes so serious that the athlete has to stop training and competing. Then we will explore why menstrual function becomes disrupted and changes that occur in the endocrine system to hormones that are vital to the health of a female athlete. Finally, we will look at measures that can be taken by athletes, and in particular the coaches and other people who support the athlete, to prevent and manage the condition.

Before then read the case study, in Box 5.1, where you are introduced to Sarah who is exhibiting typical signs of low energy availability.

BOX 5.1 SARAH (CYCLIST)

Sarah is a 24-year-old road cyclist who was a junior champion and represented Great Britain at U20 level. Since she stepped up to the senior age group, she has adopted an increasingly demanding schedule of training and competition. She trains in the early morning and in the evening six days a week. Her goal is to cycle for the senior Great Britain team at international competitions. When she can she does additional sessions that her coach is unaware of so she can gain an advantage over her competitors.

Sarah is aware that the increased intensity and duration of her training is making her lighter, and this weight loss has increased as she is not able to eat as much as she is recommended by her nutritionist. She finds that eating before training gives her stomach cramps and that she often has no appetite to eat after training. Sarah sees that her training times and performances are improving now that she is lighter. Her coach seems very pleased that she is easily achieving the goals that they have set for her. Her coach does not seem concerned about her weight loss.

However, as her weight has reduced her periods became less regular and about a year ago they stopped completely. Sarah has heard that this is common in endurance athletes, and she dismisses it as 'one less thing to worry about'. She has also started to feel really exhausted after training, needing a sleep during the day.

Her parents are concerned about her as she seems withdrawn and uncommunicative at home, and she rarely socialises with family or friends. They have asked Sarah whether she is eating properly as she looks like a 'bag of bones'. Sarah admits to her parents that she is not eating regularly and that she is missing periods. She has also had a persistent cold that does not seem to clear, so they insist that she goes to the doctor.

Sarah's doctor is really concerned and sends her for blood tests and a bone scan. The blood tests show that her hormones are out of balance and the bone scan shows that she has osteopenia, which is a precursor to osteoporosis. Sarah's doctor and parents insist that she should stop training until her period returns.

What the case study illustrates is how RED-S can develop and some of its contributing factors. A high training load and a high requirement for calories from food can often provide challenges that need to be managed. Training early in the morning can make pre-exercise eating problematic, as a meal needs to be consumed 1–2 hours before training. Training in the evening can make post-training feeding difficult as the athlete may not have a desire to eat. Also they could end up eating late in the evening giving their digestive system less time to work before the athlete goes to bed. If the athlete is also working during the day then the time needed to prepare and consume meals becomes problematic. Often RED-S is caused by a poor nutritional strategy where an athlete does not plan their nutrition carefully enough to ensure that they gain enough calories to fuel their training and other daily activities.

As we move through this chapter we will refer to Sarah's case study and you will see that she develops some signs and symptoms that are typical of the condition of RED-S. But first we will consider RED-S in more detail and the potential health and performance-related effects that can develop from low energy availability.

How does low energy availability affect the body?

Before we assess the impact of low energy availability we can take a further look at the concept of relative energy deficiency. Relative energy deficiency exists when there is insufficient energy available for normal physiological functioning of the body.

The current government recommendations are that females aged between 11–64 should eat 2000 kcals per day (Public Health England, 2016) with additional calorie intake to cover exercise and training. This energy intake is distributed to the organs and systems of the body to enable them to perform their essential functions. Table 5.1 shows how energy intake is distributed in the body, based on a female consuming 2,000 kcals a day.

TABLE 5.1 *Daily energy requirements of the organs of the human body*

Name of organ	% of energy used daily	Kcals of energy needed per day
Liver and spleen	27%	540 kcals
Brain	19%	380 kcals
Skeletal muscle	18%	360 kcals
Kidneys	10%	200 kcals
Heart	7%	140 kcals
Other (lungs, intestines, bone, fat, glands)	19%	380 kcals

Source: Adapted from Wang et al. (2010)

Table 5.1 shows that the organs of the digestive system (liver, spleen) and the brain alone require nearly 1,000 kcals, or 50 per cent of the energy consumed on a daily basis. There must be at least 2,000 kcals remaining for all the organs shown in Table 5.1 once exercise energy expenditure has been accounted for. The amount of energy remaining after exercise for normal physiological functioning is referred to as the energy availability (EA). If EA is low or there is no EA then energy is diverted away from processes that are not vital to life, such as fat storage, growth, development, and reproduction (Elliott-Sale et al., 2018). The organs shown in Table 5.1 would not receive the energy they require to function normally.

The reproductive system is particularly affected because it is the only system whose function can be lost without risking a woman's ability to sustain life. The brain will switch off the reproductive function because it assesses that there is not sufficient energy coming in to sustain a pregnancy over nine months. As a result, there is a suppression in the production of hormones associated with the menstrual cycle that are vital to the female's health. This reduction in hormones will affect the efficient functioning of many systems of the body, such as the cardiovascular, nervous, digestive, and immune systems.

RED-S refers to the health and performance consequences of low energy availability to the athlete and these are illustrated in the next section.

Health and performance-related effects of RED-S

The previous section identified several processes and systems of the body that can be impacted by RED-S. Figure 5.1 shows the breadth of these health effects to illustrate how widespread the effect of low energy availability can be on the body.

Many of these health effects caused by RED-S will disrupt the ability of a female athlete to produce optimal performance. Figure 5.2 presents how specific physiological and psychological parameters of performance are impacted by RED-S.

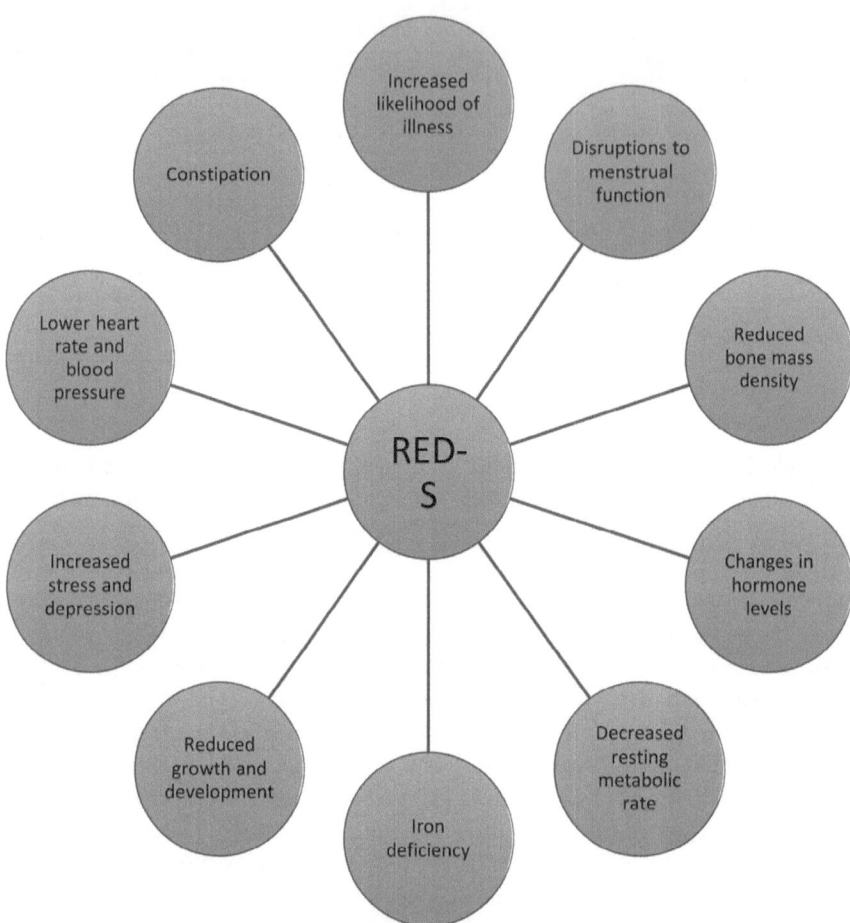

FIGURE 5.1 Potential health consequences of RED-S
Source: Adapted from Mountjoy et al. (2018)

Low energy availability can impact negatively on performance in both aerobic and anaerobic sports, as both strength and endurance are affected. Psychological problems, such as depression and irritability are also likely effects of RED-S. However, psychological problems can be both a contributory cause and an outcome of RED-S. There is a close relationship between RED-S and eating disorders, such as anorexia nervosa. RED-S is not necessarily caused by eating disorders but if an athlete has a high drive for thinness then eating disorders can become a contributing factor to its development (Mountjoy et al., 2018).

In the case study of Sarah in Box 5.1 we can see that Sarah is exhibiting some of the health consequences of RED-S as she is missing her period, and this is leading to osteopenia which is a condition characterised by bones losing their density. She is also experiencing psychological and physiological effects, as her behaviour has changed with her withdrawing socially and being exhausted after training.

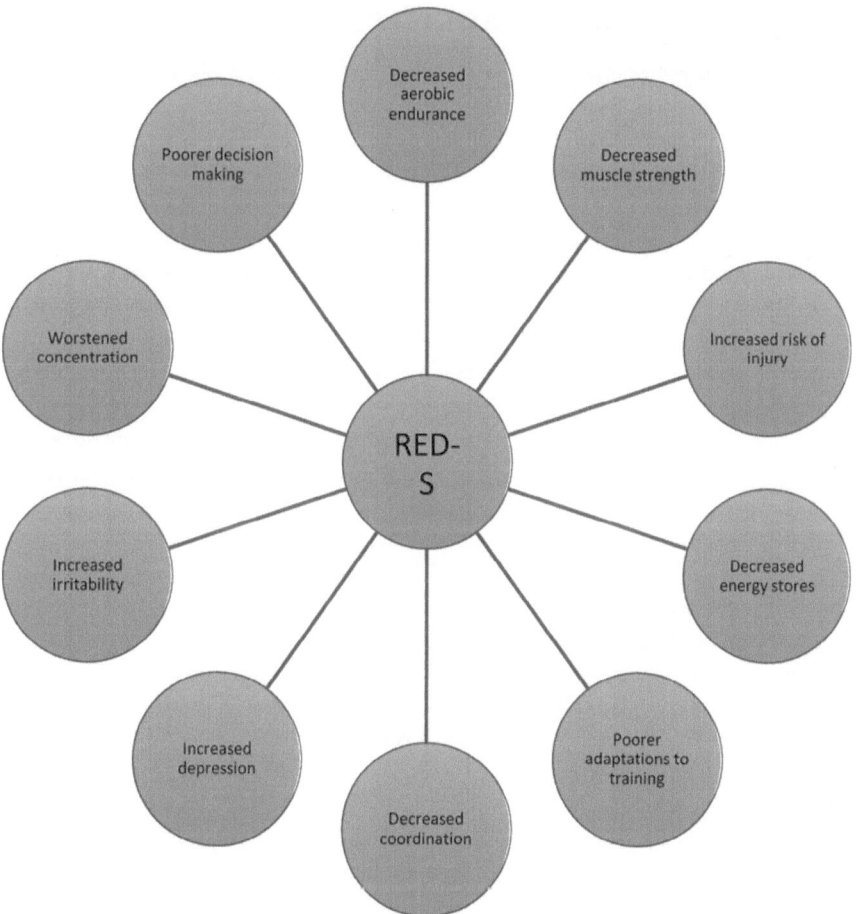

FIGURE 5.2 Potential physiological and psychological effects of RED-S
Source: Adapted from Mountjoy et al. (2018)

Causes of low energy availability in female athletes

As discussed previously the cause of RED-S is low energy availability that
occurs when an individual's dietary intake is insufficient to support the
energy required for health, function, and daily living, once the energy cost
of sport and exercise activities have been considered (Mountjoy et al., 2014).
In a recent study of 1,000 female athletes aged 15–30, it was shown that up
to 47 per cent of female athletes were at risk of low energy availability
(Ackerman et al., 2018). Before we look at several factors that contribute to
the development of RED-S, consider the following quotes in Box 5.2 from
athletes who have developed RED-S.

BOX 5.2 WHAT DO THE ATHLETES SAY?

Under fuelling became prominent within our training group and within top females; food was becoming the enemy. My under fuelled body was being forced into overtraining. Like all athletes I am obsessive. I am obsessed by athletics, with training and with being the best.

(Bobby Clay, GB International athlete)

I was proud thinking I don't have a period, that's great, it means I'm light.

(Evie Richards, GB International Cyclist)

Many athletes came forward to say that losing their periods had not been flagged. In some cases it was celebrated.

(Mary Cain, American International Athlete)

It becomes apparent that the culture around female athletes can have a powerful impact. In toxic cultures they can feel pressurised by coaches, or the athletes in their own training group, to be as light as they can irrespective of consequences. Female athletes in 'leanness sports' where thinness is thought to offer a competitive advantage, or there are weight classes, have been shown to have higher rates of low EA than those in non-leanness sports (Mountjoy et al., 2018). This does not only apply to elite performers as recreational athletes, such as regular gym users, are also at risk (de Souza et al., 2010). This may be because they are far less likely to be aware that they are energy deficient, as a result of not being monitored by a coach or undergoing regular health screening.

Loucks (2020) identified four origins of behaviours that lead to low energy availability.

1 The intentional reduction of energy availability.

Some athletes will intentionally reduce energy availability in a rational but misguided belief that it will optimise their performance in their sport (Loucks, 2020). They may believe that reducing body mass, fat mass or altering their body composition will be beneficial. This is particularly prevalent in 'leanness' sports, such as middle and long-distance running, cycling, and triathlons where the energy cost of movement is reduced by being lighter. Also, athletes in aesthetic sports such as gymnastics, trampolining and figure skating are at higher risk (de Souza, et al., 2014).

2 The presence of an eating disorder

Eating disorders are clinical mental illnesses that require specialist treatment as well as the intervention of a dietician (Loucks, 2020). However, they are characterised by similar behaviours to those taken by athletes who are intentional reducing energy availability, such as missing meals, vomiting and using laxatives. This can make it difficult to differentiate the two conditions.

Again, eating disorders are more prevalent in weight sensitive sports and where leanness has an impact on performance (Kong and Harris, 2015). However, there are other contributing factors. Disordered eating is more prevalent in athletes who are high in traits of perfectionism, competitiveness, high pain tolerance and the belief that performance is related to leanness (Stirling and Kerr, 2012). The coach-athlete relationship can also have an influence as the risk of an eating disorder is higher when the coach-athlete relationship is characterised by high conflict and low support (Shanmugam, Jowett and Meyer, 2014). Currie (2010) had found that the risk of eating disorders in young athletes was reduced in supportive sporting and coaching environments.

3 The suppression of appetite by exercise

Athletes who are partaking in exercise, whether it is prolonged or high in intensity can find that their desire to eat, or appetite, is reduced (Loucks, 2020). While being deprived of food will increase the hunger response, the same energy deficit caused by energy expenditure through exercise does not (Burgin et al., 2022). In addition, high carbohydrate diets, often favoured by athletes, can have an appetite supressing effect as well. This may be due to the bulky nature and high fibre content of high carbohydrate diets that makes an individual feel satiated for longer. When exercise and high carbohydrate diets are combined the effect is increased. To avoid the negative effect of exercise on appetite it is essential to have scheduled times for eating rather than to eat when hungry (Loucks, 2020).

This suppression of appetite is illustrated by the case study of Sarah in Box 5.1, as she finds that eating before training can give her stomach cramps. This is problematic to her as she trains early in the morning and would have to get up around two hours before to give her time to digest a pre-exercise meal. She also experiences a lack of appetite after training.

4 Young women may under-eat for social reasons rather than for sporting outcomes

Social issues, such as the expectations of females to conform to an unrealistic image of attractiveness and the pressure to present an idealistic image of oneself on social media, have contributed to more females perceiving themselves to be overweight. More adolescent female athletes reported that they dieted to improve their appearance rather than improve their sports performance (Martinsen et al., 2010). This has important implications for coaches in that actions taken in an athlete's broader life can have a significant impact on their health and sporting outcomes.

The development of RED-S from regular low energy availability is complex in nature often arising from a range of potential physiological, psychological, and sociological causes. As a result any treatment of RED-S needs to address all these diverse causes and should involve a range of professionals outside of the athletes coach. Ackerman (2018) recommends a team approach, that as well as including the athlete, parent, and coach, includes a doctor/physician, sport psychologist and sport nutritionist to ensure all bases are covered, yet for many athletes this may not always be feasible or affordable.

Low energy availability and menstrual function disruption

We have previously established that low EA causes a disruption to menstrual function as the reproductive system is suppressed with energy being diverted to processes that are vital to preserving life (de Souza et al., 2014). This suppression of menstrual function occurs as a result of changes in hormone levels.

As we saw in Chapter 3 the phases of the menstrual cycle are orchestrated by the release of several hormones across the length of its cycle. Hormones are produced by glands that make up the endocrine system. The hormones of the menstrual cycle are regulated by the hypothalamus and the pituitary gland, located in the brain. The menstrual cycle is controlled through the hypothalamic-pituitary-gonadal (HPG) axis through which the hypothalamus instructs the pituitary gland to make the ovaries (gonadal) produce and secrete reproductive hormones.

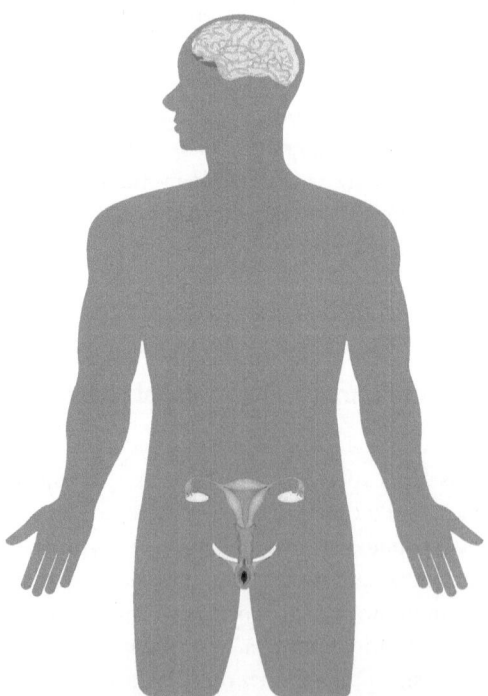

FIGURE 5.3 Hypothalamic-pituitary-gonadal (HPG) axis in females

Low energy availability will interfere with this HPG axis leading to a disruption in the menstrual cycle. The hormones that are specifically affected are follicle stimulating hormone (FSH) and luteinising hormone (LH). FSH, which is present in the early stages the cycle, stimulates follicles in the ovaries to grow and mature. LH is released around Day 13 of the cycle, just before ovulation that typically happens on Day 14. LH stimulates the maturing follicle to produce more oestrogen that in turn will make ovulation happen. LH also instructs an ovary to produce progesterone after ovulation, and this is important as progesterone controls the second half of the cycle.

As FSH and LH production are reduced the outcome is that the amounts of oestrogen and progesterone produced reduce as well. A failure to ovulate, owing to low FSH and LH levels, leads to a condition called functional hypothalamic amenorrhoea (FHA). FHA is characterised by an absence of periods for at least three months or fewer than five periods over 12 months (Gordon et al., 2017). Rather than disappearing completely periods may become irregular with intervals of 36–90 days between cycles (de Souza et al., 2010). When a female has infrequent menstrual periods it is referred to as oligomenorrhoea. Both these conditions are reversible once optimal energy requirements have returned, and there is sufficient energy available to fuel the menstrual cycle and sustain a pregnancy.

The reduction in the amount of oestrogen available has wider consequences for the body as well. For example, oestrogen is a hormone that is central to bone health and bone development as we shall see. There are also other hormones that are affected by low EA, and we shall explore how these impact on health and performance as well.

Low bone density and RED-S

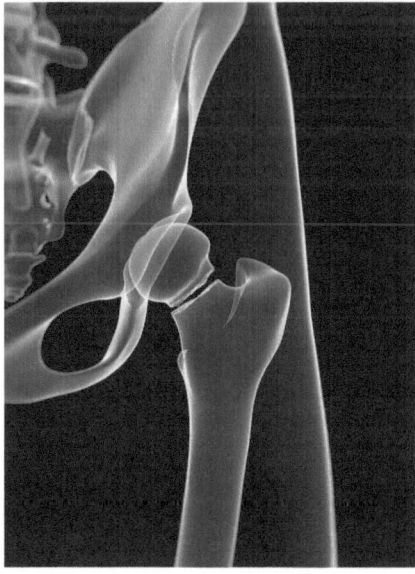

Research has shown that females with amenorrhoea or oligomenorrhoea, as well as anorexia nervosa, have lower bone mineral density, changes to structure of the bone and an impaired ability to break down old bone and build new bone (Ackerman and Misra, 2011). As a result these athletes will have lowered bone strength and increased risk of bone injuries, particularly stress fractures in the lower leg (Ackerman et al., 2015).

There are serious long term implications for athletes who experience menstrual cycle disruptions in adolescence and young adulthood. The period from puberty to around 30 years, when peak bone mass is achieved, are the prime bone building years. During this time the levels of oestrogen and other hormones are particularly high, enabling bone modelling and remodelling to occur. However, the failure to achieve an optimal peak bone mass in young adulthood can predispose women to experiencing osteoporosis, and its precursor osteopenia, in later life (de Souza et al., 2019). It is inevitable that bone mass reduces as a woman ages, particularly when they go through the menopause typically in their fifties. If peak bone mass is not achieved then there is less bone to lose before the risk of experiencing fractures increases. Osteoporosis is characterised by fractures to the hip, wrist, and spine, owing to the thinning of the bones.

Leptin and Ghrelin – the lesser known hormones

In addition to oestrogen there are other hormones important in bone building that will decrease in levels, owing to low EA. Leptin is a hormone that has several functions, including signalling to the brain when we have reached satiety during eating, thus helping to control body weight. During the menstrual cycle leptin stimulates the release of gonadotropin-releasing hormone (GnRH) which in turn releases FSH and LH to cause follicles in the ovaries to mature and for an egg to be released at ovulation. The lowering of leptin levels is another reason why the menstrual cycle is disrupted, reducing the likelihood of ovulation and its accompanying increases in oestrogen and progesterone. Leptin is also involved in bone formation as it stimulates osteoblasts to build bone, in particular the hard compact bone on the outside of bone. Reductions in leptin lead to decreases in bone mass density and less bone formation (Turner et al., 2013).

Ghrelin is a second hormone that is involved in controlling appetite. Ghrelin increases hunger and appetite, and its production increases in individuals with low EA to increase their desire to eat (Redman and Loucks, 2005). Ghrelin acts on the hypothalamus and like leptin it will disrupt the secretion of FSH and LH (Cooper and Ackerman, 2020) impacting on ovulation, oestrogen levels and bone formation.

The importance of growth hormone (GH) and insulin-like growth factor 1 (IGF-1)

Growth hormone (GH) is an anabolic hormone produced in the anterior pituitary gland and is necessary for the growth of bone and muscle (Cooper and Ackerman, 2020). GH stimulates the production of insulin-like growth factor 1 (IGF-1) which is produced mainly in the liver. IGF-1 is also involved in bone formation, in particular in the action of osteoblasts. A reduction of IGF-1, owing to low EA, will result in decreased bone formation and bone mass (Gunter and Rosen, 2013).

We can see that low EA has an effect on many hormones causing several important physiological processes to be disrupted. This is well illustrated by the case study of Sarah in Box 5.1, where changes in her hormone levels impact on her bone formation and development, leading to a lowered bone mass density (osteopenia).

BOX 5.3 SPOTLIGHT ON: EXERCISE ADDICTION – A CASE OF OVER MOTIVATION?

There are many individuals who participate in high volumes of training for sporting or recreational reasons. But when does a healthy, high volume training schedule start to present as an unhealthy exercise addiction? In both situations there are risks of injury and potential disruptions to the endocrine system as a result of low energy availability. Also, both groups may experience under performance as a result of high training volume with insufficient rest and recovery, referred to as overtraining.

The key differences in the two scenarios are attributed to psychological rather than physiological factors. Individuals with an exercise addiction are likely to have unhealthy motivating factors and an emotional connection to exercise. In particular, the exercise addict will prioritise their exercise schedule above other activities and be driven by an obsession to stick to their schedule. This can cause conflicts in social interactions where the individual may miss important family events, or social occasions, to enable them to exercise. It can also lead to negative emotional states, such as anxiety and irritability if unable to exercise. They can also feel the need to keep exercising when injured or fatigued (Hausenblas, Schreiber and Smoliga, 2017).

Two categories of exercise addiction have been identified. Primary addiction is where the individual is driven to follow an excessively high volume training schedule. Secondary exercise addiction occurs when a training programme of excessive volume is combined with a desire to control body weight (Hausenblas, Schreiber and Smoliga, 2017). It is almost inevitable that individuals with a secondary exercise addiction will develop RED-S, while those with primary exercise addiction have a significantly increased risk of developing it. Individuals with an exercise addiction may also have or develop an eating disorder.

> There is a grey area between an exercise addict and a dedicated athlete. An individual may start with healthy motivating factors to train hard and improve health and performance. This can develop into primary exercise addiction to stick to this tough training schedule rather than focus on its results. For athletes in sports where leanness offers a competitive advantage a secondary exercise addiction can develop as they are motivated by the desire to lose weight (Keay, 2017).

Preventing RED-S in female athletes

The likelihood of developing RED-S can be reduced by maintaining energy balance where energy intake matches the daily energy demands. The female maintaining health and normal functions of the body (around 2,000 kcals daily) plus the energy costs of health, training, and recovery. There may be other daily activities that an individual is involved in that need to be considered in addition to their sport. For example, they may be expending considerable energy when they are working, involved in their studies, or even socialising. Figure 5.4 gives four top tips for athletes to help them get their energy balance correct.

Coaches of female athletes can also play an important role in preventing RED-S by creating an environment or culture where important conversations around nutrition, training and recovery can take place. Coaches will be aware that the health of their athletes is central to their successful performances and nutrition plays a central role in this. However, just telling athletes to eat more is unlikely to work as eating behaviours and schedule need to be considered. Some athletes will have a dysfunctional, or emotional, relationship with food. Box 5.4 presents some ideas around how a coach can support their athletes and promote nutritional strategy of athletes.

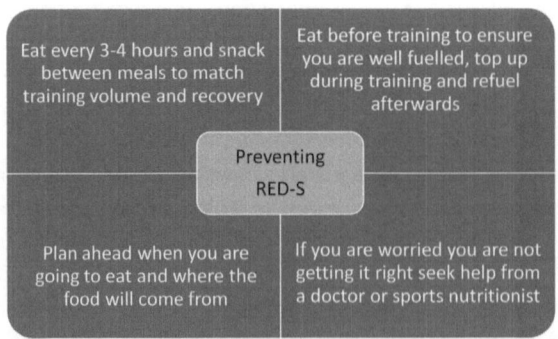

FIGURE 5.4 Tips for athletes to prevent RED-S
Source: Adapted from The Well HQ (2022)

BOX 5.4 TIPS FOR COACHES TO PREVENT RED-S

1. The coach can 'celebrate the power of food' as the fuel for performance. They can use coachable moments at the beginning of a session to ensure everyone has arrived well fuelled by asking 'what did everyone have to fuel up for today' and again at the end of the session 'what is everyone going to eat now to refuel'.

2. Use education to teach athletes about what and when to eat. While eating may seem intuitive, eating to fuel sports performance often is not and many athletes get it wrong. For example, the timing of energy delivery is as important as the number of calories consumed. Ensuring that an athlete's energy intake matches training volume, and that athletes are not training without a pre-training meal or during fasting is important. Also it is important to make certain that athletes eat soon after training.

3. Take steps to make sure that athletes stop attaching value to body shape and size. This can happen when an athlete looks at another athlete and believes their performance success is directly related to their leanness or believing that leanness will offer them a competitive advantage. It is important to understand that an under fuelled athlete, whilst being lean, is at a competitive disadvantage, owing to their shortage of energy.

4. The coach needs to be aware of any remarks they, or any other athletes, may make about an athlete's appearance, even in jest or as 'banter'. They can serve to fuel a dangerous culture of restricted eating in sport. Athletes come in all shapes and sizes, success isn't simply down to body size, and a healthy athlete is more successful than a broken one.

As well as creating an environment where athletes can comfortably discuss fuelling and refuelling coaches also need to be aware of the signs that an athlete is under fuelling and may develop RED-S. So what are the signs of RED-S that anyone working with female athletes needs to look out for?

Warning signs of RED-S

The first warning sign of RED-S is any disruption to the menstrual cycle as the period is a vital sign of health, and a measure of the levels of hormones central to female health. However, the coach or anyone else in the team around the athlete may not necessarily have access to the athlete's menstrual status unless it has been shared by the female athlete. They may also not be fully aware of the athlete's nutritional strategies as refuelling usually occurs away from the sporting environment.

Some coaches will have relationships with their athletes where these important subjects are discussed but it is not always the case. In the case of male coaches and female athletes in particular, these conversations can be difficult, owing to the sensitive nature of their content unless there is are high levels of respect and trust in the relationship.

However, there are warning signs that the coach, or anyone else supporting the female athlete can look out for:

The coach needs to be aware of the warning signs of RED-S in athletes:

Physiological
- irregular or absent periods
- difficulty staying warm in the winter and cool in the summer
- low muscle mass and inability to develop muscle
- digestive problems such as constipation or bloating

Behavioural
- pre-occupation with, and constantly talking about food and eating
- poor sleep patterns
- strictly controlling food intake
- overtraining and reluctance to take rest days

Psychological

- high levels of anxiety
- becoming withdrawn or reclusive.
- Irrational behaviour
- perfectionist tendencies

Performance
- increased prevalence of illnesses and injuries
- decrement in performance
- excessive tiredness and lethargy
- poor recovery from training sessions

(#Train Brave, 2021)

As discussed in Chapter 3, tracking cycles is an incredibly useful tool to identify any disruptions or changes to the menstrual cycles. Irregular or absent periods are a warning sign of RED-S, and the consistent tracking of cycles will enable athletes and their coaches to identify potential problems before they develop into damaging symptoms that could impact on health and performance.

Recommendations for managing RED-S in female athletes

Fortunately there is a growing awareness of the dangers of RED-S and its signs and symptoms. Coaches, who have regular contact with their athletes, are in the best position to identify any changes in their athletes' body shape or body size. However, they may have difficulty in differentiating between those athletes who body composition is appropriate for optimal performance in their sport and those who may have low EA or even an eating disorder (Plateau et al., 2014).

In 2014 the International Olympic Committee (IOC) published a consensus paper around RED-S and in 2015 these IOC authors (Mountjoy et al., 2015) developed a Clinical Assessment Tool – the RED-S CAT. This tool was developed to assist sports medicine professionals to screen for and manage cases of RED-S. The tool uses a 'red light – yellow light – green light' system of categorising athletes according to their risk.

De Souza et al. (2014) recommended that athletes at risk of the female athlete triad, which preceded the term RED-S should be screened before sports participation. This should be done using a questionnaire including information about the following: history of menstrual irregularities and amenorrhoea; history of stress fractures; history of dieting; history of depression; personality factors such as perfectionism and obsessive behaviour, and any history of receiving critical comments or inappropriate coaching behaviour (de Souza et al., 2019).

Nutritional education is essential to avoid unconscious undereating and low energy availability, owing to poor planning of meals. While the involvement of a nutritionist is important if an athlete does develop RED-S, any treatment of RED-S needs to be managed by a multidisciplinary team. This would include the athlete's coach, a sports medicine physician, sports psychologist (or mental health practitioner) and it appropriate the athlete's parents or guardian (de Souza et al., 2019). The athlete will have to be central to the process and be open to the interventions put in place by these professionals. Unfortunately for recreational athletes this support network may not be available and therefore the athlete will have to take responsibility to access the professional help they need.

BOX 5.5 REAL-WORLD APPLICATION

As a female athlete, you should:

1. Track your menstrual cycle to identify any changes in regularity or disruptions to your menstrual cycle.
2. Be aware of any changes in your energy levels, mood or psychological state, performances in training and competition, sleep patterns and digestion.
3. Know that exercise can alter the desire to eat so plan when to eat and how much based on the amount of energy you will need every day.

4. Plan ahead and develop a strategy that enables you to be well fuelled before training and be able to eat as soon as possible after training.
5. Don't be afraid to consult a nutritionist or doctor if you are concerned about any aspect of your health or performance.

As a coach, you should:

1. Develop a coaching environment where you are able to have honest conversations about an athlete's menstrual cycle and nutritional strategy.
2. Be able to identify the signs and symptoms of RED-S in your athletes.
3. Make food visible and use coachable moments to discuss what your athletes have eaten to fuel up for training and what they will eat afterwards.
4. Ensure you have a working knowledge of sports nutrition – what your athletes should be eating and when.

Develop a network of professionals around you and your athletes that you can trust and refer your athletes to if you identify any need for further help.

Summary

Having completed this chapter you will now have developed a more detailed understanding of the complex condition of RED-S. In particular you will appreciate how low energy availability impacts on the health and performance of a female athlete and some of the physiological processes that produce these effects. It is most important to understand the key role that disruptions to the menstrual cycle can have on processes in the body that are vital to health. You will also have explored the signs and symptoms of RED-S that you need to look out for and measures that can be taken to prevent RED-S and manage it once it has developed.

The key messages to take away from this chapter are:

1. Maintaining a regular menstrual cycle is vital to the health and performance of the female athlete.
2. The menstrual cycle needs to have sufficient energy available to function effectively or it will become irregular or disappear completely.
3. Being aware of the signs and symptoms of RED-S can help you to identify it in yourself and in other athletes.
4. Eating regularly and taking on sufficient calories is the basis of avoiding low energy availability and the accompanying health and physical consequences of RED-S.
5. Exercise can impact on an athlete's appetite, so it is important to develop a schedule of eating rather than relying on eating when hungry.
6. If a female athlete starts to experience changes to their menstrual cycle, increases in prevalence of illness and injury, fluctuations in performance and energy levels they should seek the help of a doctor and sports nutritionist.

End-of-Chapter Quiz

Answers can be found after the References

1. Identify why the reproductive system is particularly affected by low energy availability:

    a   Because it requires the most energy of all the body's systems
    b   Because its loss of function won't negatively affect other body systems
    c   Because it is the only system that be lost without risk to life
    d   Because it is heavily reliant on the production of hormones using energy sources

2. Identify which of the following is NOT a health consequence of RED-S:

    a   Decreased metabolic rate
    b   Decreased likelihood of illness
    c   Reduced bone mass density
    d   Reduced growth and development

3. Identify which of the following behaviours contribute to the development of RED-S:

    a   Changes in the length of the menstrual cycle
    b   Use of hormonal contraception to suppress periods
    c   Disruption to sleeping pattern after eating
    d   Suppression of appetite, owing to exercise

4. Identify why low energy availability can disrupt the menstrual cycle:

    a   Low EA will interfere with the HPG axis
    b   Low EA will cause ovaries to produce fewer hormones
    c   Low EA will cause energy to be directed away from the hypothalamus
    d   Low EA will increase adrenalin levels that suppress oestrogen action

5. Identify which of the following statements about osteoporosis is FALSE:

    a   Failure to achieve peak bone mass can predispose a female to osteoporosis
    b   Osteoporosis is characterised by fractures to the hip, knee, and spine
    c   Bone mass reduction is accelerated by the menopause
    d   As well as high levels of oestrogen, leptin and ghrelin are important in achieving peak bone mass

References

Ackerman K.E. (2018) Clinical tips from Dr Kathryn Ackerman on how to manage athletes with low energy availability. *Podcast*. Available at: https://soundcloud.com/bmjpodcasts/clinical-tips-from-dr-kathryn-ackerman-on-how-to-manage-athletes-with-low-energy-availability?in=bmjpodcasts/sets/bjsm-1 (Accessed 5 September 2022).

Ackerman, K.E., Holtzman, B., Cooper, K.M., Flynn, E.F., Bruinvels, G., Tenforde, A. S., Popp, K.L., Simpkin, A.J. and Parziale, A.L. (2018) Low energy availability surrogates correlate with health and performance consequences of Relative Energy Deficiency in Sport. *British Journal of Sports Medicine*, 53, 628–633.

Ackerman, K.E., Cano Sokoloff, N.G., De Nardo Maffazioli, G., Clarke, H.M., Lee, H. and Misra, M. (2015) Fractures in relation to menstrual status and bone parameters in young athletes. *Medicine & Science in Sports and Exercise*, 47(8), 1577–1586.

Ackerman, K.E. and Misra, M. (2011) Bone health and the female athlete triad in adolescent athletes. *Physician and Sports medicine*, 39(1), 131–141.

Burgin, A., Blannin, A.K., Peters, D.M. and Holliday, A. (2022) Acute appetite and eating behaviour responses to apparatus-free, high intensity intermittent exercise in inactive women with excess weight. *Physiology and Behaviour*, 254(1). doi:10.1016/j.physbeh.2022.113906.

Cooper, K.M. and Ackerman, K.E. (2020) Endocrine Implications of Relative Energy Deficiency in Sport. In A.C. Hackney and N.W. Constantini, *Endocrinology of Physical Activity and Sport* (3rd ed.). Switzerland: Humana Press.

Currie, A. (2010) Sport and eating disorders-understanding and managing the risks. *Asian Journal of Sports Medicine*, 1(2), 63–68.

De Souza, M.J., Koltun, K.J., Southmayd, E.A. and Aurigemma, N.C. (2019) The Female Athlete Triad. In J. Forsyth and C.M. Roberts (Eds), *The Exercising Female: Science and its Application*. Oxford: Routledge.

De Souza, M.J., Nattiv, A., Joy, E., Misra, M., Williams, N.I. and Mallinson, R. J. (2014) Female athlete triad coalition consensus statement on treatment and return to play of the female athlete triad. *British Journal of Sports Medicine*, 48(4), 289.

De Souza, M.J., Toombs, R.J., Scheid, J.L., O'Donnell, E., West, S.L. and Williams, N. I. (2010) High prevalence of subtle and severe menstrual disturbances in exercising women: confirmation using daily hormone measures. *Human Reproduction*, 25(2), 491–503. https://doi.org/10.1093/humrep/dep411.

Elliott-Sale, K.J., Tenforde, A.S., Parziale, A.L., Holzman, B. and Ackerman, K.E. (2018) Endocrine Effects of Relative Energy Deficiency in Sport. *International Journal of Sports Nutrition and Exercise Metabolism*, 28, 335–349.

Gordon, C.M., Ackerman, K.E., Berga, S.L., Kaplan, J.R., Mastorakos, G., Misra, M., Murad, M., Santoro, N. and Warren, M. (2017) Functional hypothalamic amenorrhea: and endocrine society clinical practice guideline . *The Journal of Clinical Endocrinology and Metabolism*. doi:10.1210/jc.2017-00131.

Gunter, A.R. and Rosen, C.J. (2013) IGF-1 regulation of key signalling pathways in bone. *BoneKey Reports*, 2(437). doi:10.1038/bonekey.2013.171.

Hausenblas, H.A., Schreiber, K. and Smoliga, J.M. (2017) Addiction to exercise. *British Medical Journal*, 357. doi:10.1136/bmj.j1745.

Keay, N. (2017) What distinguishes a healthy level of commitment from exercise addiction? Blog post. Available at https://blogs.bmj.com/bjsm/2017/08/03/addictio

n-exercise-distinguishes-healthy-level-commitment-exercise-addiction (Accessed 6 September 2022).

Kong, P. and Harris, L.M. (2015) The sporting body: body image and eating disorder symptomatology among female athletes from leanness focused and nonleanness focused sports. *Journal of Psychology*, 149, 141–160.

Loucks, A.B. (2020). Exercise Training in the Normal Female: Effects of Low Energy Availability on Reproductive Function. In A. Hackney and N. Constantini (Eds), *Endocrinology of Physical Activity and Sport* (3rd ed.). Cham: Humana.

Martinsen, M., Sundgot-Borgen, J. and Bratland-Sanda, S. (2010) Dieting to win or thin? A study of dieting and disordered eating among adolescent elite athletes and non-athlete controls. *British Journal of Sports Medicine*, 44, 70–76.

Mountjoy, M., Sundgot-Borgen, J.K., Burke, L.M., Ackerman, K.E., Blauwet, C., Constantini, N., Lebrun, C., Lundy, B., Melin, A.K., Meyer, N.L., Sherman, R.T., Tenforde, A.S., Torstveit, M.K. and Budgett, R. (2018) International Olympic Committee (IOC) Consensus Statement on Relative Energy Deficiency in Sport (RED-S)': 2018 Update. *British Journal of Sports Medicine*, 52, 687–697.

Mountjoy, M., Sundgot-Borgen, J.K., Burke, S., Carter, C., Constantini, N., Lebrun, C., Meyer, N.L., Sherman, R.T., Steffen, K., Budgett, R. and Ljungqvist, R. (2014) International Olympic Committee (IOC) Consensus Statement on Relative Energy Deficiency in Sport (RED-S). *British Journal of Sports Medicine*, 48(7), 491–497.

Mountjoy, M., Sundgot-Borgen, J.K., Burke, S., Carter, C., Constantini, N., Lebrun, C. Meyer, N.L., Sherman, R.T., Steffen, K., Budgett, R., Ljungqvist, R. and Ackerman, K. (2015) The IOC relative energy deficiency in sport clinical assessment tool (RED-S CAT). *British Journal of Sports Medicine*, 49(7), 421–423.

Plateau, C.R., McDermott, H.J, Arcelus, J. and Meyer, C. (2014) Identifying and preventing disordered eating among athletes: Perceptions of track and field coaches. *Psychology of Sport & Exercise*, 15(6), 721–728.

Pitchers, G. and Elliott-Sale, K. (2019) Considerations for coaches training female athletes. *Training Female Athletes*, 55, 19–30.

Public Health England (2016) Government Dietary Recommendations. Available at: https://assets.publishing.service.gov.uk/government/uploads/system/uploads/attachment_data/file/618167/government_dietary_recommendations.pdf.

Redman L.M. and Loucks A.B. (2005) Menstrual disorders in athletes. *Journal of Sports Medicine*, 35(9), 747–755.

Shanmugam, V., Jowett, S. and Meyer, C. (2014) Interpersonal difficulties as a risk factor for athletes' eating psychopathology. *Scandinavian Journal of Medicine and Science in Sports*, 24, 469–476.

Stirling, A. and Kerr, G. (2012) Perceived vulnerabilities of female athletes to the development of disordered eating behaviours. *European Journal of Sport Science*, 12, 262–273.

The Well HQ (2022) RED-S Relative Energy Deficiency in Sport. Available at: www.thewell-hq.com/category/red-s.

#Train Brave (2021) 'Risks'. *#Train Brave*. Available at: https://trainbrave.org/risks (Accessed 16 May 2022).

Turner, R.T., Kalra, S.P., Wong, C.P., Philbrick, K.A., Lindenmaier, L.B., Boghossian, S. and Iwaniec, U.T. (2013). Peripheral leptin regulates bone formations. *Journal of Bone and Mineral Research*, 28(1), 22–34.

Wang, Z., Ying, Z., Bosy-Westphal, A., Zhang, J., Shautz, B., Later, W. and Heymsfield, S.B. (2010) Specific metabolic rates of major organs and tissues across adulthood: evaluation by mechanistic model of resting energy expenditure. *American Journal of Clinical Nutrition*, 92(6), 1369–1377. doi:10.3945/ajcn.2010.29885.

Answers

1. c
2. b
3. d
4. a
5. b

6

BREAST HEALTH AND EFFECTIVE BREAST SUPPORT

Jess Pinchbeck

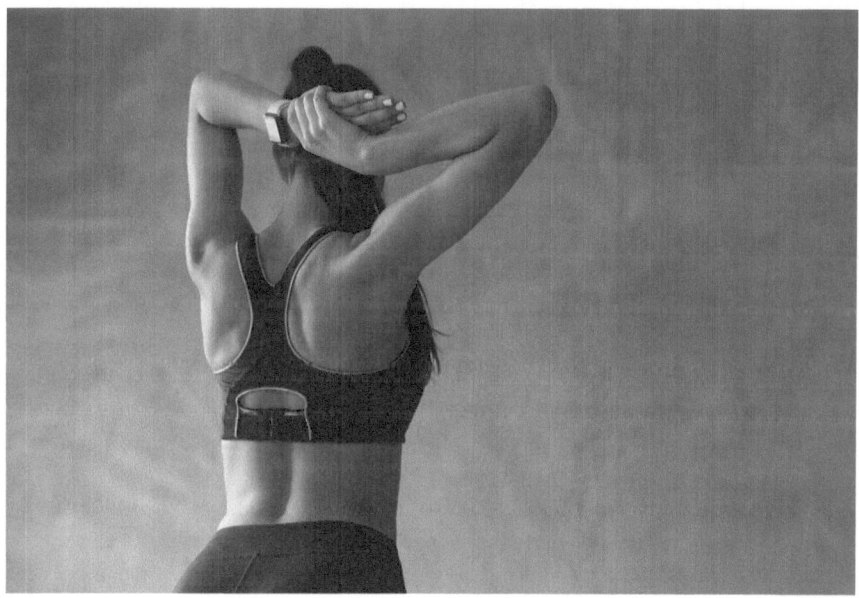

Introduction

There are a range of biological, physiological and psychological factors that make the female athlete unique and one of these is the anatomical differences between them and their male counterparts. It is crucial for both the athlete and those practitioners working with female athletes to greater understand the female body to support health and improve performance. To address this issue, more research is starting to focus on female athletes to produce specific recommendations rather

DOI: 10.4324/9781003330110-6

than generalise findings from research with male athletes. One of the key anatomical differences between male and female athletes includes the breast, and the issue of breast health has been shown to be a critical factor in participating in sport and exercise for all women. For example, research has shown that 17 per cent of women cite breasts as a barrier to participation (Burnett, White and Scurr, 2015) with 44 per cent of elite athletes experiencing breast pain when exercising (Brisbine et al., 2020).

This chapter will look at the importance of breast health for women participating in sport and fitness, and how those working with female athletes, as well as the athletes themselves, can ensure that the correct breast support for optimal performance is chosen. The chapter begins by introducing the anatomy and structure of the breast, before analysing the types of breast motion and the biomechanics of breast movement in a range of different activities. Breast bounce and breast motion are important considerations, and both can be managed through different types of sports bras, but athletes need to consider a range of factors when choosing the correct bra for their activity. The types of sports bras available and the support they offer is discussed alongside the impact of poorly fitting breast support on the breast motion and how this can potentially affect the athlete and their performance. This chapter is designed to increase the knowledge of breast health for coaches and athletes as well as to improve understanding of the challenges related to breast support that female athletes may encounter and the relationship with performance and participation.

Before then read the case study, in Box 6.1, where you are introduced to Maddie who is encountering typical issues connected with breast health and breast support.

BOX 6.1 MADDIE (EQUESTRIAN EVENT RIDER)

Maddie is a 25-year-old equestrian event rider who competes at national level on her horse Danbury. Eventing comprises three different disciplines across three days; dressage, cross country and show jumping. Maddie has been riding since she was eight years old although it is not until the last six months that she has started to wear a sports bra when riding, which has made a huge difference to both her comfort and her performance since puberty.

Throughout her teenage years Maddie was always conscious of her breasts when riding but, neither her coaches nor her parents ever talked to her about breast support or about wearing a sports bra. Maddie typically just wore any of her most comfortable normal bras but, as her breasts became larger, she became aware of the amount of movement in her breasts during riding. As a teenager Maddie was far too embarrassed to talk to anyone about this and so started wearing two bras to try and provide a bit more support to combat the movement. She always made sure her body protector was as tight as possible to help. In her late teens Maddie also started to experience some breast pain as well as discomfort and noticed that this typically occurred around the time of her period. Often she used to avoid riding completely during her period because of this, making up excuses or saying she felt unwell.

As an adult, Maddie is typically a 32DD bra size and her pain and discomfort had been getting her down as well as causing distraction during riding. This was at its worst during show jumping particularly upon landing, and, as a consequence, had started to negatively impact on her performance. Following a disappointing round at a recent competition Maddie had started chatting to a fellow competitor that she knew from the circuit and mentioned about the breast discomfort and pain she had been feeling during competition. The other rider explained to Maddie that she wore a specific type of sports bra which prevented her breasts from moving so much and was extremely comfortable. Furthermore, the other competitor described how she had been professionally fitted for her bra to make sure it was suitable.

That week, Maddie booked herself in at a local shop and was professionally fitted for a sports bra. She tried many on in a variety of styles and sizes and found one that was comfortable and seemed to reduce the breast movement when jumping up and down. Maddie wore it during training that week and was amazed at the difference. Her coach often videoed her jumping to analyse technique and Maddie could visibly see an improvement in her posture and the positive impact that wearing correct breast support had on her performance. Her shoulder blades were drawn together maintaining a much more efficient alignment of the upper body as she hadn't had to worry about any discomfort or pain. The improved posture also seemed to influence Danbury, who seemed happier and whose performance had also improved. Maddie was pleased she had found a solution but also cross that she hadn't been educated about breast support as a young rider.

What the case study illustrates is the lack of knowledge and education that many girls and women have regarding breast health. It also demonstrates the potential impact of taking part in sport and activity without appropriate breast support and the way this can affect enjoyment and performance. Women and girls should be able to participate in sport and exercise without pain or discomfort.

As we move through this chapter, we will refer to Maddie's case study and you will see that her experiences link to some of the issues reported in the research. But first we will consider breast health in more detail and the potential health and performance-related effects that can develop from poor breast support.

Why is breast health so important for sports performance?

Female participation and performance in sport and exercise has been linked to breast health and breast pain (mastalgia). Research shows that women may refrain from participation as a result of breast pain, often associated with feeling distressed or embarrassed. Furthermore, of those women who do take part in sport and exercise many often experience breast pain and discomfort, such as that described by Maddie in the case study. Figure 6.1 illustrates some of the key issues around breast health and sports participation and performance.

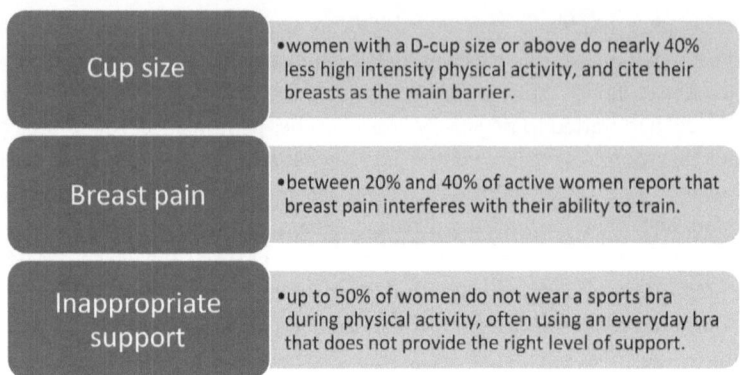

FIGURE 6.1 Key issues around breast health
Source: Adapted from The Open University (2022)

A study by Brown et al. (2014) reported that breast pain was experienced by 32 per cent of marathon runners and for 17 per cent of them it negatively affected the volume of training they were able to participate in. The study showed that the breast pain was significantly related to cup size and was greater during vigorous physical activity compared to moderate physical activity. Such findings demonstrate how inadequate breast support can have an impact upon female sports performance yet, 44 per cent of women in this study took no action to combat the discomfort experienced. The Research Group in Breast Health, based at Portsmouth University have identified, through conducting numerous studies, several implications of running with inadequate breast support. Their findings indicate that poor breast support can make exercise feel harder, increase muscle activity in the upper body causing the earlier onset of fatigue, increase ground reaction forces which raises injury risk to the lower limbs, and can reduce stride length by up to 4 cm (Research Group in Breast Health, 2022). Young females are also at risk of dropping out of sport, owing to breast issues with 73 per cent of schoolgirls reporting breast concerns impacting sport and exercise participation (Scurr et al., 2016). There are evident links with key areas discussed in other chapters within this book such as risk of injury and the adolescent female.

Understanding breast anatomy

Knowledge of the anatomy of the breast is crucial to increase understanding of breast health and breast pain and the factors associated with sport performance. As Figure 6.2 illustrates the breast is constructed mostly of fatty tissue, with some connective tissue, that provides the breast with a limited amount of internal support. This connective tissue is called the Coopers ligaments, although the term 'ligaments' is very deceptive, because

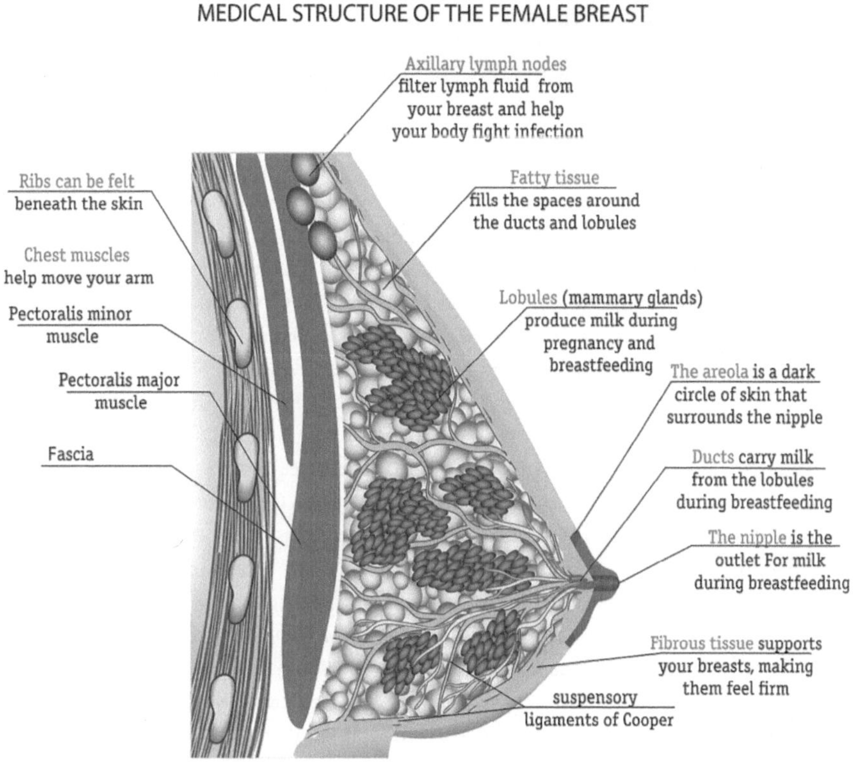

MEDICAL STRUCTURE OF THE FEMALE BREAST

Axillary lymph nodes
filter lymph fluid from
your breast and help
your body fight infection

Ribs can be felt
beneath the skin

Chest muscles
help move your arm

Pectoralis minor
muscle

Pectoralis major
muscle

Fascia

Fatty tissue
fills the spaces around
the ducts and lobules

Lobules (mammary glands)
produce milk during
pregnancy and
breastfeeding

The areola is a dark
circle of skin that
surrounds the nipple

Ducts carry milk
from the lobules
during breastfeeding

The nipple is the
outlet For milk
during breastfeeding

Fibrous tissue supports
your breasts, making
them feel firm

suspensory
ligaments of Cooper

FIGURE 6.2 Structure of the female breast
Source: Shutterstock

everywhere else in the body ligaments attach bone to bone, but Coopers ligaments are not 'real' ligaments, they are connective tissue that offers only some support for the breast mass (Page and Steele, 1999). They are positioned over the pectoralis major, or chest muscle, but these muscles offer the breasts little support and, therefore, training them has no effect.

It is the fibrous tissue of the skin that holds the breast in place on the chest wall and when the skin that supports the breast tissue stretches it can cause breast sag. Breast sag (also known as breast ptosis) can occur as a result of age, because as we age our skin reduces in elasticity, but also it can occur as a function of breast movement (The Open University, 2022). This is why it is imperative that women look after their breasts. For example, if Maddie had continued to ride without appropriate breast support, she would be at serious risk of breast sag.

The breasts also contain glands, and this is the component of the breast that has a specific job to do. This glandular tissue comprises the milk glands and ducts which are used for breastfeeding.

The biomechanics of breast movement

The anatomy of the breast is relevant to understanding the different types of breast movement when performing a range of activities. As the skin provides the one form of external support to the breast, along with limited internal support offered by the Coopers ligaments, when the body moves breast movement will also occur. Any type of movement such as walking, cycling or horse-riding, cause the breasts to move, and during high-impact activities, such as running and jumping, the breasts move even more. An average individual breast weights about half a kilogram, and when taking part in sport and exercise the movement of the breast may stretch the skin past its natural elastic range and result in permanent damage to the supporting structures (The Open University, 2022). Research shows that by wearing a correctly fitted sports bra movement of the breast can decrease by up to 74 per cent in comparison to wearing no support at all (Norris et al., 2021).

As shown in Figure 6.3 the breasts can move in three different directions; up and down, forwards and backwards and side to side. The type of activity being undertaken will determine the different movement dimensions of the breast. For example, performing a star jump would cause the breast to move in all three dimensions as a result of the take-off, moving the upper body while in the air and the impact of landing. It is likely that as a result of the range of movements involved in riding that Maddie will experiences breast movement in all three directions.

Taking part in sport and exercise while wearing incorrect breast support has been shown to cause stretching of the skin, as well as damaging the Cooper's

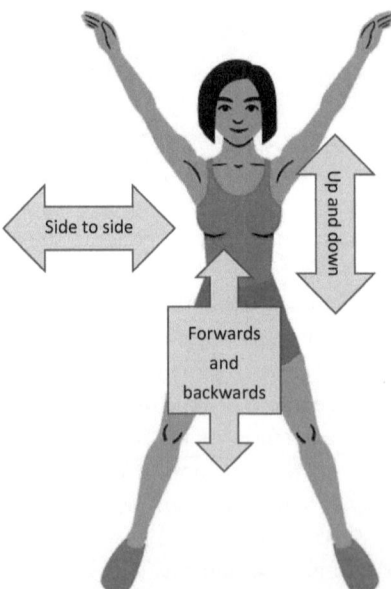

FIGURE 6.3 The three types of breast movement
Source: Shutterstock with text added by author

ligaments that support the breast (Page and Steele, 1999). The type of support that a female athlete requires is influenced by the activity they are involved in and how this impacts on breast movement.

What is the impact of poor breast support on sports performance?

Research has shown that inadequate breast support when participating in sport and exercise can have a negative impact on breast health as well as on performance. This was clearly shown in Maddie's experience, and this is the same for many athletes. Gradually more athletes are speaking out about the importance of wearing correct breast support in sport as shown in Box 6.2.

BOX 6.2 WHAT DO THE ATHLETES SAY?

You want the whole focus to be on you and your horse [...] Constantly worrying that your bra straps are falling down is not helpful. I don't think young girls are aware of breast issues. It could be very, very bad for me if I did ride in a normal bra and I wasn't aware of that as a young girl.

Natasha Baker, Paralympic equestrian rider (cited in Lewis, 2015)

If I forgot my sports bra, forget it, I just wouldn't compete. That's how integral it is to my performance.

Goldie Sayers, 11-time British javelin champion (cited in Lewis, 2015)

When I hit puberty I got larger breasts than everyone else [...] I was going into PE in the worst sports bra, having to hold my chest down and try to catch the ball with one hand because if I didn't I was in pain.

Eleanor Cardwell, England Netballer (cited in Grey, 2023)

The individual requirements of the athlete, regarding breast support, will vary according to the type of sports activity they are engaging in, and also their stage of life. This is because over the lifespan the size of a woman's breast changes, such as throughout adolescence, during the course of pregnancy, and later in life into the menopause. It is also important to note that although breast pain can be caused by movement it can also be related to hormonal changes linked to the menstrual cycle, as experienced by Maddie in the case study. For those individuals working with women in sport and for the athletes themselves, developing knowledge and awareness of how the breast moves during different sports, alongside recognising any individual needs and preferences, is vital to ensure good breast health and the best possible breast support (see Table 6.1 for examples).

In addition to some of the considerations shown in Table 6.1 there are also some sports that have added requirements such as the aesthetics of the bra. For

TABLE 6.1 Examples of different requirements for different sports

Sport/Activity	Movement considerations	Sports bra needs
Running	Breasts move in a figure of eight and over a third experience breast pain which impacted their training	Reduce breast movement and breast pain
Tennis	Upper body rotation causes a lot of lateral movement from side to side	One that supports the breast during lateral movement.
Javelin	A key concern is the range of arm movement	Shoulder straps design of the sports bra are of great importance to provide support without restricting any movement

Source: Adapted from The Open University (2022)

example, a gymnast should not wear a bra that is visible or disrupts the silhouette of the leotard and at Wimbledon female tennis players must ensure that if their bra is visible at all during play that it must be completely white.

What bras and types of breast support are available for athletes?

When participating in sport and exercise wearing poor breast support, such as an everyday bra, can damage the breast and have a negative impact on performance. Despite this, findings by the Research Group in Breast Health (2022) indicate that over 80 per cent of women wear badly-fitting bras and that many women don't even own a sports bra. As shown in Box 6.2 many sportswomen consider the sports bra as an essential piece of sports kit and this view was lobbied by the England Institute for Sport in 2021 when they provided all female GB athletes with tailor-made sports bras for the Tokyo Olympic and Paralympic games. The athletes underwent professional fittings to ensure each individual received the most appropriate size and style of sports bra to fit breast size and specific sporting movements. This was replicated by the England Roses ahead of the 2023 World Cup. However, recreational females may have neither the knowledge nor the expertise available, so it is important that education around breast support is improved.

There are typically three types of sports bras, which vary in terms of their function and how they fit. These are the compression bra, the encapsulation bra and the combination bra. Female athletes should choose the most appropriate bra based on three key factors; how it fits them, how comfortable it is and what activity they intend to wear it for. It is highly recommended that athletes are professionally fitted for a sports bra to ensure the support provided matches the needs of the individual. Table 6.2 provides a useful guide to the three types of sports bras and their suitability for different activities. Maddie opted for an encapsulation bra as, being a larger cup size and taking part in an activity that involves movement in all three directions, this provided the most appropriate support for her and her activity.

TABLE 6.2 Types of sports bras and their functions

Type of Sports bra	Compression Bra	Encapsulation Bra	Combination bra
Features	Crop top style which pulls over the head	Separates to support each breast individually	Combines features of compression and encapsulation bras.
	Compresses breast tissue against chest wall	Centre part sits flat against chest wall	Supports the breasts separately
	Suitable for smaller breasted females.	Beneficial for larger breasted women.	Compresses them against the chest wall.
Advantages	Comfortable	Offers greater support	Provides high support
	For low impact activities, i.e. yoga.	Reduces movement in all directions	For high-impact activities such as running, team games.
		For high-impact activities.	
Disadvantages	Stretchiness required to fit over the shoulder limits capability to reduce movement	Structured form and rigid material can be less comfortable than soft, stretchy fabric used in compression bras.	Back fastening bras can be difficult to put on for those with limited mobility.
Reduces Movement by	Up to 55%	Up to 73%	Up to 73%

Source: Adapted from The Open University (2022)

The Important Features of a Sports Bra

The three classifications of sports bras also possess a range of features that alter the effectiveness of the support they provide. A study by Norris et al. (2021) investigating the characteristics that impacted the effectiveness of sports bras identified five key features that helped to provide improved support: an encapsulation style, padded cups, made from Nylon, an adjustable under band and a high neckline. Figure 6.4 presents the findings from the study in more detail categorising the top five and worst five performing individual sports bras according to the reduction in breast movement (%), and the specific characteristics associated with each.

Ensuring the right fit of sports bra

Many women wear the wrong size bra which can result in inadequate support being provided. To combat this, a five-point fit technique has been developed

		Best Performing Sports Bra	Worst Performing Sport Bra
Movement	**Reduction**	Reduced movement by up to 74 %	Reduced movement by up to 36%
Characteristics		Combination Style	Compression
		Underwire Present	No Underwire
		Adjustable Shoulder	Adjustable Shoulder
		Straps	Straps
		Cross Back	Racerback
		Nylon	Polyester
		Adjustable Underband	Non-Adjustable
		Cup Padding	Underband
		Back Underband	No Cup Padding
		Closure Location	Low Neck Drop
		Hook And Eye	
		Low Neck Drop	

FIGURE 6.4 Worst-performing sports bras and their characteristics
Source: Adapted from Norris et al. (2021)

by The University of Portsmouth Breast Health Research Group to assess whether a sports bra has the best possible fit (see Figure 6.5). This technique negates the need for measuring as, owing to differences in styles and brands the same size bra can fit very differently, therefore, using only bra size to choose your sports bra can be misleading. For example, Maddie typically wears a 32DD bra but the sports bra she purchased was actually a 34E, as it was the most comfortable and provided the best fit. Instead of focussing on the size of the bra it is more effective to determine whether the bra fits well. This relies on the straps being comfortable, any underwire following the natural crease of the breast, cups that fully encase the breast, a firm and fitted underband and the front of the bra sitting between the breasts flat to the body (Research Group in Breast Health, 2022).

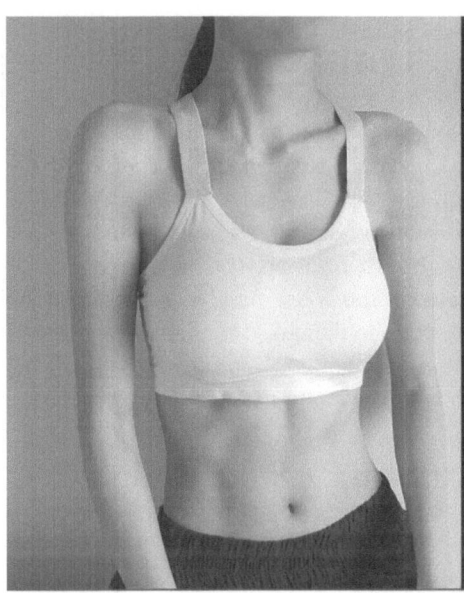

5 point Bra Fit

1. **Straps** - should be adjustable to increase comfort i.e., not dig in but also not slip.
2. **Underwire** – if a bra has underwire it should not sit on breast tissue but instead follow the natural contour of each breast.
3. **Cups** – should encase each breast without any gaping or breast spilling out of the sides or top.
4. **Underband** – should be level all the way round, sitting firmly against the chest without digging in or riding up.
5. **Front** – between the cups the lower part of the bra should sit flat against the body without gaping or lifting.

FIGURE 6.5 The Five-Point Bra Fit Technique
Source: Shutterstock
Information source: The Well HQ cited in The Open University (2022)

BOX 6.3 SPOTLIGHT ON: SELECTING A SPORTS BRA FOR HORSE-RIDING

As mentioned, different sports and activities each require specific support for the breast. If we take Maddie for instance, horse riding is an energetic and dynamic activity that can cause excessive breast movement. Research by Burbage and Cameron (2017) investigating the prevalence and impact of breast pain, bra issues and breast size on female horse riders reported that 40 per cent of women in their study experienced breast pain, and that this was significantly related to cup size and body mass. Of those who reported experiencing breast pain 60 per cent said that this was linked to their menstrual cycle, and 29 per cent felt their breast pain was a result of horse riding. In terms of severity of pain 56 per cent described their breast pain as discomforting, and 8 per cent said it was 'distressing, horrible or excruciating'. Overall, 21 per cent of riders said that breast issues negatively impacted their performance. Despite this only 35 per cent of women (14 per cent of small-breasted riders and 19 per cent of large-breasted riders) regularly ride in a sports bra. This is considerably lower than the wearing of sports bras identified within the running population. Burbage and Cameron (2017) suggest this may be due to sports bra marketing to be targeted at runners rather than other sports such as riding. Awareness and education are a positive step to help women find effective breast support solutions.

Owing to the high-impact nature of the activity, it is crucial that a suitable sports bra is worn when riding, to aid performance as well as ensure breast health is maintained. A badly fitting sports bra can detract the competitor's attention from the task in hand which can have a negative impact on performance. During competition any external distractions are not conducive to maximising performance and so falling bra straps or breast movement or pain is something that needs to be eradicated. A sports bra must be comfortable to allow for the performer to completely focus on the task in hand. As we can see from Maddie's story, a correctly fitting sports bra (following the five-point fit) can also help improve posture, which is an integral to riding as it can influence the horse.

Advice and guidance for coaches and athletes

The research presented within this chapter demonstrates how good breast support can positively impact participation and performance in sport and exercise, yet the education provided to girls and women regarding breast health and breast support is generally very poor (Brown et al., 2018). Disseminating knowledge and awareness of breast health and correct bra fit is important to empower women and girls to positively impact factors such as body confidence, participation in physical activity and overall health. Young girls and women should be educated about the significance of wearing well-fitted and appropriate breast support during sport and exercise. This should be spoken about openly rather than being seen as an embarrassing or unacceptable subject. Changing the rhetoric around the sports bra and including it as part of any essential kit list, similar to a gum shield or shin pads, is one way to overcome any social taboos. Additionally, including breast health information in any welcome talks with parents and athletes, or during any coachable moments so it occurs naturally would be appropriate. If Maddie had received this information as a junior rider, it would have saved her many years of discomfort and pain and lessened her risk of breast sag.

It is important that girls are educated about breast health at a young age, as during puberty girls will experience physical changes to their body shape, including breast development (as discussed later in Chapter 9). Adolescence is a difficult time for girls, and they can be extremely sensitive and vulnerable with regards to their body confidence. Research shows that embarrassment about breast development is a common factor associated with girls engagement in sport and exercise (Scurr et al., 2016) and so breast education plays an important role in the participation rates of girls.

During adolescence, parents, teachers and coaches should all play an important role in educating girls about the importance of breast support. It is imperative that girls and women receive advice on the importance of wearing a properly fitting sports bra, either by attending a fitting by a professional, or by following the five-point fit themselves. Parents play a role in educating their daughters and are typically responsible for taking their daughter for a bra fitting, therefore, when taking their daughter for their first bra they should include fitting for a sports bra. It should be noted that even though professional fitting is a good option, educating girls on good bra fit for themselves is also valuable.

Box 6.4 provides some useful tips for both athletes and coaches on how to maintain good breast health for optimal performance during sport and exercise.

BOX 6.4 REAL-WORLD APPLICATION

As a female athlete, you should:

1. Familiarise yourself with the anatomy of the breast and consider how the breast moves during sport and exercise.
2. Consider your individual needs such as breast size and the nature of the activity you will be taking part in, and match these requirements to the most appropriate type of sports bra.
3. Attend a fitting by a professional, or follow the 5-point fit yourself to ensure you have a properly fitting sports bra.
4. As there are many brands and styles of sports bra try a variety of bras, if possible, to find the best one that works for you.
5. Talk to your coach about breast health and breast support if you feel it is impacting your performance.

As a coach, you should:

1. Help athletes understand the importance of breast support and the need to wear a properly fitting sports bra.
2. Ensure that 'sports bra' is added to any essential kit lists that go out to players and parents.
3. Provide an environment where breast health is openly discussed and not considered an embarrassing topic.
4. Explain the connection between breast support and performance.
5. Dispel any myths surrounding breast support i.e. that two bras offer more support, as this should be discouraged as a properly fitted sports bra will be sufficient.

Summary

This chapter has provided an overview of the importance of breast health and breast support when training and competing in sport. The research presented demonstrates that although many women cite breast pain and discomfort as a common barrier to sport and exercise, through developing the knowledge and understanding of breast health, breast anatomy, breast biomechanics and appropriate support, these issues can either be eradicated completely or at least significantly reduced in terms of their impact on participation and performance.

The messages to take away from this chapter are:

1. Concerns over breast issues can deter many women from taking part in sport and exercise. Worrying about breast movement can detract an athlete's focus away from performance with potentially detrimental effects.
2. Mastalgia and discomfort are common experiences for women taking part in sport, and for female athletes such factors can impact performance.
3. Educating coaches and athletes about breast anatomy and breast movement can support and empower more women to take action to ensure they wear suitable breast support.
4. There are three types of sports bra, each appropriate for different levels of activity, and athletes should wear the correct type of bra for their individual needs.
5. The most important aspect of breast support is ensuring the bra fits correctly and female athletes should be educated about the five points to consider.

End-of-Chapter Quiz

Answers can be found after the References

1. Identify which of the following describes the term 'mastalgia':

    a Breast injury
    b Breast size
    c Breast movement
    d Breast pain

2. Identify which of the following structures provides internal support to the breast:

    a Pectoral muscle
    b Skin tissue
    c Cooper's ligament
    d Glandular tissue

3. Identify which of the following is NOT an impact of poor breast support on performance:

    a Increased muscle activity in upper body
    b Increase in stride length during running
    c Increased risk of injury to the breast

d   Increase in ground reaction forces

4.   Identify which **two** of the following are recognised types of sports bra.

a   Contraction
b   Compression
c   Cropped
d   Combination

5.   Identify whether the following statement is true or false:

When evaluating the correct fit of a sports bra, you need to consider the straps, underwiring, cups, underband and the front.

References

Brisbine, B.R., Steele, J.R., Phillips, E.J. and McGhee, D.E. (2020) 'Breast pain affects the performance of elite female athletes', *Journal of Sports Sciences*, 38(5), 528–533.

Brown, N., Smith, J., Brasher, A., Risius, D., Marczyk, A. and Wakefield-Scurr, J. (2018) 'Breast education for schoolgirls; why, what, when, and how?' *Breast Journal*, 24, 377–382.

Brown, N., White, J., Brasher, A. and Scurr, J. (2014) 'The experience of breast pain (mastalgia) in female runners of the 2012 London Marathon and its effect on exercise behaviour', *British Journal of Sports Medicine*, 48(4), 320–325.

Burbage, J. and Cameron, L. (2017) 'An investigation into the prevalence and impact of breast pain, bra issues and breast size on female horse riders', *Journal of Sports Sciences*, 35(11), 1091–1097.

Burnett, E., White, J. and Scurr, J., (2015) 'The influence of the breast on physical activity participation in females', *Journal of Physical Activity and Health*, 12(4), pp. 588–594.

Grey, B. (2023) *Sports bras: England netballer Eleanor Cardwell on finding the right fit.* Available at: https://www.bbc.co.uk/sport/netball/64786152 (Accessed: 21 March 2023).

Lewis, A. (2015) *How sports bras helped transform women's approach to sport.* Available at: https://www.bbc.co.uk/sport/athletics/32382911 (Accessed: 2 November 2022).

Norris, M., Blackmore, T., Horler, B. and Wakefield-Scurr, J. (2021) 'How the characteristics of sports bras affect their performance', *Ergonomics*, 64(3), 410–425.

Page, K.-A. and Steele, J.R. (1999) 'Breast Motion and Sports Brassiere Design: Implications for Future Research', *Sports medicine (Auckland)*, 27(4), 205–211.

Research Group in Breast Health (2022) *Experts in Breast and Bra Science.* Portsmouth University. Available at: https://www.port.ac.uk/research/research-groups-and-centres/research-group-in-breast-health#our%20researchers (Accessed: 27 October 2023).

Scurr, J., Brown, N., Smith, J., Brasher, A., Risius, D. and Marczyk, A. (2016) 'The influence of the breast on sport and exercise participation in school girls in the United Kingdom', *Journal of Adolescent Health*, 58(2), 167–173.

The Open University (2022) *Session 5: Breast health and choosing the correct breast support. Badged Open Course: Supporting female performance in sport and fitness.* Available at: www.open.edu/openlearn/mod/oucontent/view.php? id=116022 (Accessed: 14 November 2022).

Answers

1. d
2. c
3. b
4. b and d
5. True

7

PELVIC FLOOR DYSFUNCTION AND THE FEMALE ATHLETE

Simon Rea

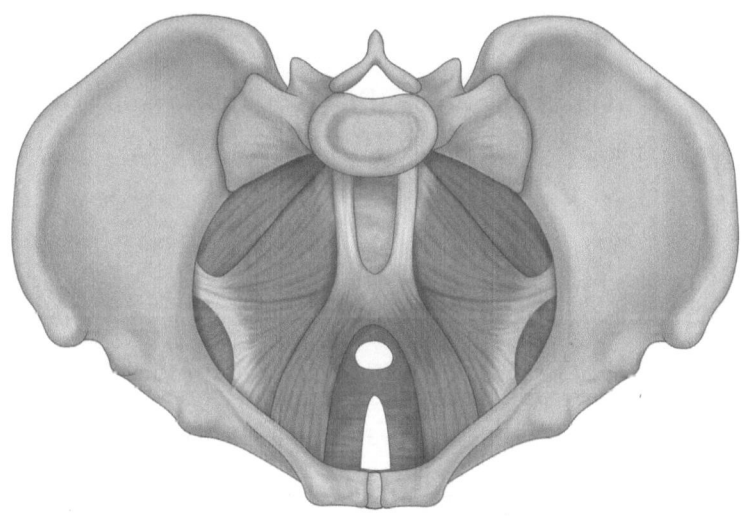

Pelvic floor dysfunction (PFD) is a collective term for a range of disorders that are caused by an impairment of the pelvic floor muscles. The pelvic floor muscles make up a broad sheet of muscle that spreads across the inside of the pelvis and are designed to support the contents of the abdomen above. They support the weight of internal organs, including the bladder, uterus, and stomach and are thus under constant stress. They also control the flow of urine from the bladder and faeces from the large intestine. Pelvic floor dysfunction is characterised by a reduced ability of the pelvic floor muscles to control the flow of urine and faeces. In particular, urinary incontinence (UI) that is defined as an involuntary leakage of urine (Haylen et al.,

DOI: 10.4324/9781003330110-7

2010), is a major symptom of PFD, along with faecal incontinence, pelvic pain, pelvic organ prolapse and sexual dysfunction (Rial Rebullido and Stracciolini, 2019).

Sport and physical activity offers many physical, social, and psychological benefits; however, pelvic floor health may be one area where the positive effect of physical activity can be questioned (Bo and Nygaard, 2020). This is because elite athletes have a high prevalence of urinary incontinence (Rodriguez-Lopez et al., 2020). While the condition may not be life threatening it presents a seriously embarrassing problem for an athlete and can negatively impact on their quality of life (de Mattos Lourenco et al., 2018). Despite the high prevalence of PFD in female athletes it is still receives relatively little attention from sports medicine clinicians and the embarrassment around pelvic issues felt by females often leads to them avoiding seeking medical attention (Rial Rebullido and Stracciolini, 2019).

In this chapter we will take a detailed look at the pelvic floor muscles, their location, the role they play, and then explore the two categories of pelvic floor dysfunction that affect athletes. These two categories are a relaxing pelvic floor and a non-relaxing pelvic floor. We will assess the symptoms and causes of each and look at how they can be treated and managed. Box 7.1 presents definitions of some of the terminology we will be using around pelvic floor dysfunction.

BOX 7.1 PELVIC FLOOR DYSFUNCTION TERMINOLOGY

Urinary incontinence: any involuntary leakage of urine

Stress incontinence: involuntary leakage of urine caused by increased effort or exertion

Urge incontinence: a type of urinary incontinence that causes a sudden, urgent need to urinate

Mixed incontinence: involuntary leakage that combines the urgent need to urinate and increased exertion and effort

---

In summary, urinary incontinence is the umbrella term for these types of incontinence, whereby urine leaks through the urethra. Stress incontinence occurs when there is a sudden, rapid loading on the pelvic floor muscles such as when sneezing or laughing.

Before we examine the pelvic floor dysfunction in detail read the case study in Box 7.2 where you will meet Shanice who is a netballer.

BOX 7.2 SHANICE (NETBALLER)

Shanice is an 18-year-old netballer who has been training since she was seven years old. She represents her club and has been competing internationally at junior levels. Her aim is to break through and gain selection for the senior international team.

Shanice plays as centre and as well as constantly running between the goal circles, she does a lot of jumping to catch the ball and twisting and turning to find space and pass. Along with her netball training she also spends several hours a week in the gym working on strength and conditioning to help her performance.

Around two years ago Shanice was warming up for a match and when she landed from jumping to catch the ball she felt that she had wet herself. She quickly went to the toilet and was surprised to see that she had leaked quite a lot of urine. She quickly changed her clothes and continued her warm up. Unfortunately she performed poorly, as she was far more worried about wetting herself again and thus unable to focus on her performance.

Over the next year she noticed that this was happening again and again. When she was in the gym and performing squats or jumping plyometric exercises she would feel the sensation that she was leaking. When she was competing she would often feel urine leakage when sprinting or landing.

However, she developed methods to deal with this leakage, such as avoiding fluids for a long time before training and completely before competition. She also made sure she went to the toilet regularly before training and competition. Unfortunately, the worry she was experiencing, and the time spent preparing, started taking up more and more of her mental energy at the expense of improving her performances.

Shanice's coach became concerned about her lack of progress and eventually Shanice confided in her coach what was happening. Her coach introduced Shanice to pelvic floor exercises and included pelvic floor exercises in her strength and conditioning work.

However, Shanice found that her symptoms got worse. She had started to experience pain in her lower back, stabbing pains in her vagina, and tingling sensations in her buttocks. She even found that she was occasionally wetting the bed at night. The exercises had no effect on her urine leakage during netball, and she was at the point where she was seriously considering quitting the sport that she loves.

The case study of Shanice shows the distress that pelvic floor dysfunction can have on an athlete and how it can destroy their confidence and impact negatively on performance. Shanice seems to be taking the correct course of action in strengthening her pelvic floor muscles, however, in some cases this can made urinary incontinence and its symptoms worse. In this chapter we will examine the two causes of pelvic floor dysfunction associated with athletes and this can help explain why Shanice's efforts to improve her condition actually caused more harm. Before that we will look at the anatomy of the pelvic floor and the musculature we are referring to.

Which muscles are we talking about? Anatomy of the pelvic floor muscles

The pelvic floor is a complex structure situated within the pelvis and running between the symphysis pubis at the anterior of the pelvis and the coccyx at the posterior. It is part of the neuromuscular system and thus consists of muscles, ligaments, and neurological tissue. Figures 7.1 and 7.2 show the position of the pelvic floor muscles from two aspects.

In Figure 7.1 we can see that the pelvic floor muscles form a cradle across the bottom of the pelvis that is approximately 1 cm thick. In a female there are three openings in the pelvic floor to allow the urethra, vagina, and anus to pass through the musculature. In the male pelvic floor there are only two openings, for the urethra and anus. Figure 7.2 shows the key structures of the pelvis and the pelvic floor. The pelvic floor muscles are not visible as they are surrounded by large global muscles, they are also complex in structure as they consist of three layers of muscle that are attached to and integrated with other body systems.

The pelvic floor muscles are the coccygeus and the levator ani. The levator ani consists of two muscles, the iliococcygeus and the pubococcygeus. They are

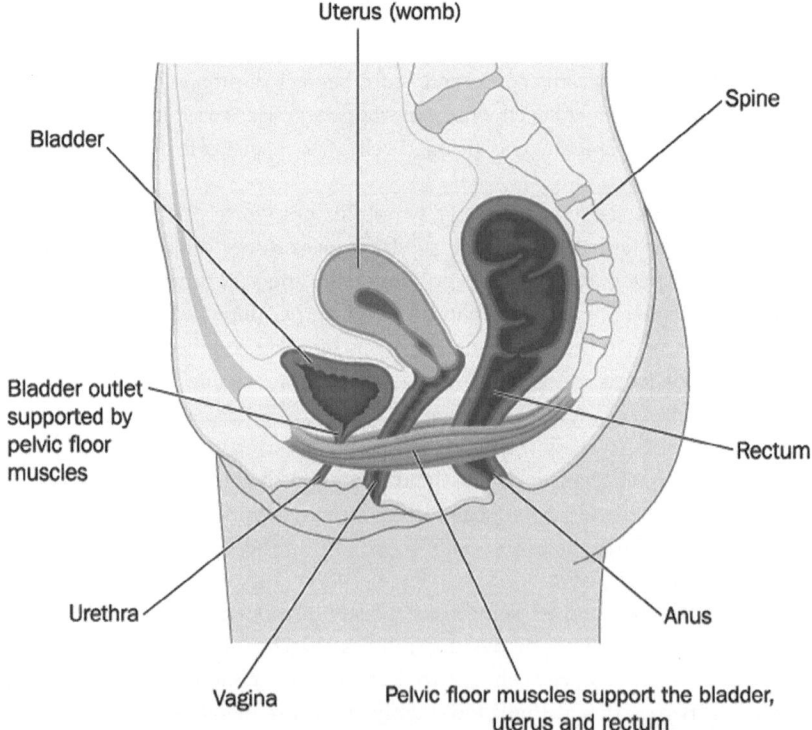

FIGURE 7.1 Pelvic floor muscles from a lateral aspect
Source: Shutterstock

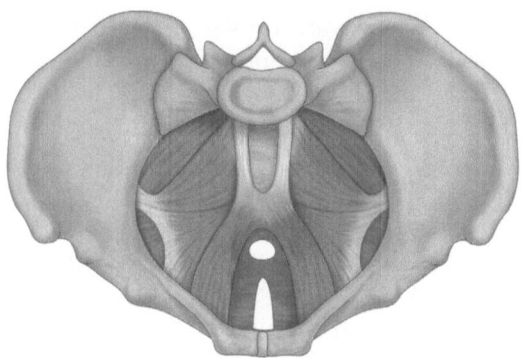

FIGURE 7.2 Pelvic floor muscles from a superior aspect
Source: Shutterstock

attached to the pelvis and coccyx via ligaments, shown in grey in Figure 7.2. Pelvic floor muscles play key roles in males and females such as continence (avoiding urine and faecal leakage), sexual function, stabilisation of the sacroiliac joint, breathing and posture (Rial Rebullido et al., 2020). In females the pelvic floor also plays a vital role in pregnancy when it supports the weight of the foetus and the placenta in the uterus, and it is also highly active in childbirth. For this reason pelvic floor issues are often related to pregnancy and childbirth, as the pelvic floor can become stretched resulting in urinary incontinence.

Pelvic floor dysfunction – symptoms and risk factors

We have already identified urine leakage and faecal leakage as symptoms of pelvic floor dysfunction. However, there are other associated symptoms, such as:

- Painful urination
- Constipation or bowel strains
- Lower back pain
- Pain in the pelvic region, genitals, or rectum
- Discomfort during sexual intercourse
- Feeling of pressure in the pelvis or rectum
- Muscle spasms in the pelvis

(Healthline, 2022)

You may have noticed that Shanice in the case study in Box 7.1 was experiencing some of these symptoms, such as lower back pain and pain in her genitals.

There are several risk factors that may predispose a female to PFD and unfortunately exercise is one of these. Teixeira et al. (2018) identified that 36 per cent of athletes had experienced urinary incontinence and that they are three times more likely to experience it when compared to non-athlete females. In addition to exercise, older age, obesity, childbirth, and the menopause are risk factors for PFD

(Teixeira et al., 2018). An additional risk factor for PFD is relative energy deficiency in sport or RED-S, a condition that was covered in Chapter 5. The relationship between RED-S and PFD is explored in Box 7.3.

BOX 7.3 PELVIC FLOOR DYSFUNCTION AND RED-S

Several studies have found that athletes in physically demanding sports that place an emphasis on leanness, such as track and field athletics, gymnastics, and dance sport, have higher rates of pelvic floor dysfunction (Teixeira et al., 2018, Rial Rebullido et al., 2020). RED-S has been shown to affect many systems of the body, including the neuromuscular system resulting in decreased strength, that may affect the proper activation of the pelvic floor (Rial Rebullido and Stracciolini, 2019).

Stress incontinence is the most common form of PFD in female athletes and having inadequate fuel sources (in the form of glycogen) may lead to early fatigue of the pelvic floor muscles and poor co-ordination of these muscles (Rial Rebullido and Stracciolini, 2019). The effect of neuromuscular fatigue on the pelvic floor muscles during strenuous competition and training has already been identified by Ree et al. (2007).

The impact of the reduced quantity of food consumed by athletes experiencing RED-S extends beyond energy input as the quantities of the micronutrients, vitamins and minerals, will also be reduced. In particular any reduction in Vitamin D can have consequences for the function of the pelvic floor. Vitamin D is essential for musculoskeletal health, strength, and function, and any insufficiency in could impact on the contractility and function of the pelvic floor muscles (Rial Rebullido and Stracciolini, 2019).

The endocrine system is also compromised in athletes experiencing RED-S as low energy availability can lead to a disruption in the hypothalamic control of the menstrual cycle and a resulting reduction in levels of sex hormones, particularly oestrogen. There are oestrogen receptors in the pelvic floor and oestrogen plays a key role in maintaining the health of the pelvic floor muscles (Copas et al., 2001). A reduction of oestrogen can lead to the thinning of the lining of the bladder and the urethra (Newson, 2019) and increases the risk of urinary incontinence.

Is pelvic floor dysfunction related to sport type?

Figures around the extent of the urinary and stress incontinence as symptoms of PFD differ between studies but all of them illustrate that is a significant problem. Early research by Nygaard et al. (1994) found that overall 28 per cent of female athletes experienced urinary incontinence with the greatest prevalence in gymnastics (67 per cent), basketball (66 per cent) and tennis (50 per cent). Another study by Nygaard et al. (1996) found that 54 per cent of female athletes experienced urinary incontinence with gymnastics again the highest with a prevalence of 70 per cent of female gymnasts.

A more recent study by Rodriguez-Lopez et al. (2020) found that 45.1 per cent of female athletes experienced urinary incontinence compared with 14.7 per cent of male athletes, making the risk of urinary incontinence in female athletes 5.45 times more likely than in male athletes. What is also concerning is that of all the female athletes experiencing urinary incontinence almost 50 per cent of them first experienced symptoms between the ages of 20–30 (Rodriguez-Lopez et al., 2020). Table 7.1 shows the prevalence of urinary incontinence in relation to sport type.

Casey and Temme (2016) concluded, based on Nygaard's research (1994, 1996), that the highest risk of urinary incontinence in young female athletes was when participating in high impact sports characterised by landing, jumping, or running, such as netball or volleyball. This is borne out in the figures in Table 7.1 and reflects the case study of netballer Shanice, in Box 7.1, who experienced urine leakage when running and landing from a jump. Owing to the ground reaction forces produced during these activities they will increase intra-abdominal pressure and exert forces directly onto the pelvic floor (Reis et al., 2011). This rapid loading of the pelvic floor produces forces that can cause it to stretch. To illustrate this further, in athletics the female athletes taking part in vertical jumps (high jump, pole vault) had much lower prevalence of urinary than those taking part in horizontal jumps (long jump, triple jump) (Rodriguez-Lopez et al., 2020). This may be because vertical jumps result in the athlete landing on a mat while horizontal jumps result in the athlete landing on their heels and with ground reaction forces of up to 16 times their body weight (Hay, cited in Bo and Nygaard, 2020).

Like any other muscle the pelvic floor muscles will fatigue during exercise as they will be constantly contracting and relaxing in response to the forces they are resisting. This may explain high prevalence of UI in endurance sports, for example

TABLE 7.1 Prevalence of urinary incontinence in selected sports

Sport type and sample size	Percentage of athletes experiencing UI
Athletics (346)	40.5%
Badminton (7)	14.3%
Boxing (16)	31.3%
Dance sport (5)	40%
Golf (7)	14.3%
Gymnastics (53)	32.1%
Hockey (23)	43.5%
Karate (11)	45.5%
Judo (49)	16.3%
Rugby (10)	80%
Soccer (63)	27%
Swimming (7)	57.1%
Weightlifting (12)	25%

Source: Adapted from Rodriguez-Lopez et al. (2020)

Rodriguez-Lopez et al. (2020) identifying high rates of UI in rugby players (80 per cent) and swimmers (57 per cent). The high rate in swimming is surprising as it is a low impact low sport and does not involve repetitive jumping and landing; however, it does include endurance events. In Rodriguez-Lopez et al.'s (2022) study of track and field athletes they found highest of stress incontinence in athletes in race walking events which last for the longest time.

It is generally regarded that urinary and stress incontinence are due to weakened pelvic floor muscles, however, this view has been disputed and there are two theories as to why female athletes experience higher incidences of UI and SI than non-athletes. We will explore this in the next section.

Pelvic floor dysfunction and female athletes – relaxing and non-relaxing pelvic floors

Pelvic floor muscles will be contracted all the time to support the weight above from the pelvic organs. There are two exceptions to this, and they are during urination and defecation (Bo, 2004). At these times the pelvic floor muscles relax to allow the urethra and anus to remain open. In addition to the constant tone of pelvic floor muscles, they can be contracted further voluntarily by lifting upwards and squeezing around the urethra, vagina, and anus. This contraction on demand is described as a 'voluntary contraction' of the pelvic floor muscles and is followed by their 'voluntary relaxation' when they relax on demand. Pelvic floor muscles can also produce an 'involuntary contraction' when they contract in response to coughing, sneezing, or laughing and prevent incontinence. The muscles can also produce an 'involuntary relaxation' during a Valsalva manoeuvre or when straining to pass urine or faeces (Casey and Temme, 2016).

Athletes may experience pelvic floor dysfunction in two ways as presented by Bo and Nygaard's (2020) two opposing hypotheses.

Hypothesis one: female athletes may have stretched and weakened pelvic floors

Exercise can stretch and weaken the pelvic floor because the muscle fibres and ligaments become damaged, as a result of the forces applied on the pelvic floor. In particular, it is exercise where the pelvic floor becomes loaded rapidly, such as when running and jumping. This type of exercise increases intra-abdominal pressure and if the pelvic floor muscles are not able to contract quickly enough or produce a strong enough contraction the muscles can become stretched and weakened leading to urinary incontinence and other pelvic floor issues.

Hypothesis two: female athletes have strong pelvic floor muscles

This hypothesis suggests that physical activity and particularly high impact activity produce a training effect to strengthen pelvic floor muscles and cause hypertrophy in muscles contained in a small space. While this may look like an advantage exercise can cause the pelvic floor muscles to become too strong. These muscles experience hypertrophy (increase in size) and may become shorter and tighter causing a reduced range of movement. These changes may mean that the muscles no longer have the flexibility required to respond to changes in pressure. Not being able to resist pressure effectively can lead to an increase prevalence in leaking of urine.

Louis-Charles et al. (2019) identify a non-relaxing pelvic floor as being problematic to female athletes. This is because the pelvic floor muscles remain in a contracted state causing increased pressure in the abdomen and resulting in abdominal or muscular pain. When assessing a non-relaxing pelvic floor it is important to be aware that the pelvic floor muscles are only one part of a kinetic chain that controls the movement of the trunk. This kinetic chain involves interaction between the hips, pelvis and spine and dysfunction at any stage of the chain may result in overcompensation by the pelvic floor muscles and result in them remaining in a state of contraction (Faubion et al., 2012).

Bo and Nygaard (2020) concluded that while there is evidence to support both hypotheses there has not been enough research in this area to make firm conclusions. In addition, this area is challenging to research because most research is invasive and it is difficult to accurately measure changes in intra-abdominal pressure, and thus pressure on the pelvic floor.

However, as knowledge in this area grows, coaches and trainers adopt more progressive approaches where pelvic floor work is becoming an integral part of an athlete's strength and conditioning work, rather than being seen as isolated work done as rehabilitation in response to dysfunction.

In the case study of Shanice, in Box 7.1, she is experiencing back pain, stabbing pains in her vagina and urinary incontinence, and this may be due to her pelvic floor becoming overdeveloped and hypertonic (unable to relax). She also explains how she was using mental energy worrying about her pelvic floor rather than focusing on her performance This is a real concern that athletes may be worrying about leaking urine during performance. It does not have to be like this, as in the next section we will see that pelvic floor muscles can be strengthened and have their normal function restored.

Treating pelvic floor muscles

Training the pelvic floor can be challenging as the muscles are not visible and they are surrounded by other muscles. Bo (2004) describes how when asked to contract pelvic floor muscles women will often contract their abdominals, gluteal and adductor muscles as well as their pelvic floor muscles. When contracting the pelvic floor muscles voluntarily the pelvic floor muscles will move upwards and contract around the urethra. The key to pelvic floor exercises is learning to isolate the pelvic floor muscles and work them on their own.

Pelvic floor muscles can be strengthened fairly quickly as it takes around 14 days of repetitive training to build up neural pathways between the brain and the pelvic floor muscles. These pathways will improve control of the pelvic floor muscles and it takes about three months of training to increase their size and strength. Pelvic floor muscles contain both slow twitch and fast twitch muscles fibre types, so it is important that there are exercise that will stimulate both these types of muscle fibre.

According to Baz Moffat (2022), a women's health coach at the Well HQ, a way to isolate your pelvic floor muscles is when you are on the toilet you contract the muscles that stop the flow of urine and then those that prevent you from passing wind. This is just a way of identifying the pelvic floor muscles, as continually stopping the flow of urine can lead to problems such as urinary tract infections. Pelvic floor exercises can be done lying, sitting, or standing and involve lifting up the muscles around the vagina and then those muscles around the anus towards the belly button and then relaxing the muscles that perform the lifting.

There are many pelvic floor exercises, but the two basic exercises are:

- Tighten and lift the pelvic floor and hold for 10 seconds, then repeat 10 times
- Tighten the pelvic floor muscles quickly and hold for 1 second before relaxing fully and repeating 10 times

(Health and Care videos, 2022)

These exercises should be done at least daily and then up to 4–5 times a day if possible. Pelvic floor exercises are supported by the NHS Squeezy app which provides prompts to remind you to do your exercises and has visual and audio content to ensure you are doing the exercises correctly. It was designed by specialist physiotherapists to allow an exercise programme to be tailored for their client.

There are also vaginally inserted pelvic floor training devices, such as Elvie and Kegel8, that are linked to apps and can monitor pelvic floor strength as muscles contract and relax. These are useful as they provide feedback to the about both the contraction and the relaxation. Moffat (in Tomas, 2022) recommends that it is best to learn pelvic floor exercises on their own initially without a device, and that contacting a women's health physiotherapist to learn how to do the exercises should be the first priority.

For female athletes these exercises are only the start of the process as they need to progress and integrate pelvic floor work into their strength and conditioning training, and in particular into their core work. This will involve the coach or trainer in getting the female athlete to activate their pelvic floor muscles before performing key lifts such as squats and lunges, and then focusing on keeping these muscles contracted during the exercise.

BOX 7.4 SPOTLIGHT ON: TREATMENT FOR A NON-RELAXING PELVIC FLOOR

A non-relaxing pelvic floor is also referred to as a hypertonic pelvic floor, meaning abnormally high muscle tone. Women with a hypertonic pelvic floor can experience a range of symptoms including an inability or difficulty to pass urine and faeces, constipation, pain during sexual intercourse, pelvic pain, and low back pain (Faubion et al., 2012). Unfortunately the pain experienced can worsen with physical activity and increases from walking to more vigorous activity (Louis-Charles et al., 2019).

Once a hypertonic pelvic floor has been diagnosed it can be treated in several ways:

1. Teaching pelvic floor relaxation exercises. The individual will focus their attention on relaxing the pelvic floor muscles and combine this with diaphragmatic breathing.
2. Manual manipulation of the pelvic floor muscles, including trigger point massage and myofascial release. This is often done by the therapist inserting their finger into the vagina or anus to give them access to these deep pelvic floor muscles (coccygeus and levator ani). They must only be done by a woman's health physiotherapist with the consent of the female to undertake this treatment.
3. Physical therapist can prescribe exercise to stabilise the pelvis and strengthen core muscles.
4. A doctor may prescribe medication to treat chronic pelvic pain, such as nerve block injections or analgesics (Louis-Charles, 2019).

The treatment of a hypertonic pelvic floor may take a considerable amount of time as a result of muscle memory causing relaxed muscles to return to their original hypertonic state (Louis-Charles, 2019). However, it may be that a multidisciplinary approach needs to be adopted with specialists in gastroenterology, gynaecology, sexual medicine, and urology becoming involved (Faubion et al., 2012).

BOX 7.5 REAL-WORLD APPLICATION

As a female athlete, you should:

1. Appreciate that urine leakage is not acceptable and should never be ignored.
2. Understand that certain types of sports can predispose you to pelvic floor dysfunction and take steps to minimise the risk.
3. Seek support as soon as you recognise symptoms of pelvic floor dysfunction, such as urinary incontinence, faecal incontinence, pelvic pain, or back pain.
4. Practice pelvic floor exercises daily and integrate them into strength and conditioning training.
5. Be aware that pelvic floor dysfunction is not always caused by a weak pelvic floor but may be the result of muscles becoming too strong and tight and unable to work through their full range of movement.
6. Minimise other risk factors for pelvic floor dysfunction such as relative energy deficiency in sport (RED-S), smoking and drinking carbonated drinks.

As a coach, you should:

1. Be aware of the types of sport and activities where pelvic floor dysfunction is most prevalent and be able to recognise the signs and symptoms.
2. Appreciate that leakage of urine and faeces is an embarrassing issue that needs to be dealt with sensitively and avoid humour around the subject.
3. Learn how to teach pelvic floor exercises and be able to integrate them into training at the appropriate time.
4. Source a trustworthy physiotherapist who specialises in women's health and can effectively treat pelvic floor dysfunction.

Summary

Having completed this chapter you will now have developed a more detailed understanding of why pelvic floor dysfunction is such a critical issue to female athletes who are focused on producing their optimal performance, and the physical and psychological problems it can present. You will have an appreciation of the location and anatomy of the pelvic floor muscles and the signs and symptoms that occur when these muscles are not functioning correctly. In particular you will be aware that pelvic floor dysfunction is complex because it may be caused by muscles that are either too weak to withstand changes in intra-abdominal pressure or so strong that they are not able to function correctly in response to this pressure. It is important to point out that this is an area where there has been limited research and our understanding, especially when related to sport, needs to develop further.

The key messages to take away from this chapter are:

1. Pelvic floor dysfunction is a collective term for a range of disorders caused by an impairment to the function of pelvic floor muscles, including urinary incontinence, stress incontinence and faecal incontinence.
2. Pelvic floor health is one condition that may not be improved through exercise, and it may actually be a cause of pelvic floor dysfunction.
3. Pelvic floor dysfunction is most prevalent in high impact sports characterised by running, jumping, and landing.
4. Figures differ but between 36–45 per cent of female athletes will experience urinary incontinence.
5. There are two hypotheses about pelvic floor dysfunction in female athletes, that it may be caused either by a stretched, weakened pelvic floor or one that is too strong, or hypertonic.
6. Learning pelvic floor exercises can help to train the pelvic floor to avoid urinary incontinence, while a hypertonic pelvic floor may need to be treated by a physiotherapist specialising in women's health.

End-of-Chapter Quiz

Answers can be found after the References

1. Identify what is meant by the term 'stress incontinence':

    a   Involuntary leakage of urine caused by a sudden need to urinate
    b   Involuntary leakage of urine caused by pelvic floor pain
    c   Involuntary leakage of urine caused by increased exertion
    d   Involuntary leakage of urine caused by anxious thoughts

2. Identify which of the statements about the pelvic floor is false:

    a   The pelvic floor muscles support the bladder, uterus, and rectum
    b   The pelvic floor muscles run from the symphysis pubis to the sacrum
    c   The pelvic floor in a female has three openings for the urethra, vagina, and anus
    d   Pelvic floor muscles are about 1cm thick and consist of three layers of muscle

3. Identify which sport is most likely to have the highest percentage of athletes that experience urinary incontinence:

    a   Athletics
    b   Badminton
    c   Judo
    d   Golf

4. Identify why high impact exercises can cause urine leakage:

    a   Because it is a type of high intensity exercise
    b   Because it increases the rate of pelvic muscle fatigue
    c   Because the body is not always supporting its own weight
    d   Because of the effect of ground reaction forces produced on landing

5. Identify which is the correct way to train pelvic floor muscles:

    a   Use slow and fast muscle contractions during the exercises
    b   Contract all the muscle groups around the pelvis
    c   Always train by stopping and starting the flow of urine
    d   Exercises for the pelvic floor muscles need to be done three times a week

References

Bo, K. (2004) Urinary incontinence, pelvic floor dysfunction, exercise and sport. *Sports Medicine*, 34(7), 451–464.

Bo, K. and Nygaard, I.E. (2020) Is physical activity good or bad for the female pelvic floor? A narrative review. *Sports Medicine*, 50(3), 471–484.

Casey, E.K. & Temme, K. (2016) Pelvic floor muscle function and urinary incontinence in the female athlete. *The Physician and Sports Medicine*, 45(4), 399–407.

Copas, P., Bukovsky, A., Asbury, B., Elder, R. and Caudle, M. (2001) Estrogen, progesterone, and androgen receptor expression in levator ani muscle and fascia. *Journal of Women's Health and Gender-Based Medicine*, 10, 785–795.

de Mattos Lourenco, T.R., Matsuoka, P.K., Baracat, E.C. and Haddad, J.M. (2018) Urinary incontinence in female athletes: a systematic review. *International Urogynecology Journal*, 29(12), 1757–1763.

Faubion, S.S., Shuster, L.T. and Bharucha, A.E. (2012) Recognition and management of non-relaxing pelvic floor dysfunction. In *Mayo Clinic proceedings*, Vol. 87, pp. 187–193.

Haylen, B.T., de Ridder, D., Freeman, R.M., Swift, S.E., Berghmans, B., Lee, J., Monga, A., Eckhard, P., Rizk, D.E., Sand, P.K. and Schaer, G.N. (2010) An International Urogynecological Association (IUGA)/International Continence Society (ICS) joint report on the terminology for female pelvic floor dysfunction. *International Urogynecological Journal*, 21(1), 5–26.

Health and Care Videos (2022) Pelvic Floor Strengthening. Online at: https://healthandcarevideos.uk/bladder?videoId=1595 (Accessed 14 November 2022).

Healthline (2022) Pelvic Floor Dysfunction. Online at: www.healthline.com/health/pelvic-floor-dysfunction (Accessed 3 November 2022).

Louis-Charles, K., Biggie, M.D., Wolfinbarger, A., Wilcox, B. and Kienstra, C.M. (2019) Pelvic floor dysfunction in the female athlete. *American College of Sports Medicine*, 18(2), 49–52.

Moffat, B. in Rea, S.Pinchbeck, J. and Ross, E. (2022) Session 4: Pelvic floor muscles: out of sight and often overlooked. *Badged Open Course: Supporting female performance in sport and fitness*. Online at: www.open.edu/openlearn/mod/oucontent/view.php?id=116023&section=6 (Accessed 14 November 2022).

Newson, L. (2019) *Menopause; all you need to know in one concise manual*. Yeovil: Haynes.

Nygaard, I.E., Glowacki, C. and Saltzman, C.L. (1996) Relationship between foot flexibility and urinary incontinence in nulliparous varsity athletes. *Obstetrics and Gynecology*, 87(6), 1049–1051.

Nygaard, I.E., Thompson, F.L., Svengalis, S.L. and Albright, J.P. (1994) Urinary incontinence in elite nulliparous athletes. *Obstetrics and Gynecology*, 84(2), 183–187.

Ree, M.L., Nygaard, I.E. and Bo, K. (2007) 'Muscular fatigue in the pelvic floor muscles after strenuous physical activity. *Acta Obstetricia et Gynecoligica Scandinavica*, 86, 870–876.

Reis, A.O., Camara, C.N.S., Santos, S.G. and Dias, T.S. (2011) Comparative Study of the Capacity of Pelvic Floor Contraction in Volleyball and Basketball Athletes. *Revista Brasiliera de Medicine do Esporte*, 17(2), 97–101.

Rial Rebullido, T.C., Chulvi-Medrano, I., Faigenham, A.D. and Stracciolini, A. (2020) Pelvic floor dysfunction in female athletes. *Strength and Conditioning Journal*, 42, 82–92.

Rial Rebullido, T.C. and Stracciolini, A. (2019) Pelvic floor dysfunction in female athletes: Is relative energy deficiency in sport a risk factor? *American College of Sports Medicine*, 18(7), 255–257.

Rodriguez-Lopez, E.S., Acevedo-Gomez, M.B., Romero-Franco, N., Basas-Garcia, A., Ramirez-Parenteau, C., Calvo-Moreno, S.O. and Fernandez-Dominguez, J.C. (2022) Urinary incontinence among elite track and field athletes according to their event specialization: a cross-sectional study. *Sports Medicine – Open*, 8(78), 1–10.

Rodriguez-Lopez, E.S., Calvo-Moreno, S.O., Basas-Garcia, A., Gutierrez-Ortega, F., Guodemer-Perez, J. and Acevedo-Gomez, M.B. (2020) Prevalence of urinary incontinence among elite athletes of both sexes. *Journal of Science and Medicine in Sport*, 24, 338–344.

Teixeira, R.V., Colla, C., Subruzzi, G., Mallman, A. and Paiva, L.L. (2018) Prevalence of urinary incontinence in female athletes: a systematic review with meta-analysis. *International Urogynecology Journal*, 29, 197–204.

Tomas, F. (2022) 'Special Report: There was urine flying through the air' – the incontinence crisis blighting elite women's sport. *The Telegraph*. Online at: www.telegraph.co.uk/womens-sport/2022/02/23/special-report-urine-flying-air-incontinence-crisis-blighting/ (Accessed 14 November 2022).

Answers

1.   c
2.   b
3.   a
4.   d
5.   a

8

INJURIES AND THE FEMALE ATHLETE

Simon Rea

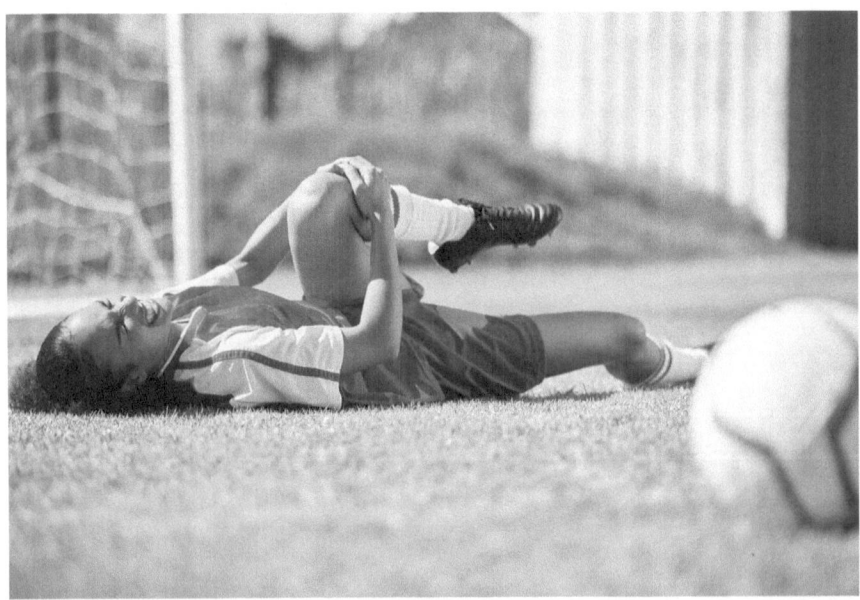

Introduction

Owing to the increased visibility and celebration of sports women in the media it may be becoming difficult to remember that there was a time when women and girls were generally not involved in or encouraged to play sport. However, in the UK the Football Association had banned women from playing football between 1921 and 1969. The FA Women's Super League in the UK became the first fully professional league in the world only as recently as 2018. In the USA

DOI: 10.4324/9781003330110-8

the passing of Title IX in 1972 created equal access for women to participate in sports and educational activities and receive federal funding. Title IX has been credited with dramatically increasing female participation in sport in the USA.

Unfortunately, the surge in females participating in sport and exercise has been accompanied by an upturn in the in the occurrence of musculoskeletal injuries in female athletes. For example, at the UEFA Women's Euro 2022 football tournaments three high profile players, Alexia Putellas of Spain, Simone Magill of Northern Ireland, and Marie-Antoinette Katoto of France all suffered serious knee injuries. In netball 25 per cent of major injuries involve rupture of the ACL (Hewitt, 2023). But it's not just an increased prevalence of knee injuries, ACL ruptures in particular, as female athletes are more at risk of shoulder injuries, knee pain, ankle sprains and stress fractures (Wolf et al., 2015). Worryingly females are also more susceptible to concussions, experience worse symptoms, and take longer to recover (McGroarty, Brown and Mulcahy, 2020).

In this chapter we will explore the myriad of factors that are contributing to an increased susceptibility of female athletes to certain injuries. In particular, we will look to see which sports these injuries are occurring in and what it is about these sports that are increasing the risk. We will examine musculoskeletal, physiological, and biomechanical differences between males and females that may be playing a role and also ask whether the changing hormones levels during the menstrual cycle are also a contributing factor. We will also question whether there are other subtle social reasons why female athletes may be experiencing specific injuries, and we will look at what measures can be taken to reduce the prevalence of injury and make sports safer for female athletes.

Before then read the case study, in Box 8.1, where you are introduced to Elena who has experienced a range of injuries in her sport of skiing.

BOX 8.1 ELENA (SKIER)

Elena is 21 years old and has been skiing since the age of three when her parents taught her how to snowplough. By the age of six she was skiing down full slopes and started competing in downhill races aged 11. She has been part of the British Junior Alpine Team and has competed in the Senior British Alpine Ski Championships. However, here she tells us about the serious injuries she has suffered during her career.

My first major injury was when I was 15, and I was decelerating at the end of a downhill run. I didn't see it but there was a rock that had become exposed by other skiers stopping. When my skis hit the rock I was jolted sideways and as I fell I put my arms out to break my fall. I was still travelling quite fast and when I hit the ground I felt something go in my right shoulder and then just incredible pain. I had actually dislocated the joint between my sternum and clavicle and as the clavicle dislocated it tore my trapezius muscle. I had to have surgery to set the clavicle and sternum back in their correct position and to repair the trapezius and other damaged muscles.

My second serious injury happened when I was travelling at full speed during a competition, and I went through a dip on the course too quickly. As I came out of the dip I lost control and flipped backwards landing on the back of my head. As I was wearing a helmet I thought I was probably okay. Although I was a bit dazed when I realised that I hadn't hurt anything I thought I was fine and ready to compete in the next event. However, over the next few days I developed a terrible headache and often felt dizzy and nauseous. These symptoms carried on for about a month after which I did start training again.

The third injury happened during training, and I was not travelling very fast. I was skiing on a lower slope where the snow was a bit patchy, and my left ski got stuck in a patch of slushy snow. As my right ski was still going fast my left knee got twisted suddenly. I heard a definite pop in my knee followed by a tingling sensation. I knew from the sound that it was serious, and it turned out that I had torn my anterior cruciate ligament (ACL) in my left knee. It's strange because I had just started my period that day and nearly didn't go training. The doctor said that that may have been a contributing factor. It took me about nine months to recover from this injury and I am still wary of my left knee.

The case study illustrates three injuries that are typically suffered by female athletes as there are factors that predispose females to shoulder injuries, concussions, and ACL injuries. As we move through this chapter we will assess what these factors are and explore ways that the risks of these injuries can be reduced. We will start by examining musculoskeletal differences between males and females.

Which injuries commonly affect female athletes?

Female participation in sport has increased steadily over the last 50 years, but in particular the last ten years have seen a rapid rise in participation in sports such as football, rugby, and cricket, that were previously seen as being 'masculine'. The demands placed on sportswomen as a result of the increasing professionalisation of team sports have contributed to a greater risk of specific injuries in women when compared with men. For example, overuse injuries, such as tendinitis, bursitis, and stress fractures, are more common in female athletes while traumatic injuries are more common in male athletes (Frank et al., 2017). Injuries that are most prevalent in female athletes are shoulder instability, ankle sprains and instability, knee pain and anterior cruciate ligament (ACL) ruptures (Gianakos et al., 2022).

Female athletes sustain ankle sprains twice as often as male athletes, and this is partly down to females having looser ligaments around the ankle. As ligaments restrict movement this increased range of movement at the ankle can make it more prone to sprains and long term instability (Wolf et al., 2015). Ankle injuries to females are common in sports that demand multidirectional movement and quick changes of direction, such as football, basketball, netball, volleyball, and track and field events (Swenson et al., 2013).

The reason for increased shoulder injuries is that, similar to the ankle, the joint is slightly looser. In addition men will typically have more musculature at the shoulder and stronger rotator cuff muscles giving it added stability. The looser shoulder joint in females does offer a greater range of movement but also makes it more at risk of subluxations (partial dislocations) and dislocation (Wolf et al., 2015). Female athletes in sports that demand repetitive overhead movements, such as volleyball, baseball and javelin throwing, were most at risk of this type of injury (Frank et al., 2017).

Female athletes are over two times more likely to experience knee pain at the front of the knee between the femur and the patella (Boling et al., 2010). There are several anatomical and biomechanical variations between the males and females at the knee joint that predispose females to knee pain. Female athletes have a greater Q-angle (the angle between the pelvis and patella at the knee), increased knee valgus (where the knee buckles inwards), greater quadriceps dominance and weaker hamstrings in comparison to men (Frank et al., 2017). These differences also make female athletes between two to eight times more at risk to ACL injuries (Sutton and Bullock, 2013). Before we look at ACL injuries in depth we need to examine the musculoskeletal differences between males and females.

Musculoskeletal differences between males and females

While there can be large variations in male and female physiques there are several inherent differences in their respective musculoskeletal systems. There are also differences in the endocrine system and the combination of these factors can account for variations in sports performance and crucially differences in the types of injuries sustained by males and females. In terms of purely appearance there are three factors that influence the shape of the male or female body. They are skeletal differences, muscle size and development, and subcutaneous fat distribution.

The most significant skeletal difference relates to the wider pelvis in females post puberty. This wider pelvis allows for potential childbearing and results in the femur, and the quadriceps muscle at the front of it, sitting at a greater angle in females when compared to men. Specifically, in females it causes an increase in the Q-angle which is the angle between the anterior iliac spine and the patella, as seen in Figure 8.1. Figure 8.2 illustrates that in females the Q-angle is around 16 degrees compared to 11 degrees in men. This difference in angle can affect the way that forces are transmitted through the leg from ankle to hip and hip to ankle causing potential dysfunction in the knees and ankles (Zumwalt, 2019). Females with wider Q-angles can often appear 'knock-kneed', and also become prone to maltracking of the patella contributing to increased knee pain at the patella-femoral joint (Zumwalt, 2019). There is also an increased risk of the knees collapsing inwards when landing from a jump or quickly changing direction of movement.

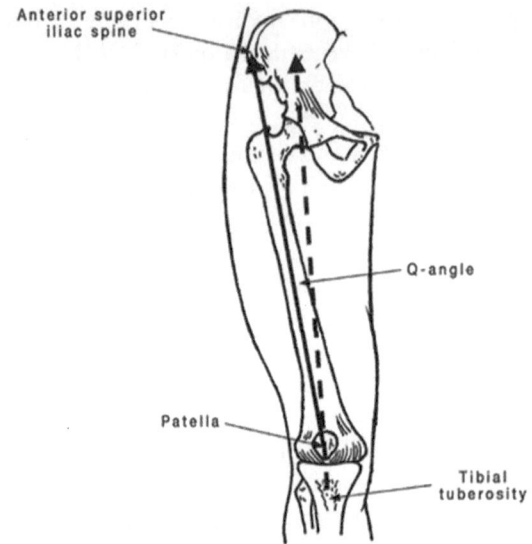

FIGURE 8.1 The Q-angle

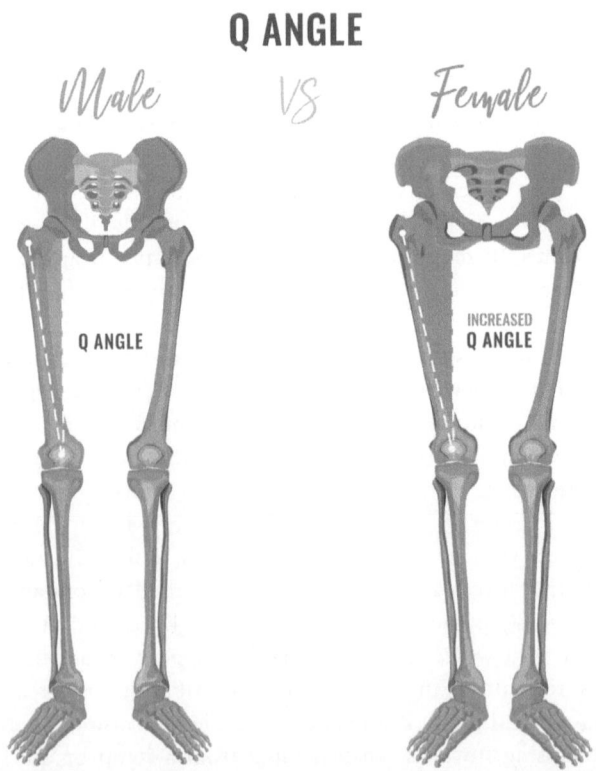

FIGURE 8.2 The differing Q-angle in females and males
Source: Shutterstock

This difference in Q-angle is a factor in ACL injuries (Hewett et al., 2016), as potentially are the differences in shape and size of the intercondylar notch in males and females. As shown in Figure 8.3 the intercondylar notch is a space in the knee at the distal end of the femur where the ACL and PCL (posterior cruciate ligament) cross over. In females the intercondylar notch is generally narrower, and as a result the ACL may be smaller in size and thus weaker in females (Wolf et al., 2015), although this difference has been disputed.

There are also differences in upper limb anatomy between males and females. Males tend to have wider shoulders and females have a slightly wider angle at the elbow at the hinge joint between the humerus and ulna. This wider angle, referred to as the carrying angle, develops at puberty in response to the widening of the hips so that the hands rest beside the hips rather than risking contact with hips while walking.

The significant difference in the upper limb between males and females is the increased musculature around the shoulders in males. This is evident in the pectoralis major, trapezius, deltoids and the rotator cuff muscles and can offer males potentially greater shoulder stability. Females will experience a greater incidence of multidirectional shoulder instability and have greater joint laxity (Wolf et al., 2015). However, there is little difference in the incidence of shoulder dislocation between males and females (Owens et al., 2007). We can see that Elena, in the case study in Box 8.1, suffered this injury as a result of a putting her arms out during a fall.

Reference female, which was developed as a theoretical model for comparing body composition, as identified by Behnke in McArdle, Katch and Katch (2022) has significantly less muscle (20.4 kg) than reference male (31.3 kg). The strength and stabilising effect of muscle at both the shoulder and around the knee can also raise the risk of injury in female athletes at both joints (MacMillan, 2020). Also, owing to the changing mechanics of how the femur and tibia function there is more stress on the muscles around the knee in females (MacMillan, 2020).

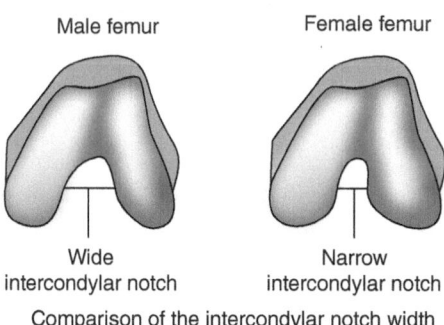

Male femur   Female femur

Wide   Narrow
intercondylar notch intercondylar notch
Comparison of the intercondylar notch width

FIGURE 8.3 The location of intercondylar notch and differences in intercondylar notch width in males and females

Women naturally have more fat than men; Behnke's reference man typically has a body fat percentage of 15 per cent compared with the female fat percentage of 27 per cent (McArdle, Katch and Katch, 2022). The additional body fat is referred to as sex-specific essential fat and serves biological functions such as childbearing and the production of hormones. Sex-specific essential fat is stored at the pelvis, buttocks, thighs, and breasts and contributes to the shape of the female body. There is an energy cost to females in transporting this additional fat and unlike muscle it does not contribute to the development of movement so becomes a reason why female athletes may not produce performances in endurance events equivalent to male athletes. Successful female endurance athletes will typically have fat percentages as low as 12–20 to minimise the energy cost of movement (McArdle, Katch and Katch, 2022). However, because some hormones are produced in body fat when it becomes lowered the reduction in the production of hormones, such as leptin and oestrogen, can become a risk factor in female health.

ACL injuries and why they are so prevalent in female athletes

Figures differ on ACL injury rates between males and females but Hewett et al. (2016) identify that females in sports involving jumping and cutting are two to ten times more at risk of sustaining an ACL injury. Cutting sports are those sports where the athlete plants their foot and then suddenly changes direction, for example when side stepping in basketball. Silvers-Granelli (2021) showed that collegiate females in the USA were three times more likely than their male counterparts to suffer the injury. Elena, the skier in Box 8.1, suffers an ACL injury when her leg becomes stuck, and the forward force of her body causes the knee to twist suddenly and with force.

What is the ACL?

The anterior cruciate ligament (ACL), as shown in Figure 8.4, is a ligament inside the knee that attaches the femur to the tibia. Its role is to provide stabilisation to the knee, and it does this along with the posterior cruciate ligament (PCL). The term 'cruciate' refers to the cross shape they make in the knee.

How is the ACL injured?

According to Khadavi and Fredericson (2019), there are several contact and non-contact causes of ACL injuries.

Contact causes include:

1. When the knee is hit directly, particularly when it the leg is extended or bent slightly inwards.
2. When the knee is bent backwards or twisted during a fall or awkward landing.

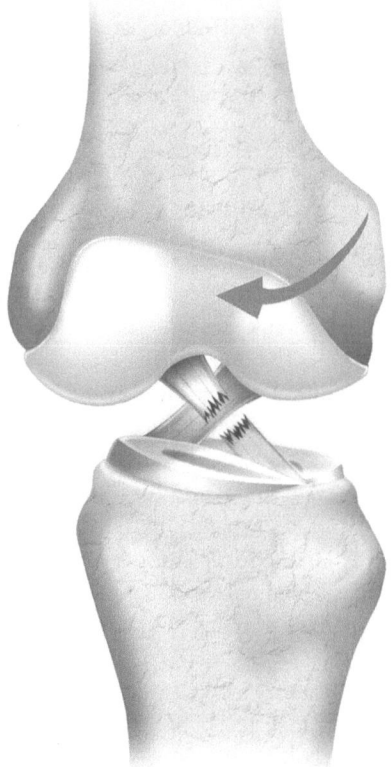

FIGURE 8.4 Anterior cruciate ligament experiencing a tear, as a result of torsion forces
Source: Shutterstock

For example, in netball a significant number of contact ACL injuries occur when the netballer is unbalanced during a jump and lands in an unfamiliar position.

Among non-contact causes of the injury are:

1. Cutting or pivoting movements where the athlete plants their foot and suddenly changes direction or moves sideways.
2. When an athlete lands on one leg, such as when jumping in basketball or volleyball.
3. Suddenly slowing down or stopping while running as it can cause the knee to hyperextend rapidly.

More than 70 per cent of ACL injuries in females are non-contact injuries where there is no direct impact on the knee (Kiapour and Murray, 2014). The sports that seem to incur most risk are basketball, football/soccer, volleyball, downhill skiing, and tennis (Khadavi and Fredericson, 2019). These

sports are all characterised by jumping, cutting, pivoting, sudden deceleration, and landing on one leg. In particular, females are more at risk of ACL
injury when they are in defending or find themselves in unanticipated positions, and they are more likely to injure the knee of their non-dominant leg
(Silvers-Granelli, 2021).

Contributing factors in ACL injuries

As identified previously the differences in Q-angle and the size of the intercondylar notch may play a role in increasing the risk to female athletes, as
is the relatively less muscle bulk around the female's knee. This increased
muscle bulk is due to males having higher levels of the sex hormone, testosterone. There are also differences in how males and females stabilise their
knee joints. Females will predominantly use the quadriceps to stabilise their
knee while males will use co-contractions of both hamstrings and quadriceps. Also, when compared to males, there is a greater imbalance in the
strength of quadriceps and hamstrings in females, as their quadriceps are
significantly stronger. This quadriceps dominance places more pressure on
the ACL to be involved stabilising the knee and contributes to an increased
likelihood of the ACL being stretched and torn (Hewett et al., 2016; Smith
and Smith, 2002).

There are physiological factors as well that may contribute to ACL injuries.
Specifically, changes in hormone levels across the menstrual cycle may lead to
increased ligament and tendon laxity. More musculoskeletal injuries occur in
the first half of the cycle (follicular phase), particularly in Days 1 and 2, and
during the ovulatory phase (around Days 10–14), owing to high levels of oestrogen circulating (Zumwalt, 2019) causing ligament laxity. The risk of injury
drops during the second half of the cycle when progesterone dominates, and
oestrogen levels are lower. The hormone relaxin, which is present in pre and
post-natal females, adds another complication. Relaxin's role is to relax soft
tissue, such as muscle and ligaments, to allow the joints of the pelvis (sacroiliac joint and symphysis pubis) to increase their range of movement during
childbirth. As a result exercising when pregnant, and for a short period
afterwards, can raise the risk of knee injuries, owing to increased ligament
laxity (Wolf et al., 2015).

Musculoskeletal and physiological differences are central to our understanding of certain injuries in females; however, are there may be more subtle
social factors in play as well. Silvers-Granelli (2021) questions whether females
are more vulnerable to ACL injuries, or are they the outcome of gender based
social and environmental decisions? She highlights the disparities in training,
coaching and competitive resources available to female sports.

Fox et al. (2020) suggest the root cause of ACL injuries in female athletes
may be due to 'gendered environmental disparities' where females have different
experiences in sport and less access to training facilities. The result of this is

that not all females start in their chosen sport with adequate skill and the necessary physical development to protect against injury (Parsons, Coen and Bekker, 2021). Other causes of increased ACL injury rates could include women's teams often being allocated artificial surfaces, or poorer grass surfaces to train and compete on than men (Braun, Wasterlain and Dragoo, 2013).

Measures to reduce prevalence of ACL injuries in females

An analysis of studies into training for ACL prevention by Webster and Hewett (2018) showed that ACL prevention training programmes could reduce the number of injuries by 50 per cent and non-contact ACL injuries by 67 per cent. However, there are many factors that must be considered when developing environments to minimise the risk of ACL injury. A strength and conditioning programme needs to be centred around improving neuromuscular control. Neuromuscular control weaknesses include low muscular strength and power, low core muscle strength, poor co-ordination, and faulty muscular activation patterns (Hewett et al., 2016). But the neuromuscular system is responsive to potentially preventative training methods (Voskanian, 2013). In particular it is important to address the quadriceps dominance and ligament dominance when stabilising the knee that is prevalent in female athletes.

Additionally there is a need to train the neuromuscular system in a way that replicates movement patterns found in any chosen sport and for correct 'landing techniques' so that forces can be shared between muscle groups and joints. Figure 8.5 shows examples of effective and ineffective landing techniques.

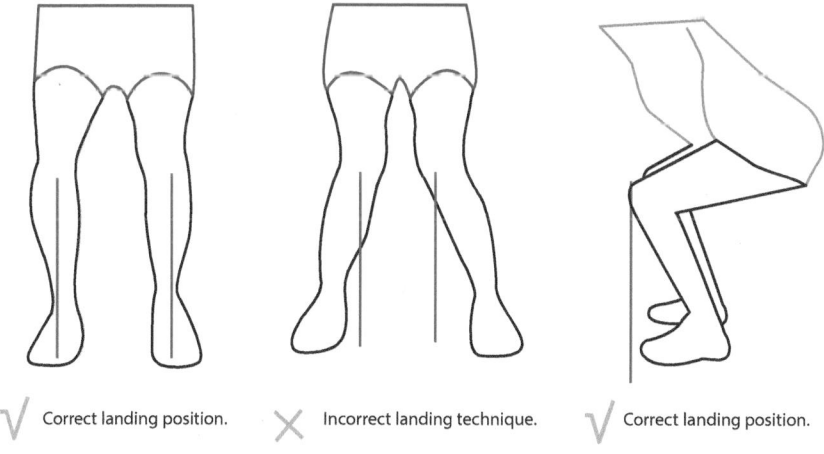

√ Correct landing position. ✕ Incorrect landing technique. √ Correct landing position.

FIGURE 8.5 Effective and ineffective landing techniques

The first image in Figure 8.5 shows the hips, knees, and ankles all in line during landing with the feet at hip width apart. This will ensure all forces are absorbed without additional pressure on the knee joint. This is in contrast to the second image where the knees are buckling inwards causing increased risks of ligaments becoming stretched and ruptured. The third image shows a landing with 90 degrees angle at the knee and around 90 degrees flexion at the hip. This is a much more effective way for the body to absorb forces than if the knees and hips were more fully extended. Many sports such as netball, basketball and tennis involve landing on one leg and if this is the case training must replicate the range of possible landings.

Preventing ACL injuries

As stated before prevention training programmes, such as the PEP programme, which was designed to prevent ACL injuries in footballers, can reduce injury risk by around 50 per cent and enhance athletic performance in females (Hewett et al., 2016). The PEP programme is outlined in Box 8.2.

BOX 8.2 SPOTLIGHT ON: PREVENT INJURY AND ENHANCE PERFORMANCE (PEP) PROGRAMME

The PEP programme was designed by the Santa Monica Orthopaedic and Sports Medicine Research Foundation to specifically reduce ACL injuries in footballers. There are 20 exercises that fall into five categories: avoidance, flexibility, strengthening, plyometrics and agilities.

1 Avoidance
The first step acts as a warm up and involves running with good technique. The aim is to keep the knees flexed, and the hips and knees over the ankles. The three exercises are:

- Jogging
- Shuttle run with sidestepping
- Backwards run

Each exercise is done twice over 40 metres

2 Stretching
After using avoidance exercises as a warm up, static stretches can be performed to improve range of motion, reduce muscle stiffness and any post-exercise soreness. Static stretches to include:

- Calves
- Quadriceps
- Hamstrings
- Adductors (inner thigh)
- Hip flexors

Each stretch is a static stretch held for 30 seconds and repeated twice

3 Strengthening

To increase the strength of lower limb muscles and increased stability at the knee, hip, and ankle.

- Walking lunges
- Russian hamstring
- Single toe leg raise

Each exercise is repeated 30 times.

4 Plyometrics

Explosive exercises to build up power, strength, and speed. There must be a particular focus on correct landing technique by landing as softly as possible on the balls of the feet, rolling onto the heel with a bent knee and straight hip.

- Side to side hops over cones
- Frontward and backward hops over cones
- Single leg hops over cones
- Vertical jumps with headers
- Scissor jumps

Each exercise is repeated 20 times

5 Agilities

Agilities involve proprioceptive training to improve a player's sense of where their joints are positioned in space. The exercises replicate movements that will be encountered in a match situation.

- Shuttle runs with backward and forward running
- Diagonal runs
- Bounding runs

There is more detail about how to perform PEP exercises online by searching for 'A Practical guide to PEP Programme'.

(Adapted from LA84 Foundation, PEP Practical Guide, 2021)

In summary, the anatomical, physiological, and biomechanical differences between males and females predispose female athletes to an increased risk of knee joint and particularly ACL injuries. This is particularly apparent in team sports involving multidirectional movements where jumping is also a feature. To mitigate against ACL injuries, it is advisable to include specific strength and conditioning training to prepare the neuromuscular system for the demands of the sporting activity. This should include developing relevant motor skills patterns, core strengthening, and exercises to develop lower body strength. Also, female athletes need to learn how to land safely and transfer this learning into their sporting activity.

Stress fractures in female athletes

Stress fractures are a common injury in female athletes and account for around 13 per cent of all injuries seen in sports medicine clinics (Abbott et al., 2020). They are most common in the tibia and metatarsals but are also seen in the femur. Stress fractures are most common in sports involving running and jumping, extreme endurance events, such as long distance running and triathlons, as well as aesthetic sports where athletes are required to maintain a lean physique (Beck and Drysdale, 2021). Running and jumping sports are characterised by repeated loading of the lower limb and these forces can produce stress fractures. However, extreme endurance sports and aesthetic sports are associated with a prolonged negative energy balance and an increased risk of developing RED-S (as covered in Chapter 5).

Stress fractures become more common when periods are disrupted, owing to insufficient energy availability. The disruption of the period affects the production of the hormone oestrogen that is vital to the development and replacement of bone. The story of Bobby Clay, who won European 1500m gold in, 2015 illustrates this well. She was underfuelling and overtraining and by the age of 19 had never had a period. She suffered a stress fracture to her foot while swimming and her tibia snapped when she sat down in the gym. She was diagnosed with osteoporosis in her hips and spine.

Concussion and the female athlete

A concussion is a brain injury caused by a direct blow to the head, either from another player, a ball or other sporting object, or from contact with the playing surface. Concussions also occur when the head is shaken violently. Concussions are synonymous with rugby as it involves heavy collisions, shoulder barges and illegal high tackles. However, athletes in football/soccer, hockey and basketball are also at risk.

Unfortunately research shows that female athletes are almost twice as likely to experience a sport-related concussion than male athletes (Bretzin et al., 2021), sustain more serious concussions, have worse symptoms, and take longer to recover (McGroarty, Brown and Mulcahy, 2020). The mechanisms of injury are also different for male and female athletes. There is also a wide gender gap in the research as historically female players have been excluded from rugby-based concussions analysis (Tomas, 2020). This is illustrated by the 2020 concussion consensus statement produced by World Rugby that failed to include any analysis from elite women's rugby despite female players accounting for 28 per cent of players globally.

BOX 8.3 WHAT IS A CONCUSSION, ITS SYMPTOMS, AND LONG TERM IMPLICATIONS

A concussion is a brain injury that is not visible because there is not necessarily any blood or a fracture. The damage is more subtle and occurs because the brain, and the thin layer of fluid that surrounds it, have very limited space to move within the intercranial cavity. After a head impact the head will decelerate rapidly and the brain will be forced against the inside of the cranium. This force produced is transmitted deep into the brain and cause structural damage to nerve cells called axons.

It is a misconception that you need to be knocked out to sustain as only around 10 per cent of concussions involve loss of consciousness. The immediate symptoms are feeling dazed and confused to the extent that you may not know where you are or what day it is. There may also a lack of co-ordinated movement. As the concussion develops symptoms include headaches, fatigue, dizziness, nausea and problems with concentration and memory. In the long term repeated blows to the head can lead to disorders, such as dementia, characterised by memory loss and confusion.

Box 8.2 presents the typical symptoms of a concussion injury, and these are common across males and females. Elena, the skier in Box 8.1 suffered some of these symptoms when she sustained a concussion after a fall. However, there are complex reasons that females are more at risk of sustaining concussions and suffer more serious symptoms.

First, females generally have smaller heads and necks than males. The female neck is on average 30 per cent smaller than the male neck (Tomas, 2020), and, owing to less musculature around the neck, it can be up to 47 per cent weaker than males' necks (Sanderson, 2021). This smaller skull with less support will be accelerated more quickly when hit; there will be an increased 'whiplash' effect potentially causing more damage to the brain. However, the strength of neck muscles can be developed through an appropriate strength and conditioning programme and while this is common in the elite game it is less so in the community game (Tomas, 2020).

Second, there are differences in the mechanism of injury or how concussions are sustained. Research on female rugby players shows that more than 50 per cent of concussions were caused by contact between the head and the ground, compared to only 4 per cent of male rugby players (Sanderson, 2021). This may be due to different techniques male and female players use when falling to the ground. The main cause of concussions in male rugby and football players was contact with another player. In football, 42 per cent of concussion injuries in females were caused by contact with the ball or equipment (Bretzin et al., 2021).

Thirdly, the different outcomes of concussions in females may be due to structural differences in their brains. Every nerve cell in the brain has a major fibre, called the axon, that transmits messages between cells in the brain. In each axon there are tiny protein tunnels called microtubules and in females these microtubules are smaller in size and number. These smaller structures predispose the brain of a female to a greater risk of injury when the brain moves and stretches (Dollé et al., 2018).

Fourthly, the phases of the menstrual cycle play a role. Research by Wunderle et al. (2014) showed that women who experienced concussion during the luteal phase (second half of their menstrual cycle) suffered worse outcomes than those women experiencing head injury during the follicular phase (the first half of their cycle). Progesterone levels are high during the luteal phase and the disruption to the HPG causes progesterone levels to fall rapidly (Snook et al., 2017).

Additionally, concussion injuries can cause disruption to the menstrual cycle, including irregular bleeding patterns and amenorrhea (McGroarty, Brown and Mulcahy, 2020). This is because the menstrual cycle is controlled by the Hypothalamus-Pituitary- Gonadal axis (HPG axis) that originates in the brain, and its function is affected by head injuries. Any changes in the hormones produced during the menstrual cycle can also have implications for fertility and bone development in young females.

Research into the menstrual cycle and concussion is still emerging but tracking when concussions occur in the cycle might provide helpful information in the complex evaluation of brain injuries.

BOX 8.4 THE ACCUMULATIVE DANGERS OF SUBCONCUSSIONS

While there are protocols in place to protect athletes who have experienced concussions, there is still a risk to brain cells every time there is impact between the head and an object. When a concussion is suffered there will be acute symptoms like headaches, slowed reaction times and brain fog; however, lower force impacts can damage brain cell function but without producing any acute symptoms. These are referred to as subconcussions and as they are asymptomatic they will not be recorded, and they are up to 500 times more frequent than concussive events. While damage to brain cells from single events is significant the risk and severity of brain damage is increased by the accumulation of these smaller sub concussive events that go unrecorded.

BOX 8.5 REAL-WORLD APPLICATION

As a female athlete, you should:

1. Become aware of the types of injury that female athletes in your chosen sport are most prone to and how these injuries are caused.
2. If you participate in a sport involving jumping, pivoting, and cutting movements regularly practice a preventative programme, such as PEP, to minimise your risk of injury.
3. Ensure that your nutritional and rest strategies are appropriate to prevent low energy availability and protect against stress fractures in your lower limbs.
4. Learn how you might experience a concussion injury in your chosen sport and how you might feel if concussed.
5. Track menstrual cycles so that you can be prepared to take measures to mitigate against the risk of ACL injuries or concussions at specific times during your cycle.

As a coach, you should:

1. Spend time educating your female athletes about the causes of injuries that females are more likely experience in the sports activity you coach.
2. Ensure that all athletes have undergone appropriate strength and conditioning training to prepare for the demands of a sport and reduce their risk of injury. If you are unable to deliver this type of training then you could bring a strength and conditioning coach into their team.
3. Be aware of the different mechanisms through which female athletes can suffer concussions and know the signs and symptoms of a concussion so you can help to identify them. Direct athletes to medical help if you have any concerns around an athlete who has experienced a blow to the head.

Develop an environment where you can discuss the menstrual cycles of your athletes and be able to adapt training to reduce risks of ACL injuries and concussions at specific stages in their cycle.

Summary

Having completed this chapter, you will be much more aware of the types of injuries that female athletes are more susceptible to, and in which sports there may be risks of injury to the active female. Understanding the anatomical, physiological, and biomechanical differences between males and females will help you appreciate why female athletes have an added risk in sports involving jumping, pivoting and sideways movements. To be able to protect against injuries to the knees, ankles, and shoulders in particular it is vital to have access to strength and conditioning programmes. Understanding that female athletes may experience more concussions and more serious symptoms is essential in ensuring the short and long term health safety of female athletes.

The key messages to take away from this chapter are:

1. The musculoskeletal, physiological, biomechanical and endocrinological differences between male and female athletes have an impact on the different ways that they can become injured.
2. Being aware of the types of injury and different mechanisms of injury experienced by female athletes can inform the development of female-centric training programmes.
3. The risk and severity of all injuries and in ACL injuries in particular can be protected against by a specific strength and conditioning programme that focuses on neuromuscular control, core strength, body co-ordination and muscle activation patterns.
4. Adapting training methods and schedules can help to mitigate against any increased risk of injuries at specific points of the menstrual cycle.
5. Developing an awareness of the short term and long term signs and symptoms of concussion is vital to protect the health of female athletes.

End-of-Chapter Quiz

Answers can be found after the References

1. Identify which types of injury female athletes are more susceptible to:

    a   Knee and ankle injuries
    b   Traumatic contact injuries
    c   Muscle and tendon tears
    d   Bone fractures

2. The Q-angle is located between:

    a   Symphysis pubis and sacroiliac joint
    b   Patella, tibia, and fibula
    c   Anterior iliac spine and patella
    d   Quadriceps and hamstrings

3. Identify which of the following may be a contributory factor to higher ACL rates in females:

    a   Females have a wider intercondylar notch
    b   Females are more quadriceps dominant
    c   Females have tighter ligaments and tendons
    d   Females use hamstrings as knee stabilisers

4.   Females sustain more concussions because they have:

   a   Slower reaction times
   b   More collisions per game
   c   Thinner bones in the skull
   d   Weaker neck muscles

5.   Identify which of the following statements about concussion is true.

   a   Males are more likely to suffer a concussion from a fall than females
   b   Females are more likely to lose consciousness after a serious head impact
   c   Structural differences in the brain cause females more serious concussions
   d   Males will experience concussion symptoms for longer after a head impact

References

Abbott, A., Bird, M.L., Wild, E., Brown, S.M., Stewart, G. and Mulcahey, M.K. (2020) Part I: epidemiology and risk factors for stress fractures in female athletes. *The Physician and Sports medicine*, 48(1), 17–24. doi:10.1080/00913847.2019.1632158A.

Beck, B., and Drysdale, L. (2021) Risk Factors, Diagnosis and Management of Bone Stress Injuries in Adolescent Athletes: A Narrative Review. *Sports*, 9(4), 52. doi:10.3390/sports9040052.

Boling, M., Padua, D., Marshall, S., Guskiewicz, K., Pyne, S. and Beutler, A.(2010) Gender differences in the incidence and prevalence of patellofemoral pain syndrome. *Scandinavian Journal of Medical Science and Sports*, 20, 725–730.

Braun, H.J., Wasterlain, A.S. and Dragoo, J.L. (2013) The use of PRP in ligament and meniscal healing. *Sports Medicine Arthroscopy Review*, 21(4), 206–212.

Bretzin, A.C., Covassin, T., Wiebe, D.J. and Stewart, W. (2021) Association of sex with adolescent soccer concussion incidence and characteristic. *JAMA Network Open*, 4 (4). Available at: https://jamanetwork.com/journals/jamanetworkopen/fullarticle/2779117 (Accessed September 2022).

Dollé, J.P., Jaye, A., Anderson, S.A., Ahmadzadeh, H., Shenoy, V.B. and Smith, D.H. (2018) Newfound sex differences in axonal structure underlie differential outcomes from in vitro traumatic axonal injury. *Experimental Neurology*, 300, 121–134. doi:10.1016/j.expneurol.2017.11.001.

Fox, A., Bonacci, J., Hoffman, S., Nimphius, S. and Saunders, N. (2020) Anterior cruciate ligament injuries in Australian football: should women and girls be playing? You're asking the wrong question. *BMJ Open Sport and Exercise Medicine*, 9(6). Available at: https://bmjopensem.bmj.com/content/6/1/e000778 (Accessed 21 September 2022).

Frank, R.M., Romeo, A.A., Bush-Joseph, C.A., Charles, A. and Bach, B.R. (2017) Injuries to the Female Athlete in 2017. *The Journal of Bone and Joint Surgery*, 5(10). doi:10.2106/JBJS.RVW.17.00017.

Gianakos, A.L., Abdelmoneim, A., Kerkhoffs, M.D. and Mulcahey, M.K. (2022) Rehabilitation and Return to Sport of Female Athletes. *Arthroscopy, Sports Medicine and Rehabilitation*, 4(1), 247–253.

Hewett, T.E, Myer, G.D., Ford, K.R., Paterno, M.V. and Quatman, C.E. (2016) Mechanisms, prediction, and prevention of ACL injuries: Cut risk with sharpened and validated tools. *Journal of Orthopaedic Research*, 34(11), 1843–1855.

Hewitt, B. (2023) Knee Injuries in Netball. Online at: *Knee Injuries in Netball – Dr Benjamin Hewitt* (Accessed 6 April 2023).

Khadavi, M. and Fredericson, M. (2019) ACL Tear: Causes and Risk Factors. *Sports Health*. Online at: www.sports-health.com/sports-injuries/knee-injuries/acl-tear-ca uses-and-risk-factors (Accessed 21 September 2022).

Kiapour, A.M. and Murray, M.M. (2014) Basic science of anterior cruciate ligament injury and repair. *Bone and Joint Research*, 3(2), 20–31.

LA84 Foundation (2021) PEP Practical Guide. Online at: *A Practical Guide to the PEP Program – LA84 Foundation* (Accessed 21 September 2022).

McArdle, W., Katch, F.I. and Katch, V.L. (2022) *Exercise Physiology: Nutrition, Energy and Human Performance* (9th ed.). Philadelphia: Wolters Kluwer.

McGroarty, N.K., Brown, S.M. and Mulcahey, M.K. (2020) Sport-related concussion in female athletes: a systematic review. *Orthopaedic Journal of Sports Medicine*, 16(8). Available at: https://journals.sagepub.com/doi/10.1177/2325967120932306?icid=int. sj-full-text.citing-articles.3 (Accessed 12 September 2022).

MacMillan, C. (2020) Are ACL tears really more common in women? *Yale medicine*. Online at: Are ACL Tears Really More Common in Women? > News > Yale Medicine (Accessed 15 September 2022).

Owens, B.D., Duffey, M.L., DeBerardino, T.M, Taylor, D.C. and Mountcastle, D.C. (2007) The incidence and characteristics of shoulder instability at the United States Military Academy. *American Journal of Sports Medicine*, 35(7), 1168–1173.

Parsons, J.L., Coen, S.E. and Bekker, S. (2021) Anterior cruciate ligament injury: towards a gendered environmental approach. *British Journal of Sports Medicine*, 55, 984–990.

Sanderson, K. (2021) Why concussions are worse for women. *Nature*. Available at: www.nature.com/articles/d41586-021-02089-2 (Accessed 26 September 2022).

Silvers-Granelli, H. (2021) Why female athletes injure their ACLs more frequently? What we can do to mitigate their risk. *International Journal of Sports Physical Therapy*, 16(4), 971–977.

Smith, F.W. and Smith, P.A. (2002) Musculoskeletal differences between males and females. *Sports Medicine and Arthroscopy Review*, 10, 98–100.

Snook, M.L., Henry, L.C., Sanfilippo, J.S., Zeleznik, A.J. and Kontos, A.P. (2017) Association of Concussion with Abnormal Menstrual Patterns in Adolescent and Young Women. *JAMA Pediatrics*, 171(9), 879–886. doi:10.1001/jamapediatrics.2017.1140.

Sutton, K.M. and Bullock, J.M. (2013) 'Anterior cruciate ligament rupture: Differences between males and females'. *Journal American Academy of Orthopaedic Surgery*, 21, 41–50.

Swenson, D.M, Collins, C.L., Fields, S.K. and Comstock, R.D. (2013) Epidemiology of U.S. high school sports-related ligamentous ankle injuries. *Clinical Journal of Sports Medicine*, 23, 190–196.

Tomas, F. (2020) Special Report: the hidden concussion crisis in women's rugby. *The Telegraph*. Online at Special report: The hidden concussion crisis in women's rugby (telegraph.co.uk) (Accessed 26 September 2022).

Voskanian, N. (2013) ACL injury prevention in female athletes: review of literature and practical considerations in implementing an ACL prevention program. *Current Reviews in Musculoskeletal Medicine*, 6(2), 158–163.

Webster, K.E. and Hewett, T.E. (2018) Meta-analysis of Meta-analyses of Anterior Cruciate Ligament Injury Reduction Programs. *Journal of Orthopaedic Research*, 36, 2696–2708.

Wolf, J.M., Cannada, I., Van Heest, A.E., O'Connor, M.I. and Ladd, A.I. (2015) Male and female differences in musculoskeletal disease. *Journal of the American Academy of Orthopaedic Surgeons*, 23(6), 339–347.

Wunderle, K., Hoeger, K.M., Wasserman, E. and Bazarian, J.J. (2014) Menstrual phase as a predictor of outcome after mild brain injury in women. *Journal of Head Trauma Rehabilitation*, 29(5), 1–8.

Zumwalt, M. (2019) Musculoskeletal injury and the exercising female. In J. Forsyth and C.M. Roberts (Eds), *The Exercising Female: Science and its Application*. Oxford: Routledge.

Answers

1. a
2. c
3. b
4. d
5. c

9

THE ADOLESCENT FEMALE

Supporting the Transition from Girl to Woman

Jess Pinchbeck

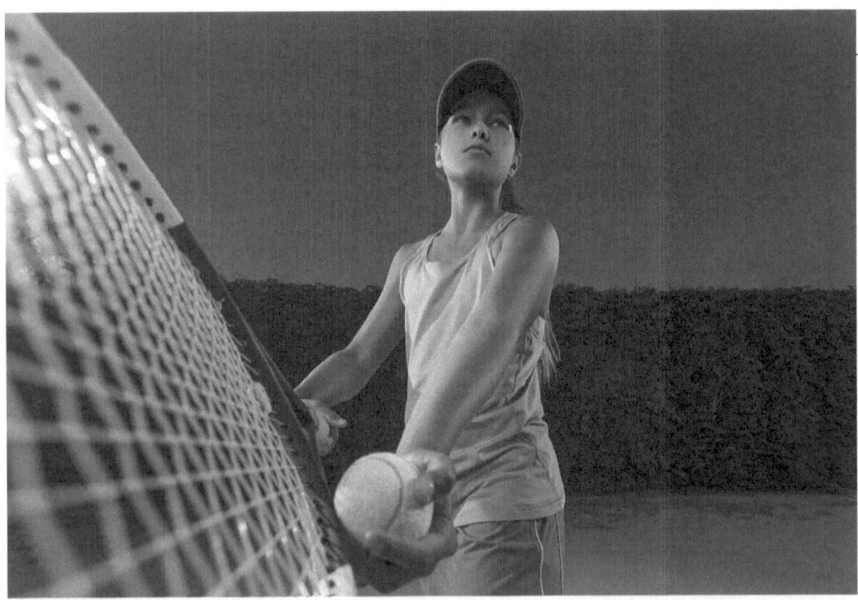

Introduction

Adolescence describes the transition period between childhood and adulthood. It is a time where an individual experiences intense bouts of physiological and psychological growth and development, which for females includes the onset of the menstrual cycle. The body changes considerably as does the importance and value placed on social relationships, including a powerful quest to establish an identity (Lundvall and Walseth, 2014). During this time there are many

DOI: 10.4324/9781003330110-9

pressures placed on females that can result in a reduction of activity and even withdrawal. Such pressures that arise can be linked to body image, perceived competence and intricacies surrounding gender stereotypes and ideologies. This chapter revisits concepts raised in previous chapters such as menstruation, prevalence of injury and breast health but specifically applies them to the adolescent athlete. The ways that adolescent females can be supported while navigating the challenges of this life stage is also examined.

The case study, in Box 9.1, introduces you to 15-year-old Akachi, a talented young netballer, who is experiencing some doubts about whether to continue playing.

BOX 9.1 AKACHI (NETBALLER)

Akachi is a 15-year-old netballer who has recently been successful in U17 trials at a super league club. This means she is part of their performance hub which involves training twice a week, playing friendlies against other hubs and playing fixtures in the Netball Performance League between September and April. In addition to her netball training at the club Akachi also has to follow a strength and conditioning programme and, now over eight weeks into the programme, she can see the benefits this additional training is having on her game. However, as a result of the training Akachi's body is becoming more athletic and muscular, and she has encountered some cruel comments from some of the girls at school about looking 'manly', which is making her feel very self-conscious about the changes to her body. On the other side, the club provided the girls with some excellent education around sports bras and for the first time Akachi now has a sports bra that reduces the breast bounce when playing and is far more comfortable than any she has worn before.

Akachi has made some good friends at the netball academy and has fun and is comfortable there but in contrast she feels that she is drifting away from her school friends. Akachi has training on Friday evenings and often misses out on social events that her schoolfriends go to. She has had to refuse invites so many times that now they stop asking. Her boyfriend is also getting fed up with her netball schedule, which makes it harder for them to spend time together outside of school, to the point where Akachi has pretended to be injured a couple of times to get out of training to see him. She has also had to miss a couple of school netball fixtures due to performance hub commitments and the school team have made comments that she thinks she is too good to play for them, which is not the case at all.

Akachi also has to make sure her diet includes enough calories and sufficient nutrients to accommodate her training, especially her iron intake as she suffers from low iron levels, more so during her period. Initially she was prescribed iron supplements for six months, however, now Akachi manages her iron levels largely by her diet.

Akachi loves playing performance netball and is proud of her achievements and would love to play for England one day but, she also wonders how much

> easier her life would be if she didn't play performance netball. It is so hard to fit in her studies, her friends, and her netball, and she doesn't have time to play any other sports which she used to enjoy.

What the case study illustrates is some of the issues that adolescent females face when participating in sport and physical activity. As we move through this chapter, we will refer to Akachi's case study to highlight some of the practical steps that can be taken to support her, and teenage girls in general, to continue playing. But first we will consider adolescence and the potential issues that can impact the participation and performance of adolescent females.

What is adolescence?

The World Health Organisation (2022) classes an adolescent as anyone between the ages of ten to nineteen, describing it as 'the phase of life between childhood and adulthood'. Though, such a transition from girl to woman, is a unique experience and may start later or earlier for some individuals (Lundvall and Walseth, 2014). Yet, age is only one element of this classification of human development and Eime et al. (2013) express adolescence to be a time in one's life where biological, environmental, social, and psychological (e.g. self-worth, body image) transformations take place. These changes in the brain and body can influence how an individual feels, thinks and acts and within physical activity and sport it is a crucial stage of participation and performance. It is also during adolescence that puberty takes place.

Puberty

Puberty is 'the process of maturation that occurs during adolescence and includes acquisition of secondary sexual characteristics, rapid bone maturation, and acceleration of growth' (Bradley et al., 2020, p. 1). It is a time where developmental changes contribute to noteworthy shifts in stature, body composition, and the Neuroendocrine Axis (the structure for interactions between the brain, hormones and glands) (Gerber, Pienaar and Kruger, 2021). It is during puberty that the body reaches its full potential in terms of fitness, physical strength and reproductive capacity (Viner, 2012). The impact of these changes can affect the participation and performance of girls in sport.

Physical changes are of particular significance including, breast development. As Figure 9.1 illustrates, breast development has been shown to influence adolescent participation in sport and fitness. The study by Scurr et al. (2016) revealed that for 46 per cent of girls aged 11–17 years their breasts had some effect on their participation in sports and exercise. This was more prevalent in girls aged 13–14 years (51 per cent) and in larger-breasted girls (63 per cent). The study concluded that overall breast concerns during sports were high with

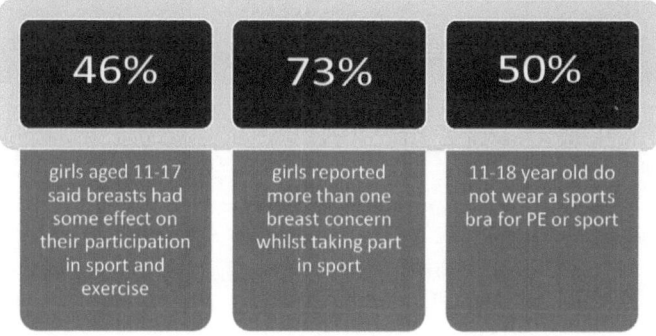

FIGURE 9.1 Breast development and participation
Source: Adapted from Scurr et al. (2016)

73 per cent of girls reporting more than one concern. Yet research also shows that 50 per cent of 11–18-year-olds do not wear a sports bra for PE or sport (Scurr et al., 2016). This suggests that girls and parents need to be educated about the importance of breast health and breast support during sport and exercise. The practicalities of such issues also need to be considered with some girls not wanting to change their bras in front of others, as described by England netballer Eleanor Cardwell in Box 9.2.

BOX 9.2 ATHLETE STORIES

I remember all too well the experiences I went through as a younger girl with bigger breasts, who'd be too shy to get changed at school. So I'd either go into PE (wearing a regular bra) and be in pain, or sit in a sports bra all day and be really uncomfortable in it, as it was the wrong size.

Eleanor Cardwell, England netballer (cited in Sinclair, 2022)

Stages of adolescence

It is important that both the family and those working with young female athletes understand the changes experienced by adolescent females and their potential impact on performance and participation. Figure 9.2 identifies the three stages of adolescent development and the breadth of changes a young athlete may be experiencing.

Identity formation during adolescence

Transitions at key life stages and the reorientation of identity during these transitions pose key barriers to participation, particularly when applied to

Early Adolescence 10-15 years	Middle Adolescence 14-17 years	Late Adolescence 16-19 years
Are developing physically	Physical changes almost complete	Completed physical development and achieved adult height
Breast development	Regular periods	
Menstruation begins	Interest in romantic and sexual relationships	Stronger sense of individuality
Curiosity and anxiety around physical changes		Identify their own values
May question their gender identity	May spend less time with family and more time with friends	Increased stability of friendships and romantic relationships
Increased need for privacy	Increased concern with appearance	More emotionally and physically independent from family
Increased independence from family	Susceptible to peer pressure	
May push boundaries	Brain developing and maturing but decisions still influenced by strong emotions	

FIGURE 9.2 Stages and characteristics of female adolescence
Source: Adapted from Allen and Waterman (2019)

teenage girls and young women (Allender, Cowburn and Foster, 2006). The physical and psychological changes that take place during puberty are also accompanied by socialisation and identity formation (Lundvall and Walseth, 2014). Adolescence is viewed as a critical time in an individual's identity formation (Erikson, 1968) and the pursuit for an identity is at its most powerful (Lundvall and Walseth, 2014). It often involves a period of conflict in which individuals wrestle with doubts and insecurities. Overcoming such conflict enables young people to become more aware of their strengths and weaknesses, increase in confidence and arrive at a more consistent and logical sense of identity that they are comfortable with (Buckingham, 2008). It should be noted that throughout this period of conflict, adolescents typically reduce the time spent within the family and gain more independence, developing independent social competence, often through involvement with their peers who can also exert influence on this identity formation (Buckingham, 2008). This is a period of exploration and conflict where adolescents socialise with people from a variety of backgrounds and engage in a range of activities. It is an essential stage that provides individuals with experiences and information to enable informed choices to be successful in adult life (Brewer and Petitpas, 2017) making sports participation a valuable pursuit.

Adolescents can also develop an athletic identity and this is 'the degree to which an individual identifies with the athlete role' (Brewer, Van Raalte and Linder, 1993, p. 237). This is shaped by how strongly the individual identifies with the athlete role, how they respond to setbacks or failures as an athlete, and whether they have any other roles. As athletes begin to perform at higher levels their athletic identity can become their only identity, which can cause issues if their athletic identity is threatened. Akachi is experiencing significant identity conflict in her roles as a schoolfriend, as a girlfriend and as a netballer. Her athletic identity is currently being formed and shaped as part of her wider environment as she begins to focus more on her netball and starts to play at a higher standard. It is this transition to investing more time into her sport that is causing the conflict.

Sport participation: sampling, specialising and investing

Sports participation is a multifaceted and complex concept as people engage in sport in a variety of different ways involving different motives and aspirations. Models of sports participation and development are used to provide a framework that enables a better understanding of the complex way in which people engage in sport. There are several models of sports participation, each used in different ways and with different levels of empirical evidence to support them. One influential model of participant development is the Developmental Model of Sport Participation (DMSP) (Côté, 1999).

The DMSP, although based around psychological theories and on parental support, provides a useful narrative of the different pathways of sports participation for young athletes. This model was developed drawing upon a range of research with elite performers, recreational participants and individuals who have dropped out of sport. In summary, the model proposes three stages of participation: sampling, specialising and investment. The sampling years typically occur between the ages 6–13 years where children sample a variety of sport activities for fun and enjoyment. The specialising years occur between the ages of 13 and 15, and during this stage the athlete typically makes a commitment to one or two sports. The investment years, typically occur beyond the age of 15, and is where an athlete has the goal of becoming an elite sportsperson and commits to one sport, such as Akachi is doing. Yet not everyone is aiming to become an elite performer and it is important that girls' participation in sport is not lost between these phases, and they remain in recreational participation where elite performance is not the goal.

Sport performance has also been shown to be impacted by a girl's stage of physical development. For example, Gerber, Pienaar and Kruger (2021) found that the onset of the menstrual cycle significantly influenced the rate of anthropometric growth of girls as those reaching maturity earlier were taller and heavier at a younger age with longer body portions (e.g. arm spans), which contributed to improved sports performance. However, these physiological differences typically even out towards the end of puberty, by age 16, suggesting that the potential for talent can only be evaluated realistically at this time in a girl's development. This suggests that talent identification and pathways should select from 16 years onwards rather than the younger selection ages that currently occur in many sports.

There is also the issue of early specialisation, particularly in sports such as gymnastics and swimming. Although there are a range of different definitions, the general consensus is that early specialisation involves 'engagement in a single sport to the exclusion of all others' (Baker, Mosher and Fraser-Thomas, 2021, p. 179) and that this often occurs at an age much younger than the adolescent specialising years suggested by the DMSP. The risks associated with early specialisation are discussed further in Box 9.3.

BOX 9.3 SPOTLIGHT ON: EARLY SPORT SPECIALISATION

Early specialisation was defined by Mosher, Fraser-Thomas and Baker (2020) to include year-round, intense training in a single sport to the exclusion of other sports. Early specialisation is typically classified as focusing on one sport prior to 12 years of age, although there is some debate by Jayanthi et al. (2019) that a specific age range cannot be stated. Research evidence collated over the years has highlighted both psychological and physiological concerns with specialising in one sport prior to adolescence but despite this, certain sports, such as gymnastics, retain a culture of early specialisation.

Gymnastics is a sport that is associated with early specialisation due to peak performance typically occurring during adolescence or early adulthood (Feeley, Agel and LaPrade, 2015). Yet, there is compelling evidence linking the prevalence of injury in female gymnasts to those who specialise at an early age. For example, Sweeney, Horan and MacNamara (2021) reported that young gymnasts who specialised earlier than age 14 were twice as likely to sustain a gymnastics-related injury that required surgery. Research by Nusman et al. (2011, p. 929) proposed that it was the excessive training regimes combined with a fast-growing skeleton, that provided a significant risk factor for overuse injuries, such as stress fractures in young adolescents. In addition to the physiological risks Kruse and Lemmen (2009) also raised concerns regarding psychosocial stress in the occurrence of injury, as for most gymnasts' high-level competition takes place in the adolescent years, with young gymnasts experiencing the stress of training and competition.

Due to the young age at which gymnasts enter elite performance training, and the aesthetic and strength-based demands of competitive gymnastics, Tan et al. (2014) suggest that elite gymnasts may be at particular risk of developing eating disorders. This was supported in findings by Sweeney, Horan and MacNamara (2021) whereby 34 per cent of former female college gymnasts, where the mean age of specialisation was 8 years, reported disordered eating.

Early specialisation has also been linked to burnout and overtraining causing girls to withdraw from sports completely, however there are many other factors that contribute to non-participation and withdrawal in girls.

Participation drop-off

It is widely reported that regular participation in organised sports can help adolescents to achieve their physical activity recommendation as well as to develop their physical literacy and socialise with others yet research has consistently found that the greatest dropout from organised sport occurs during adolescence (Lundvall and Walseth, 2014). In particular, female adolescents are more likely than their male counterparts to withdraw from sport and reduce their physical activity (Hopkins and Hopkins, 2022). A key question arising from research is whether the inactivity of adolescence can be attributed to biological changes as well as behavioural or environmental changes (Metcalf et al., 2015). Figure 9.3 shows key findings from The Women's Sport Foundation, Keeping Girls in the Game Report by Zarrett, Veliz and Sabo (2020) on factors linked to the dropout or non-participation of female adolescents.

In the case study of Akachi, we can see that she is experiencing some of the issues associated with being an adolescent female, and this is leading her to question whether to continue participating in her sport. Many of these factors that contribute to withdrawal of adolescent female athletes can be prevented through appropriate support and education, particularly working with coaches, parents and educators. The next sections look at some of these factors in more detail.

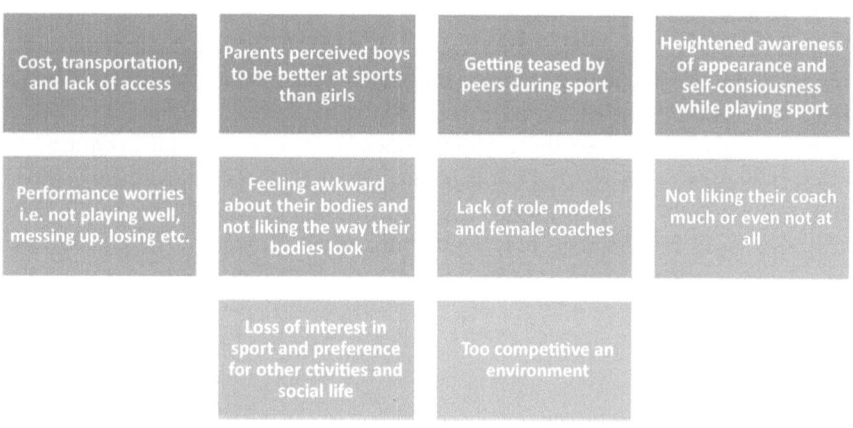

FIGURE 9.3 Factors contributing to non-participation and dropout of adolescent females
Source: Adapted from Zarrett et al. (2020)

Body perception in adolescent female athletes

The social environment is one of great importance for adolescent girls, and girls often feel pressure to 'fit in' and conform to social norms (Spencer, Rehman and Kirk, 2015). In a systematic review of dropout from organised sport Crane and Temple (2015) found evidence that gender stereotypes and the pressure to appear feminine contributed to the dropout of adolescent girls. The societal implications of femininity and bodily ideals and the performing body is a factor in female sports participation, influencing not only the type of activity engaged in but whether girls and women have the confidence to engage at all. During adolescence, gender identity is constructed within the context of social and cultural values including what is defined as the embodiment of masculine and feminine (Lundvall and Walseth, 2014). Undoubtedly, stereotypes are continuously being challenged regarding social conformity of femininity and masculinity in relation to the sporting body, yet, contradictions in society still exist. For instance, Lunde and Gattario (2017) found that young Swedish women who played sport had a complex view of themselves, with their bodies viewed for performance as being strong, fast and agile but also that they wanted their bodies to fit the societal cultural standards. There was a contradiction between lifting weights to become stronger for their sport without becoming muscularly bulky, similar to those experienced by Akachi. This is termed the 'female athlete paradox', where women feel conflicted about being an athlete, which is synonymous with strong, masculine traits and which contradict those associated with being a woman and femininity (Krane et al., 2004).

A sport such as netball, which is considered to be a feminine appropriate sport, as the requirements of the sport align more with the societal notion of femininity (Devonport et al., 2019) has remained relatively unchanged over the years, with women and girls still expected to wear netball attire that reflects feminine conventions, such as dresses or a skirt and top (Marfell, 2017). However, these are now extremely short in length and made of lycra, producing a body-hugging effect (Treagus, 2005). This in itself can cause females stress in relation to how their bodies may look in tight fitting uniforms, to the extreme that some girls may not even attempt a sport because of how they look in the required dress (Staurowsky, 2016). Indeed, research by Slater and Tiggemann (2011) reported that teasing and concerns over body image may contribute to the lower participation rates of adolescent girls in sport and physical activity. Some sports are beginning to address this by providing a choice of kit i.e. in netball, girls can often choose dresses, skirts and tops and tops and leggings.

Consider the following quotes in Box 9.4 from athletes discussing their bodies.

BOX 9.4 WHAT DO THE ATHLETES SAY?

I was teased for looking like a boy because I was pretty muscular even before I started lifting weights. I've always had an athletic build so even now sometimes people say, "Oh, you look like a boy, you don't have boobs".

Natasha Hastings, Olympic gold medalist, track and field

When I was transferring from gymnastics to wakeboarding, I was a little self-conscious. There's not a huge difference going from a leotard to a bathing suit, but you'd see these beautiful girls in bikinis, and I'm only 13 or 14 years old with this buff little body. I grew into being really proud of it, knowing that that's what has enabled me to do what I do.

Dallas Friday, X Games Champion Wakeboarder

There was a time where I didn't feel incredibly comfortable about my body, because I felt like I was too strong [...] And then I had to take a second and think, who says I'm too strong? This body has enabled me to be the greatest player I can be and I'm not going to scrutinize that. This is great. I mean, this is amazing.

Serena Williams, Tennis player

It becomes apparent that the culture around female athletes and their bodies can have a powerful impact. Often this can be pressurised by coaches, other athletes, peers, and social media to present their bodies in a certain way. This applies not only to female athletes but young girls in general. Research by Jankauskiene and Baccviciene (2019) found that adolescents involved in sports demonstrated greater body image satisfaction and did not seem to present a greater risk for disturbed eating attitudes and behaviours (DEABs) than those who were not involved in sports activities. However, girls participating in weight-sensitive leisure sports (such as dancing, gymnastics, swimming) showed greater body image concerns and higher prevalence of DEABs. Therefore, the type of sport may be an influential factor in how adolescent girls feel about their bodies.

It's not cool to sweat

In addition to body image societal perceptions of female athletes can also influence why young girls may not think it's cool to play sports. For example, Gorely et al. (2009), found that some UK schoolgirls held traditional views regarding gender-appropriate sports. While the identity of being sporty was perceived by most to be acceptable, it was still portrayed as contradicting the norms associated with femininity. Further evidence of a gender influence was presented by Carlin, Murphy and Gallagher (2015) who revealed that 11–13-year-old British males preferred more intense and competitive forms of physical activities, for instance structured sport, whereas females showed preference for activities like dance. Gender stereotypes such as these in the context of sport conveyed from the social environment have been linked to dropout in female adolescents (Boiché et al., 2014). Therefore, those involved in female sports need to work together to change the narrative around such stereotypes. One such example of this is the 'This Girl Can' campaign by Sport England, which celebrates women taking part in all types of sport and physical activity. The rise in popularity of women's football, rugby and cricket are also helping to break such gender stereotypes.

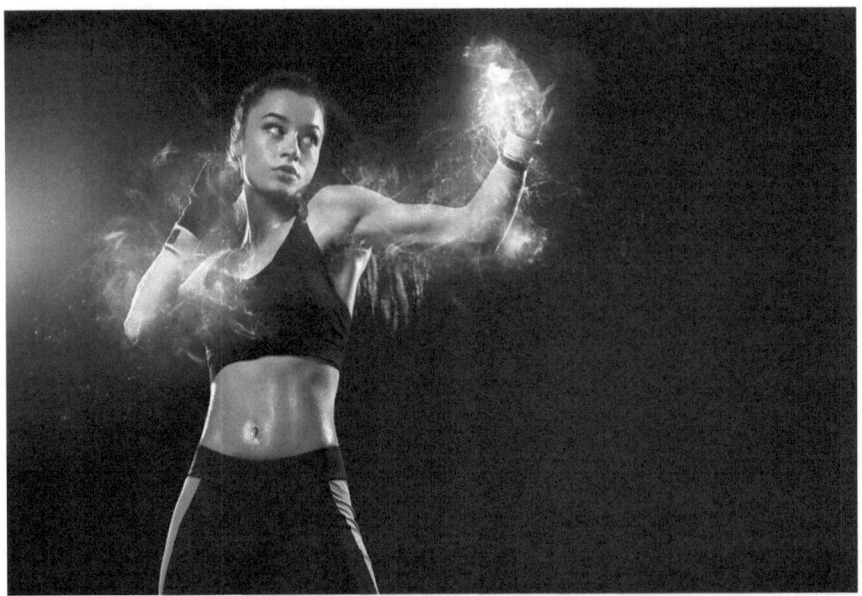

Fuelling the adolescent body

Body image also has strong links to diet and nutrition, and nutrition is particularly important for youth female athletes. During adolescence females experience a pubescence growth spurt, which increases their energy and nutrient requirements, and if these requirements are not adequately met then the athlete becomes at risk of hormonal irregularities, delayed development, poor bone health, and increased risk of injury (Sharples, Baker and Black, 2020). Inadequate nutrition could lead to a range of problems and stress injuries can be an indicator of poor nutrition (Gastrich et al., 2020). This is linked to low energy intake (discussed in Chapter 5), therefore, optimal nutrition is a key requirement for adolescent females who are training and competing on a regular basis. One of the most frequent nutrient deficiencies among female athletes is iron depletion. This is typically due to low dietary iron intakes, menstrual losses, raised hepcidin (a protein that regulates iron into the circulation), erythropoiesis (the production of red blood cells), and foot strike hemolysis (when red blood cells burst due to repeated striking of the foot on the floor) (Sharples et al.,

2020). Akachi experienced low iron levels and now manages this largely through her diet with the occasional iron supplements where necessary.

All athletes will have their own unique nutritional requirements and so it is not feasible within this chapter to provide specific information and guidance. However, education is vital to ensure that adolescent athletes are provided with the appropriate information, skills and support to foster a positive and enduring relationship with food (Desbrow et al., 2019). Some girls may engage in disordered eating, such as cutting out certain food groups or focusing only on one source of food, without being an eating disorder like anorexia. Gastrich et al. (2020) identified a lack of general nutrition knowledge among athletes, sports teams, and coaches. It is also important that the coach and family keep an eye on an athlete's nutritional intake to identify early any potential disordered eating or eating disorders and to prioritise dealing with those before worrying about performance.

Injuries and the adolescent body

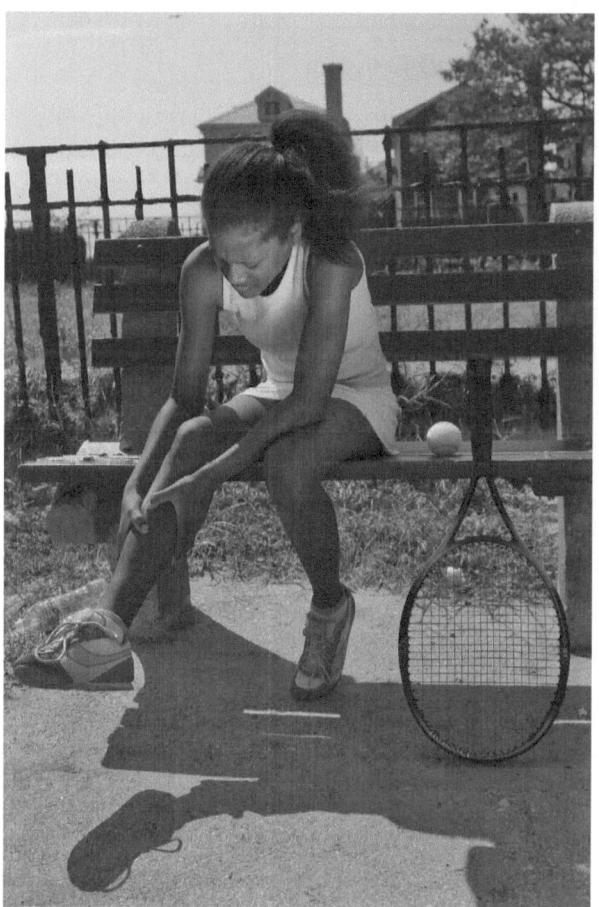

As discussed in Chapter 8, research has shown that adolescent females are more at risk of ACL injury. This is particularly evident between 11 and 17 years of age where the ACL injury risk is increasing at a greater rate in girls than in boys due to sex differences in physical characteristics (Shultz et al., 2022). Female athletes, following the onset of puberty, are 3.5 times more likely to experience anterior cruciate ligament (ACL) injuries, and so, early maturing girls yet to develop expertise in sport-specific techniques, may be particularly at risk (Voskanian, 2013). Early sport specialisation has also been linked to female injury risk. A study by DiCesare et al. (2019) showed that female athletes who specialised early in a sport demonstrated altered lower extremity co-ordination which can lead to less stable landings and an increased injury risk. They suggested that participating in multiple sports could facilitate improved co-ordination in youth female athletes and as a consequence lessen the injury risk. Engaging in strength and conditioning is also a useful strategy to mitigate against the risk of knee injuries and as such is incorporated in many youth development programmes.

Balancing demands and pressures

For those athletes that are performing at a high level, not all are able to sustain such consistently high levels of performance and athletes do drop out of sport at various stages of their athletic development. It is important to recognise that during adolescence individuals will be experiencing various demands and pressures on their time including academic, social, sporting and even work commitments for some. Most sport during adolescence takes place within the community which often means limited resources and expertise with less access to high quality coaching and medical services, and so it is important to understand how to balance the benefits of participation with the risks (McKay, Cumming and Blake, 2019). Due to these competing demands young female athletes are at risk of overtraining and burnout, as discussed further in Chapter 11.

Maintaining the well-being of adolescent females

As this chapter has identified, adolescent females are at risk of dropping out of sport completely due to the factors discussed. Parents are often key to maintaining their daughter's participation and aid their performance (as discussed in Chapter 11), however, as well as the family it is important for all those working with adolescent female athletes to consider all factors relating to the wellbeing of each athlete. Grounded in literature and consultations Ross et al. (2020, p. 473) defined adolescent well-being as:

> ... the support, confidence, and resources to thrive in contexts of secure and healthy relationships, realizing their full potential and rights.

Alongside this definition Ross et al. (2020) also proposed five inter-connected domains for adolescent well-being including the requirements for adolescents to achieve well-being within each of these domains (see Figure 9.4). This definition of adolescent well-being and its five domains applies in all contexts and is relevant for all adolescents, and therefore can be used as a framework when considering the wellbeing of female adolescent athletes.

Maintaining good physical and mental health alongside optimum nutrition are important aspects of sports performance. Athletes should ensure they eat well, hydrate effectively and get enough sleep. The coaching environment must also be one that does not place psychological stress on the athlete. This links with the domain of safety and a supportive environment, not only maintaining a safe physical environment but also ensuring that young female athletes are treated fairly and not discriminated against. Athlete voice is particularly important within the sport domain. In the modern world the safe environment also extends to the digital environment and the use of social media. Most National Governing Bodies have safeguarding rules around the use of social media with under-18s that must be adhered to by coaches. Connectedness and the sense of belonging that girls experience within sport play a vital role in their continued participation. The value of team sports and fostering social identity with one's sport team may con-tribute to greater enjoyment of sport and reductions in sport dropout in

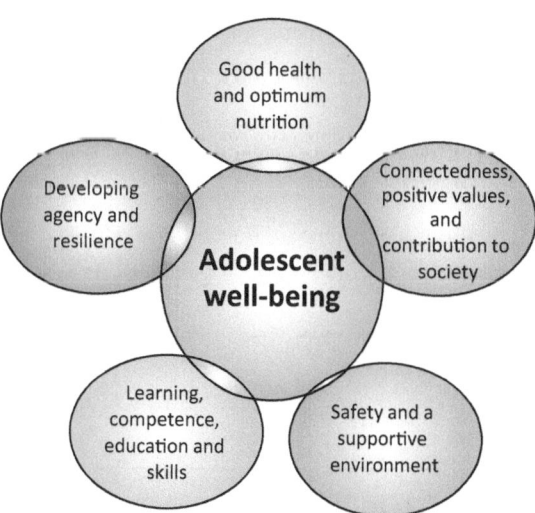

FIGURE 9.4 Five Domains of Adolescent Wellbeing
Source: Adapted from Ross et al. (2020)

adolescent girls (Murray and Sabiston, 2021). Furthermore, maintaining respect for others in the sporting environment and developing interpersonal skills also allows the athlete to contribute positively to the sporting society they are part of. Learning and mastering new skills have been shown by the Women's Sport Foundation (2020) to be important to girls playing sport, with competitiveness increasing as the girls increased in age. Yet, those girls that had dropped out from sport were less confident in their performance and worried about not being good enough. This illustrates that personal development, fun and enjoyment should be a priority to keep girls involved and that confidence is a vital factor in the continued participation of girls. Developing agency and resilience in youth female athletes is vital to their wellbeing and sporting interactions with peers have been shown to help female adolescent athletes to develop their emotional and intellectual, social, and physical selves (MacPherson, Kerr and Stirling, 2016). Box 9.5 provides some useful tips for both athletes and coaches to maintain athlete wellbeing.

BOX 9.5 REAL-WORLD APPLICATION

As an adolescent female athlete, you should:

1. Ensure you have the right nutrition and sleep and general health.
2. Utilise the support available to you from coaches, family and peers.
3. Feel empowered to make your own decisions.
4. Develop positive relationships with peers and teammates.
5. Focus on your own development, learning and skills rather than that of others.

As a coach of an adolescent female athlete, you should:

1. Understand the complexities of adolescence and the challenges girls may face.
2. Educate girls about fuelling before training and refuelling after training.
3. Provide a positive environment for empowering girls to develop agency and resilience.
4. Encourage and support peer relationships and friendships between athletes.
5. Focus on learning and individual development to develop confidence in female athletes.

Coaches of female athletes can also play an important role in encouraging the continued participation of their young female athletes. Box 9.6 presents some ideas around how a coach can support their athletes to prevent dropout and 'keep them in the game'.

BOX 9.6 TIPS FOR COACHES TO PREVENT DROPOUT

1. The coach can provide a supportive and encouraging environment for females to facilitate emotional, social, and physical development.
2. Use education to help girls understand the changes in their bodies and how this may impact performance, and the importance of optimal nutrition and sleep.
3. Take steps to break down gender stereotypes and work with parents where appropriate.
4. The coach needs to be aware of any other commitments on the athlete's time such as academic pressures and other activities.

Summary

Having completed this chapter, you will now have developed a more detailed understanding of the complex issues faced by adolescent females in relation to sports participation. In particular you will appreciate how participation can often decline in the adolescent years and some of the reasons for this. It is most important to understand the societal pressures that face adolescent female athletes and the support that they will require. You will also have explored the physiological risk of injury and the importance of maintaining a young athlete's physical and mental wellbeing.

The key messages to take away from this chapter are:

1. Puberty involves key physiological and psychological changes that can impact sports participation and performance.
2. During adolescence young girls are going through the process of identity formation and often role conflict can arise.
3. There are physiological and psychological risks involved with early specialisation.
4. Body perception is a key contributor to female participation and performance.
5. Fuelling the adolescent body appropriately and avoiding injury are important factors
6. There are five factors that contribute to an adolescent female's overall wellbeing.

End-of-Chapter Quiz

Answers can be found after the References

1. Identify what ages the World Health Organisation class to be an adolescent:

    a 10–20
    b 13–21

c   10–19
d   11–18

2. Identify which are the three stages of adolescence:

    a   Early adolescence, middle adolescence, late adolescence
    b   Young adolescence, teenage adolescence, older adolescence
    c   Pre-pubescent, pubescent, post pubescent
    d   Pre-menstrual, menstrual, post menstrual

3. Identify the most appropriate age for talent development in female athletes:

    a   14
    b   16
    c   18
    d   20

4. Identify which injury is 3.5 more common in female athletes between 11–17 years:

    a   Hamstring tears
    b   ACL injuries
    c   Achilles tendon injuries
    d   Plantar fasciitis

5. Identify which of the following statements about adolescent female athletes is true:

    a   Female adolescent athletes are more likely to withdraw from competitive sport as they hate all forms of competition
    b   Female adolescent athletes are more likely to participate in individual activities as they don't like team sports
    c   Female adolescent athletes are more likely to participate when the environment is fun and the focus is on personal development
    d   Female adolescent athletes are more likely to participate in sport that is highly competitive and based on winning

References

Allen, B. and Waterman, H. (2019) *Stages of Adolescence*. Available at: https://www.healthychildren.org/English/ages-stages/teen/Pages/Stages-of-Adolescence.aspx (Accessed: 20 January 2023).

Allender, S., Cowburn, G, and Foster, C. (2006) 'Understanding participation in sport and physical activity among children and adults: a review of qualitative studies', *Health Education Research*, 21(6), 826–835.

Baker, J., Mosher, A. and Fraser-Thomas, J., (2021) 'Is it too early to condemn early sport specialisation?', *British Journal of Sports Medicine*, 55(3), 179–180.

Boiché, J., Plaza, M., Chalabaev, A., Guillet-Descas, E. and Sarrazin, P. (2014) 'Social antecedents and consequences of gender-sport stereotypes during adolescence', *Psychology of Women Quarterly*, 38(2), 259–274.

Bradley, S.H., Lawrence, N., Steele, C. and Mohamed, Z. (2020) 'Precocious puberty', *British Medical Journal*, 368. Available at: doi:10.1136/bmj.l6597 (Accessed: 15 October 2023).

Brewer, B.W. and Petitpas, A.J. (2017) 'Athletic identity foreclosure', *Current Opinion in Psychology*, 16, 118–122.

Brewer, B. W., Van Raalte, J. L., and Linder, D. E. (1993) 'Athletic identity: Hercules' muscles or Achilles heel?', *International Journal of Sport Psychology*, 24(2), 237–254.

Buckingham, D. (2008) 'Introducing Identity', *Youth, Identity, and Digital Media*, 1–24. Available at: doi:0.1162/dmal.9780262524834.001 (Accessed: 15 January 2023).

Carlin, A., Murphy, M.H. and Gallagher, A.M. (2015) 'Current influences and approaches to promote future physical activity in 11–13 year olds: a focus group study', *BMC Public Health*, 15(1), 1–12. Available at: doi:10.1186/s12889-015-2601-9 (Accessed: 15 January 2023).

Côté, J. (1999) 'The influence of the family in the development of talent in sport', *The Sport Psychologist*, 13(4), pp. 395–417.

Crane, J. and Temple, V. (2015) 'A systematic review of dropout from organized sport among children and youth', *European Physical Education Review*, 21(1), 114–131.

Desbrow, B., Burd, N.A., Tarnopolsky, M., Moore, D.R. and Elliott-Sale, K. J. (2019) 'Nutrition for special populations: Young, female, and masters athletes', *International Journal of Sport Nutrition and Exercise Metabolism*, 29(2), 220–227.

Devonport, T.J., Russell, K., Leflay, K. and Conway, J. (2019) 'Gendered performances and identity construction among UK female soccer players and netballers: a comparative study', *Sport in Society*, 22(7), 1131–1147.

DiCesare, C.A., Montalvo, A., Foss, K.D.B., Thomas, S.M., Hewett, T.E., Jayanthi, N. A. and Myer, G.D. (2019) 'Sport specialization and coordination differences in multi-sport adolescent female basketball, soccer, and volleyball athletes', *Journal of Athletic Training*, 54(10), 1105–1114.

Eime, R.M., Harvey, J.T., Sawyer, N.A., Craike, M.J., Symons, C.M., Polman, R.C. and Payne, W. R. (2013) 'Understanding the contexts of adolescent female participation in sport and physical activity', *Research Quarterly for Exercise and Sport*, 84(2), 157–166.

Erikson, E.H. (1968) *Identity: Youth and crisis*. WW Norton & Company.

Feeley, B.T., Agel, J. and LaPrade, R.F. (2015) 'When Is It Too Early for Single Sport Specialization?', *The American Journal of Sports Medicine*, 44(1), 234–241. Available at: doi:10.1177/0363546515576899 (Accessed: 6 October 2023).

Gastrich, M.D., Quick, V., Bachmann, G. and Moriarty, A.M. (2020) 'Nutritional risks among female athletes', *Journal of Women's Health*, 29(5), 693–702.

Gerber, B., Pienaar, A.E. and Kruger, A. (2021) 'Two-year follow-up on differences in anthropometric growth between pre-and post-menarcheal girls: implications for sport participation', *Journal of Physical Education and Sport*, 21, 3252–3264.

Gorely, T., Atkin, A.J., Biddle, S.J. and Marshall, S. J. (2009) 'Family circumstance, sedentary behaviour and physical activity in adolescents living in England: Project STIL', *International Journal of Behavioral Nutrition and Physical Activity*, 6(1), 33–40.

Hopkins, C. and Hopkins, C.S. (2022) 'Applying Theory Of Planned Behavior To Examine Adolescent Female Athletes' Intentions Of Continued Sport Participation: 521', *Medicine & Science in Sports & Exercise*, 54(9S), 130.

Jankauskiene, R. and Baceviciene, M. (2019) 'Body image and disturbed eating attitudes and behaviors in sport-involved adolescents: the role of gender and sport characteristics', *Nutrients*, 11(12), 3061.

Jayanthi, N.A., Post, E.G., Laury, T.C. and Fabricant, P.D. (2019) 'Health consequences of youth sport specialization', *Journal of Athletic Training*, 54(10), 1040–1049.

Krane, V., Choi, P.Y., Baird, S.M., Aimar, C.M. and Kauer, K.J. (2004) 'Living the paradox: Female athletes negotiate femininity and muscularity', *Sex roles*, 50(5–6), 315–329.

Kruse, D. and Lemmen, B. (2009) 'Spine injuries in the sport of gymnastics', *Current Sports Medicine Reports*, 8 (1), 20–8.

Lunde, C. and Gattario, K.H. (2017) 'Performance or appearance? Young female sport participants' body negotiations', *Body Image*, 21, 81–89.

Lundvall, S. and Walseth, K. (2014) 'From girl to woman: Becoming an adult; socio-cultural factors and sports participation during adolescence', Women and Sport: Scientific Report Series.

MacPherson, E., Kerr, G. and Stirling, A. (2016) 'The influence of peer groups in organized sport on female adolescents' identity development', *Psychology of Sport and Exercise*, 23, 73–81. Available at: doi:10.1016/j.psychsport.2015.10.002 (Accessed: 10 October 2023).

Marfell, A. (2017) '"We wear dresses, we look pretty": The feminization and hetero-sexualization of netball spaces and bodies', *International Review for the Sociology of Sport*, 54(5), 577–602.

McKay, C.D., Cumming, S.P. & Blake, T. (2019) 'Youth sport: friend or foe?', *Best practice & research Clinical rheumatology*, 33(1), 141–157.

Metcalf, B.S., Hosking, J., Jeffery, A.N., Henley, W.E. and Wilkin, T.J., (2015) 'Exploring the adolescent fall in physical activity: a 10-yr cohort study (EarlyBird 41)'. *Medicine and Science in Sports and Exercise*, 47(10), 2084–2092.

Mosher, A., Fraser-Thomas, J. and Baker, J. (2020) 'What Defines Early Specialization: A Systematic Review of Literature', *Frontiers in Sports and Active Living*, 2. Available at: doi:10.3389/fspor.2020.596229 (Accessed 15 October 2023).

Murray, R.M. and Sabiston, C.M. (2021) 'Understanding relationships between social identity, sport enjoyment, and dropout in adolescent girl athletes', *Journal of Sport and Exercise Psychology*, 1, 1–5.

Nusman, C., van Rijn, R., Lim, L. and Maas, M. (2011) 'An 11-year-old high-level competitive gymnast with back pain', *British Journal of Sports Medicine*, 47(14), 929–32.

Ross, D.A., Hinton, R., Melles-Brewer, M., Engel, D., Zeck, W., Fagan, L., Herat, J., Phaladi, G., Imbago-Jácome, D. and Anyona, P. (2020) 'Adolescent well-being: A definition and conceptual framework', *Journal of Adolescent Health*, 67(4), 472–476.

Scurr, J., Brown, N., Smith, J., Brasher, A., Risius, D. and Marczyk, A. (2016) 'The influence of the breast on sport and exercise participation in school girls in the United Kingdom', *Journal of Adolescent Health*, 58(2), 167–173.

Sharples, A., Baker, D. and Black, K. (2020) 'Nutrition for Adolescent Female Team Sport Athletes: A Review', *Strength & Conditioning Journal*, 42(4), 59–67.

Shultz, S., Cruz M., Casey, E., Dompier T., Ford, K., Pietrosimone, B., Schmitz, R. and Taylor, J. (2022) 'Sex-Specific Changes in Physical Risk Factors for Anterior Cruciate Ligament Injury by Chronological Age and Stages of Growth and Maturation From 8 to 18 Years of Age', *Journal of athletic training*, 57(9–10), 830–876.

Sinclair, J. (2022) *NS EXCLUSIVE: The superpowers of Eleanor Cardwell*. Netball Scoop. Available at: https://netballscoop.com/ns-exclusive-the-superpowers-of-eleanor-cardwell/ (Accessed: 15 January 2023).

Slater, A. and Tiggemann, M. (2011) 'Gender differences in adolescent sport participation, teasing, self-objectification and body image concerns', *Journal of Adolescence*, 34 (3), 455–463.

Spencer, R.A., Rehman, L. and Kirk, S.F. (2015) 'Understanding gender norms, nutrition, and physical activity in adolescent girls: a scoping review', *International Journal of Behavioral Nutrition and Physical Activity*, 12(6).

Staurowsky, E. (2016) 'Women's Sport in the 21st Century', in E. Staurowsky (Ed.), *Women and Sport: Continuing a Journey of Liberation and Celebration*, pp. 37–54. Leeds: Human Kinetics.

Sweeney, L., Horan, D. and MacNamara, Á., (2021) 'Premature professionalisation or early engagement? Examining practise in football player pathways'. *Frontiers in Sports and Active Living*, 3, p. 660167.

Tan, J., Bloodworth, A., McNamee, M. and Hewitt, J. (2014) 'Investigating eating disorders in elite gymnasts: conceptual, ethical and methodological issues', *European Journal of Sport Science*, 14, 60–8.

Treagus, M. (2005) 'Playing Like Ladies: Basketball, Netball and Feminine Restraint', *The International Journal of the History of Sport*, 22(1), 88–105.

Viner, R. (2012) 'Chapter 8: Life stage: Adolescence'. *Annual Report of the Chief Medical Officer 2012, Our Children Deserve Better: Prevention Pays*, Available at: https://assets.publishing.service.gov.uk/government/uploads/system/uploads/attachment_data/file/252658/33571_2901304_CMO_Chapter_8.pdf. (Accessed: 15 January 2023).

Voskanian, N. (2013) 'ACL Injury prevention in female athletes: review of the literature and practical considerations in implementing an ACL prevention program', *Current reviews in musculoskeletal medicine*, 6(2), 158–163.

Women's Sport Foundation (2020) 'Keeping Girls in the Game: Factors That Influence Sport Participation'. Available at: https://files.eric.ed.gov/fulltext/ED603915.pdf (Accessed: 5 January 2023).

World Health Organisation (2022) *Adolescent health*. Available at: https://www.who.int/health-topics/adolescent-health#tab=tab_1 (Accessed: 27 September 2023).

Zarrett, N., Veliz, P. and Sabo, D. (2020) 'Keeping Girls in the Game: Factors That Influence Sport Participation'. New York: Women's Sports Foundation.

Answers

1. c
2. a
3. b
4. b
5. c

10

EXERCISE CONSIDERATIONS FOR THE FEMALE ATHLETE IN PREGNANCY

Simon Rea

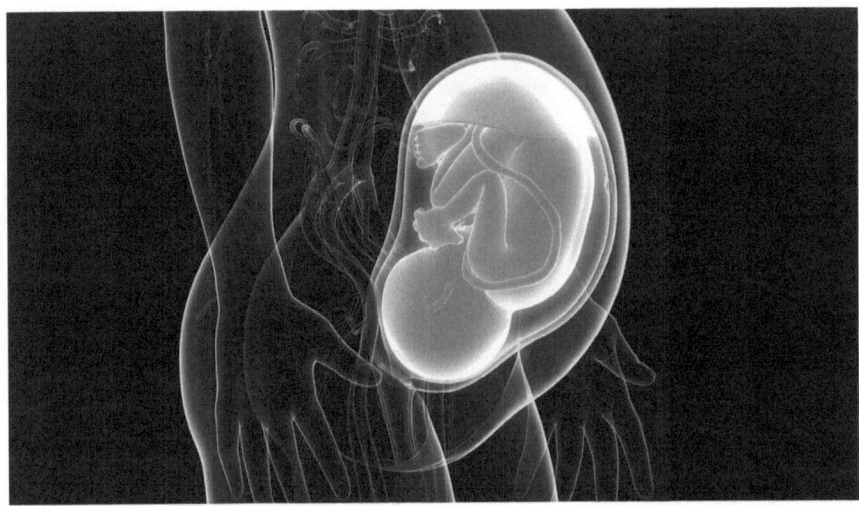

Introduction

Many athletic careers coincide with the time when the female is at her most fertile, and thus pregnancy is something the female athlete may have to consider during their career. There is also a growing awareness within the health and fitness industry of the benefits to both mother and child of exercising through pregnancy. However, pregnancy is a time of rapid physiological and hormonal changes for women and there may be some risks if exercise isn't managed appropriately during this nine-month period. Traditionally in the UK, sports organisations and pregnancy advisory groups have taken a conservative approach to training during pregnancy, with particular

DOI: 10.4324/9781003330110-10

concern around contact sports where the baby could be injured through physical contact with another person or object.

These somewhat dated views are starting to change as advice from the UK Chief Medical Officer (2019) states that if you are active then keep going, or if you were previously sedentary then start exercising gradually. UK Sport (2021) has produced pregnancy guidance to inform National and Home Country governing bodies on how to best support pregnant elite athletes. Much of this guidance is how to practically manage this stage of a female's athletic career but the English Institute of Sport (EIS) offers specialist support through their SmartHER programme.

Pregnant females may have differing motivations for exercise such as making their pregnancy more comfortable, preparing for labour and birth, having a healthy baby, and staying in shape during pregnancy. In contrast female athletes may want to continue participating in their sport for as long as they can and protect their pre-pregnancy levels of cardiovascular and muscular fitness as much as possible to facilitate a smooth return to sport post-partum. However, there can be risks and complications associated with pregnancy, so it is important that pregnant women of all fitness levels consult their doctor before either starting or continuing exercise and continue to do so through the course of the pregnancy.

In addition to physical concerns around pregnancy female athletes may have practical worries such as loss of income and availability of childcare. Some sportswomen may experience either a reduction in, or removal of, funding during and after pregnancy while they are unable to compete (Roberts and Kenatta, 2018).

This chapter explores the benefits of exercise, and assesses the physiological, muscular, and hormonal changes that occur across the three trimesters of pregnancy. The focus then moves to exercise prescription and assesses what exercise may be appropriate, and what should be avoided. Finally, training during the post-natal period is examined to help the mother recover from the birth, manage changes to their body, and return them to full participation in their sport or physical activity.

Before exploring the benefits of exercise read the case study, in Box 10.1, where you are introduced to Emily and her experiences of pregnancy.

BOX 10.1 EMILY (TRIATHLETE)

Emily is a 35-year-old competitive triathlete who came to the sport relatively late after competing solely as a swimmer for 15 years. She has also being trying for a baby with her partner but was concerned that her low body weight and high activity level may make conception problematic. This concern proved to be unfounded as she became pregnant within six months of stopping oral contraception.

Emily was aware that at age 35 she was a relatively older mother and that carried an increased risk of miscarriage. She was also keen to maintain her level of fitness so that she could return to competition quickly after the birth.

Emily was determined to keep training for as long as she could during the pregnancy but found that in the early weeks she felt so sick that she was often not able to leave the house. She was aware of morning sickness, but quickly found out that the sickness was not just present in the morning and often lasted all day. Owing to her nausea she also found that eating was problematic and that she was steadily losing weight and she knew this was not a good thing during pregnancy. Swimming was the only one of her disciplines that Emily could participate in without feeling nauseous and while it was a struggle to get to the pool she found that it did reduce her symptoms making her feel a bit better.

Once Emily had passed the 12-week mark she started to feel less nauseous and more energised. She decided that she would try running and cycling again as she could do those fairly comfortably. After about five months Emily's pregnancy was really showing and she was finding that the baby was increasingly pressing down on her pelvic floor. She got to the point where frequent urination interrupted her running and so decided that it was time to stop running and try brisk walking. She also stopped cycling as she found it uncomfortable and was producing pain in her pelvis.

By the time Emily reached her third trimester she was still able to do some swimming and brisk walking. She had to change the stroke she was doing in the pool as breaststroke was causing pelvic pain and she felt a moving sensation in her pelvis. She was still able to swim front crawl and enjoyed that the water would support the weight of her stomach. This gave her some relief from the back pain that had developed through her pregnancy and was now really uncomfortable.

Emily kept on swimming and walking up until the birth of her son, Zachary, and had a relatively quick albeit incredibly painful labour. Once she had recovered from her labour she started exercising lightly again. Initially she focused on pelvic floor and abdominal exercises but after six weeks she started building up her running and swimming again.

Benefits of exercise in pregnancy

As long as exercising females follow guidelines from their doctors and exercise recommendations there are considerable benefits for their baby and themselves from training during pregnancy. However, the pregnant female, and their coach or trainer, may initially have some concerns about exercise, owing to their own preconceptions, or things they may have heard.

Some pregnant women may feel that exercising in the early stage of pregnancy may increase risk of miscarriage. While around 1 in 8 pregnancies will result in miscarriage (NHS, 2023), it is very unlikely that exercise is a risk factor. A meta-analysis of over 100 studies on physical activity and pregnancy showed that less than 1 per cent of 'adverse events' during pregnancy were related to exercise (Verdière et al., 2017). This review even concluded that vigorous exercise could not be linked to increased risk of miscarriage.

Doctors recommend exercise during pregnancy because it has benefits for both pregnant women and their babies as shown in Figure 10.1.

Pre-eclampsia,, which is characterised by high blood pressure and the presence of proteins in the urine, is a particular concern as it is among the leading causes of maternal mortality (Roberts et al., 2003). Pre-eclampsia can also affect the foetus with an increased risk of early birth and foetal death. If pre-eclampsia is diagnosed then often an early delivery is the only treatment. While the research is not conclusive exercise has been shown to act as a protective mechanism against the development of pre-eclampsia (Kuhrt et al., 2015).

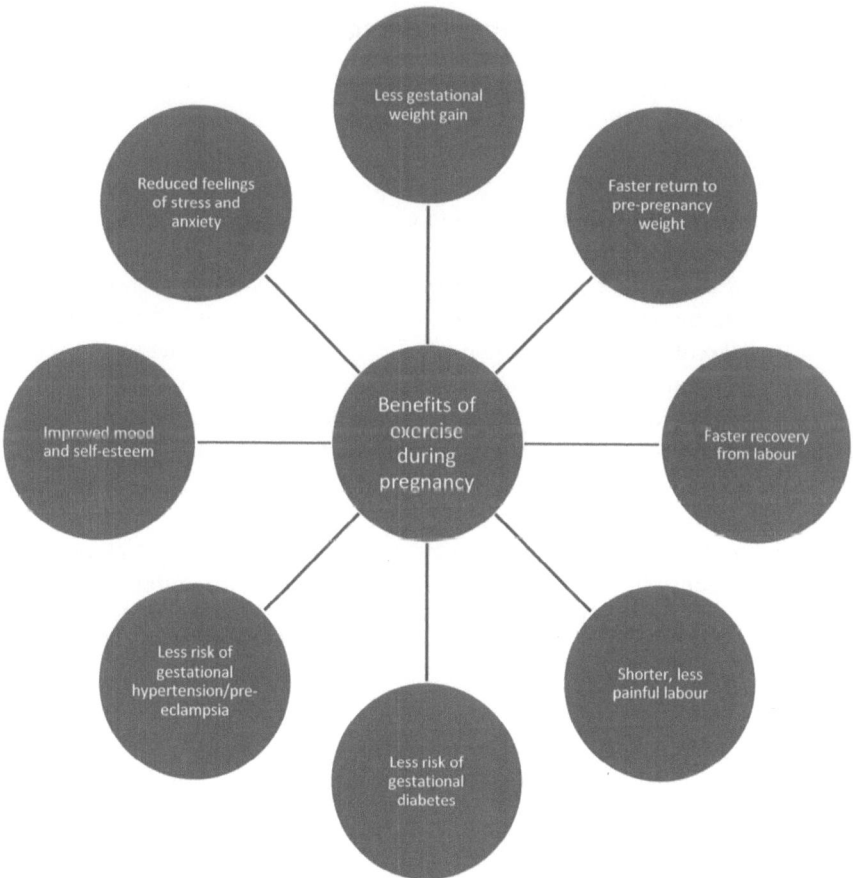

FIGURE 10.1 Benefits of exercise during pregnancy
Source: Adapted from Westcott and Faigenbaum, 2021 and Berghella and Saccone (2017)

Gestational diabetes is glucose intolerance that occurs specifically in pregnancy and then dissipates after delivery. Pregnant women who gain more than 10 per cent of their pre-pregnancy weight are at risk of developing gestational diabetes, along with an increased risk of pre-eclampsia (Kuhrt et al., 2015). Owing to the glucose intolerance of the mother, increased amounts of glucose ingested in the diet will flow to the foetus and can result in a larger baby. This offers complications at birth with potential concern for both mother and baby. Regular exercise can have a positive effect on insulin secretion, insulin sensitivity and glucose uptake and as a result reduce the risk of developing gestational diabetes (Westcott and Faigenbaum, 2021).

These benefits indicate that in the absence of medical or pregnancy related complications healthy pregnant women should be encouraged to exercise daily for the length of their pregnancy. However, they do need to be aware of what type of exercise is and what should be avoided.

BOX 10.2 PREGNANCY-RELATED TERMINOLOGY

There is specific terminology associated with pregnancy that is used in this chapter.

Pregnancy is considered to have reached full term at 40 weeks, but it has three **trimesters:**

First trimester: covers the first three months or weeks 1–12.

Second trimester: cover months 4 to 6, or weeks 13–26.

Third trimester: covers months 7–9, or weeks 27–40

During the first trimester the developing baby is referred to as an **embryo**, while in the second and third trimesters it is referred to as a **foetus** (fetus in US).

The **placenta** attaches the embryo/foetus to the wall of the uterus and acts to provide nutrients, exchange waste, and as a protective barrier against disease. The placenta will also produce hormones needed to maintain pregnancy.

The embryo/foetus itself develops within a sac filled with **amniotic fluid**. The amniotic fluid helps to provide shock absorption for the foetus and regulate its temperature.

The **corpus luteum** is responsible for producing hormones, such as oestrogen and progesterone, in the early stages of pregnancy. The corpus luteum is formed in an ovary from the ovarian follicle responsible for releasing the egg that was fertilised.

Across the three trimesters of pregnancy the female's body will adapt and go through significant changes. These changes are to support the health, development and growth of the foetus and they will have a significant effect on how the pregnant female feels and functions. The cardiovascular, respiratory, and muscular systems are all impacted by changes in hormones produced to support the pregnancy from conception through to birth. The next section looks at hormonal changes and how they affect the cardiovascular, respiratory, and muscular systems function to support pregnancy.

Hormonal changes during pregnancy

The hormones, oestrogen, and progesterone, associated with the menstrual cycle and fertility also play a significant role in maintaining pregnancy (Reese and Casey, 2015). The body will also produce other hormones, such as relaxin, specific to pregnancy. For the first 6–8 weeks the corpus luteum will be the main source of pregnancy-related hormones. After this period the placenta takes over responsibility for the production of hormones. These hormones will interact with and influence body systems central to pregnancy.

Oestrogen

Oestrogen levels rise steadily throughout pregnancy and then fall after birth when the mother is lactating. Oestrogen acts to promote foetal growth and wellbeing (Draca, 2006). In the mother it will stimulate breast growth and increase production of prostaglandins (hormone like substances) and the hormone, oxytocin, which assist in labour (Wylie, 2005). However, increasing oestrogen levels also contribute to increases in joint laxity, particularly in the cartilage and ligaments at the knee and pelvis (Reece and Casey, 2015). The increased levels of oestrogen during pregnancy also stimulate bone development in the female and helps to protect against the development of osteoporosis in later life. In the case study in Box 10.1 Emily experiences pelvic pain when she is cycling and swimming breast stroke. This may be due to increased mobility of the joints in her pelvis and hips.

Progesterone

During the menstrual cycle progesterone is produced by the corpus luteum, but after the first trimester of pregnancy it is predominantly produced by the placenta. Progesterone levels initially fall but in the second and third trimesters they rise steadily (Ahrens et al., 2014). Progesterone is essential for the pregnancy to develop in its early stage as it prevents overgrowth of the uterus lining encouraged by oestrogen. This ensures the fertilised egg is able to implant into the uterus wall and afterwards it helps to maintain the pregnancy by keeping the uterus relaxed (Reese and Casey, 2015). Progesterone also causes blood vessels to dilate and carry more blood. This increase in blood volume helps control body temperature and prevent the foetus from overheating (foetal hyperthermia).

Relaxin

Relaxin is a key hormone in pregnancy that appears in the first trimester. It peaks around week 12 and then starts to fall through the second and third trimester. Relaxin's role is often misunderstood as it was assumed that it was responsible for increasing joint laxity and range of movement in the symphysis pubis and sacro-iliac joints of the pelvis, in preparation for the passage of the foetus through the pelvis at birth (Dehghan et al., 2014). However, oestrogen and progesterone are mainly responsible for the softening of ligaments around the pelvis, and other joints, to increase their range of movement. Relaxin's role is to remodel the ligaments around the pelvis before birth and to promote relaxation of the uterus while it is carrying the foetus (Reece and Casey, 2015).

Testosterone

Testosterone is present during all phases of the menstrual cycle and during pregnancy its levels rise steadily through the three trimesters. Testosterone exerts a controlling influence on the development of the foetus's bone, muscle, ligament, and cartilage (Reece and Casey, 2015).

Although there other hormones involved during pregnancy these are the most significant ones that work together to produce physiological changes and support pregnancy and birth.

Cardiovascular system changes during pregnancy

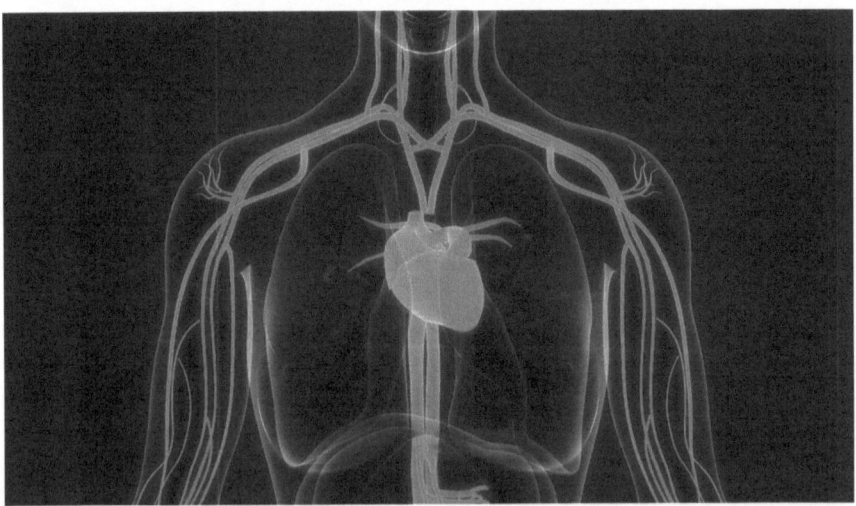

The cardiovascular system goes through changes during all three trimesters. During the first trimester progesterone will cause blood vessels to expand and dilate. This causes blood pressure to drop by around 10 per cent as there is the same volume of blood contained in a larger blood vessel (American College of Obstetricians and Gynecologists, 2020). This is referred to as vascular underfill and contributes to the feelings of nausea, fatigue and light headedness experienced in the early stages of pregnancy. To compensate for the lower blood pressure the heart rate will increase by between 3–5 per cent at rest and during exercise (American College of Obstetricians and Gynecologists, 2020). This can be problematic when using heart rate to assess the intensity of exercise during training and it is advised that rating of perceived exertion (RPE) is used during the first three months of pregnancy rather than relying on heart rate (Westcott and Faigenbaum, 2021).

Towards the end of the first trimester blood volume will start to rise, however, this increase is mainly plasma rather than additional blood cells (Soma-Pillay et al., 2016). During the second trimester this increase in blood volume will start to increase blood pressure, and heart rate can rise by up to 10–15 per cent. As a result there will be increases in cardiac output and stroke volume (American College of Obstetricians and Gynecologists, 2020).

The increased ability of the pregnant female to dissipate heat is accompanied by a lowering of the sweat point (temperature where sweat response is initiated) and can make them feel that they are sweating more easily or constantly sweating slightly (Charkoudian and Stachenfeld, 2016). This is vital to prevent foetal hyperthermia. There is a concern that the rise in body temperature of exercising pregnant females will affect the foetus, but these mechanisms make this unfounded.

One common concern about exercising during pregnancy is a reduction in blood supply to the foetus (foetal hypoxia). This could be caused by exercising on the back (supine lying) after the first trimester. Exercising in the supine position increases intra-abdominal pressure and can cause the uterus, that is increasing in size, to block the passage of blood through the vena cavae and reduce venous return. In turn this reduces cardiac output and potentially blood flow to the foetus. After four months of the pregnancy any exercise on the back should be avoided (Westcott and Faigenbaum, 2021). This includes exercises such as bench press, sit ups and other supine abdominal exercises, also stretches from the supine position should be avoided.

By the third trimester blood volume will have increased again causing blood pressure to rise (American College of Obstetricians and Gynecologists, 2020). At this time, the doctors will continually monitor blood pressure amid concerns around the development of hypertension and pre-eclampsia. The increased blood volume, vasodilation and lowered sweat point often give pregnant females in this trimester a rosy glow as well as a feeling that they are constantly sweating slightly.

Respiratory system changes during pregnancy

The respiratory system is relatively unaffected during the first trimester, although during the second and third trimesters the expanding uterus starts to push up into the diaphragm at the base of the rib cage. As this causes a restriction in the depth of breathing in response oestrogen and relaxin act to relax the cartilage between the ribs enabling the ribcage to push upwards and outwards. While depth of breathing becomes shallower the chest cavity actually becomes larger resulting in increases in tidal volume and minute volume of up to 50 per cent (Westcott and Faigenbaum, 2021). This contributes to increased blood flow to the foetus and again protects against foetal hypoxia.

The restriction in the depth of breathing can become a significant issue during the third trimester as the expanding foetus and placenta can make breathing a real effort and this will impact on the female's ability to exercise comfortably. Pregnant women should be encouraged to maintain regular breathing during exercise rather than holding their breath as this can increase pressure on the pelvic floor muscles.

Musculoskeletal system changes during pregnancy

As a pregnancy advances the female's uterus and breasts become larger and this causes changes in their centre of mass. The centre of mass moves forwards, and along with the effect of the hormones increasing joint laxity, can affect their balance and body control in movements such as changes in direction or where high levels of stability are needed (Pitchers et al., 2020). Any exercise that challenges the pregnant female's balance should be avoided during the third trimester as a fall or any abdominal trauma may have serious consequences for the foetus. In the case study in Box 10.1 Emily complained of back pain during her pregnancy and this is a common feature of pregnancies as the weight of the uterus produces postural changes as shown in Figure 10.2.

One significant postural change is an exaggeration of the lumbar curve that causes lumbar lordosis. This change in spinal position produces an anterior tilt of the pelvis, as indicated in Figure 10.2. The anterior pelvic tilt has a significant impact on muscles of the abdominals, lower back and those that attach

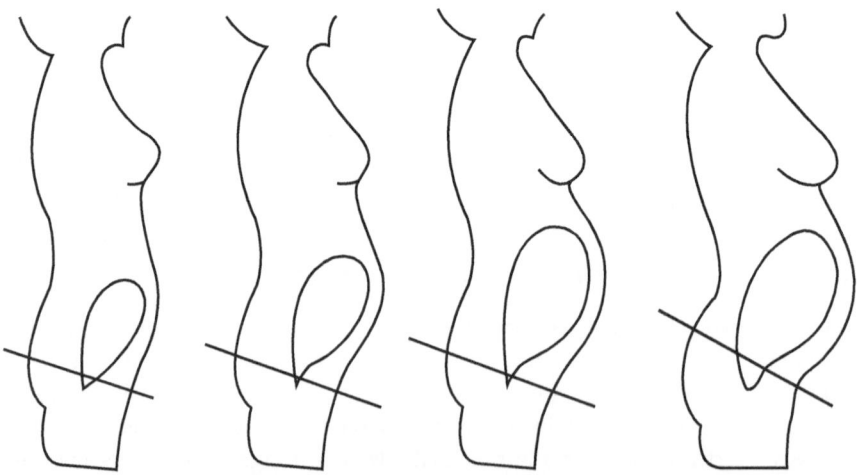

FIGURE 10.2 Postural changes to the spine and pelvis across the length of a pregnancy

to the pelvis. Each muscle will undergo change by either becoming stretched or tightened. Stretched muscles will become weakened and painful, owing to the increased load they are supporting, while shortened muscles will also become painful, as a result of being overworked. Table 10.1 indicates whether a muscle will become stretched or tighter.

In addition to these changes as pregnancy progresses into the second trimester there will be increased flexion in the cervical spine and depression of the shoulder girdle to support the weight of the breasts (Soma-Pillay et al., 2016).

The set of muscles that will come under the most strain during pregnancy are the pelvic floor muscles as pregnancy can lengthen, weaken, or overload these muscles (Pitchers et al., 2020). As shown in Figure 10.3, the pelvic floor muscles support the contents of the abdomen which includes the uterus containing the developing foetus, the placenta, and the amniotic sac.

The pelvic floor muscles are located within the pelvis, and they control the flow of urine through the urethra and faeces from the anus. Stretched and weakened pelvic floor muscles can make control of urine flow particularly problematic and lead to stress incontinence, or urine leakage. As a result pelvic floor exercise (Kegels) should be performed as soon as the female knows she is pregnant, during their pregnancy and if possible for the rest of their lives. These exercises involve tightening and relaxing of the muscles within the pelvis, and with training women can learn how to contract these muscles and strengthen them to support loading from the abdomen above. Women can also learn how to relax these muscles so the baby can be delivered more easily (Westcott and Faigenbaum, 2021). Advice on how to perform pelvic floor exercises is presented in Chapter 7.

Once there is increased stress on the pelvic floor, probably starting in the second trimester, it is advisable to avoid activities that raise stress on the pelvic floor even further. In particular high-impact exercise like jumping or changing direction quickly should be avoided. Emily in the case study in Box 10.1 found that running was problematic as the increased stress on her pelvic floor was causing her to urinate frequently. Although this was the case for Emily some athletes find that they can still run without discomfort well into their third trimester, although they may already have well developed pelvic floor muscles.

TABLE 10.1 Muscular changes during pregnancy

Muscle name	Change during pregnancy
Rectus abdominus (abdominals)	Stretched
Erector spinae (lower back)	Tight
Hip flexors	Tight
Glutes	Stretched
Quadriceps	Tight
Hamstrings	Stretched

Source: Adapted from Fiat et al. (2022)

PELVIC FLOOR MUSCLES

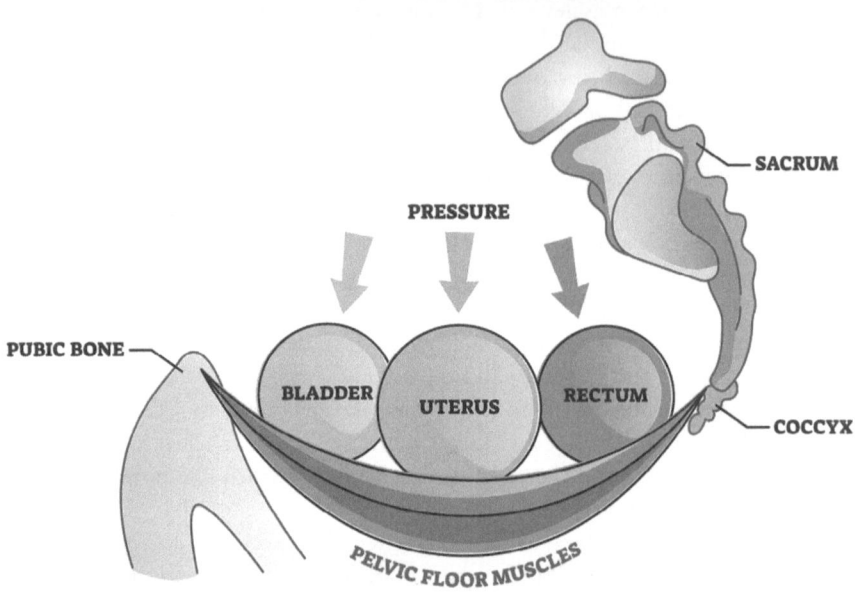

FIGURE 10.3 Pelvic floor muscles and the structures they support
Source: Shutterstock

Guidelines for exercising pregnant females

The physiological changes discussed should be taken into account when planning training programmes and while exercise can bring huge benefits to both the future mother and the foetus there are some conditions where exercise should be avoided (absolute contraindications), or participated in with caution and after specialist advice (relative contraindications) as shown in Table 10.2.

In the UK, the Royal College of Obstetrics and Gynaecology (RCOG) offer guidance to women with uncomplicated pregnancies who exercise. The guidance, developed by the UK Chief Medical Officer (2019), is that they should aim for 150 minutes of moderate intensity exercise every week, or 30 minutes every day. This includes activities such as walking, cycling, swimming, and dancing, as well as aiming for muscle strengthening exercises twice a week. Additional advice is to listen to your body, adapt any activities if necessary and be careful to avoid bumping the bump.

Tillet et al. (2019), of the Royal College of Nursing, stress three things to consider when exercising during pregnancy. First, the problem with increasingly mobile joints as a result of relaxin and oestrogen, avoiding exercising in the supine position after 16 weeks, and the increasing strain on the back and pelvic floor muscles as the pregnancy develops. Box 10.3 presents further considerations to exercise guidelines during each trimester and some general considerations as well.

TABLE 10.2 Absolute and relative contraindications

Absolute contraindications to exercise

- *Heart disease that significantly affects blood flow (atherosclerosis, hypertension, heart failure, peripheral artery disease)*
- *Restrictive lung diseases*
- *Multiple pregnancy with risk of early labour*
- *Persistent bleeding through second and third trimesters*
- *Placenta previa (where the placenta covers the opening of the cervix) after 26 weeks*
- *Premature labour during previous pregnancy*
- *Pre-eclampsia*
- *Severe anaemia*
- *Ruptured membranes of the amniotic sac*
- *Incompetent cervix (cervix starts opening early in pregnancy)*

Relative contraindications to exercise

- Anaemia
- Cardiac arrhythmia
- Chronic bronchitis
- Poorly controlled type 1 diabetes
- Hypertension
- Morbid obesity (BMI >40)
- Severe underweight (BMI <12)
- History of extreme sedentary lifestyle
- Foetus is not growing at expected rate in the uterus
- Orthopaedic limitations
- Heavy smoker

Source: Adapted from American College of Obstetricians and Gynecologists Guidelines, 2015.

BOX 10.3 EXERCISE CONSIDERATIONS IN EACH TRIMESTER

First trimester

- May feel nauseous - vomiting, and light headedness may cause drop in performance level
- Vascular underfill leads to low blood pressure and higher heart rates
- Avoid hyperthermia (overheating) and high altitude training
- Choose moderate intensity aerobic exercise
- Use RPE to monitor intensity rather than heart rate
- Resistance training to focus on postural muscles that will become load bearing later in pregnancy
- Avoid contact sports, sky diving, scuba diving and sports with a high risk of falling e.g. ice skating (Bø et al., 2018)

Second trimester

- May be feeling more energised and motivated and may want to do too much but intensity and duration should decrease as pregnancy develops (Barakat et al., 2015)
- Relaxin is present so stretch and exercise from a stable base and avoid using a stability ball
- Changes in centre of gravity may start to cause instability
- Limit movement involving rapid changes of direction, high amounts of stability and high impact
- No supine lying after 16 weeks
- Moderate intensity aerobic exercise
- Keep resistance training at low intensity/high repetitions and modify exercises to account for bump
- Avoid contact sports through second and third trimesters

Third trimester

- Mother will have gained weight, and the size and position of the bump varies significantly between individuals
- May be constantly breathless, have pressure on their bladder and back pain
- They may find it difficult getting up and down from the floor so limit changes of exercise position
- Blood pressure may be rising, and they may have to be trained as a hypertensive
- Balance and stability will be considerably affected
- Training may need to be scaled down

All trimesters

- Ensure an additional 300 kcals are eaten per day and carbohydrate intake before exercise to cover energy cost of exercise (Kuhrt et al., 2015)
- Avoid excessively hot or humid environments
- Keep hydrated at all times by constantly sipping water
- If there are any adverse signs such as vaginal bleeding, abdominal pain, painful contractions, dizziness, headaches, chest pain or calf pain then stop exercise immediately and consult a doctor

In 2017 US tennis player Serena Williams won the Australian Open while in the first trimester of her pregnancy which showed athletes that it is safe and reasonable for pregnant women who already participate in high intensity activities to continue when pregnant (Gregg and Ferguson, 2017). To ensure they are exercising safely they will need to follow the guidelines presented in Box 10.3 and exercise under advice and supervision from their doctors. Despite being highly conditioned their bodies will still experience the physiological adaptations that occur during pregnancy, so precautions need to be taken to minimise the risk of injury.

There is a scarcity in literature with pregnant elite females as participants, but it is recommended that if they wish to continue strenuous exercise then they need to have a clear understanding of the risks and consider reducing training load during resistance training. Any activities where there is a risk of injury to the foetus need to be avoided and caution needs to be taken to avoid over-heating (American College of Obstetricians and Gynecologists, 2020).

Post-natal exercise

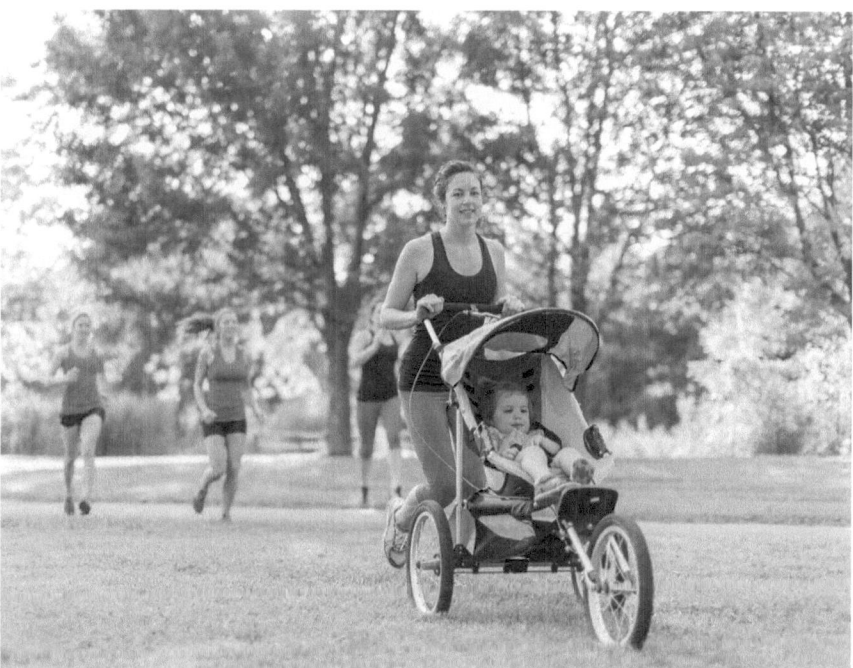

UK Sport (2021) offer guidelines to female athletes who are intending to return to training and competition post-partum and EIS support post-natal athletes through their SmartHER programme. There are also guidelines for women who wish to return to, or start, exercising. However, there are currently limited amounts of national or international guidelines available to health professionals, such as physiotherapists working with women who wish to return to sport after having a baby (Goom, Donnelly and Brockwell, 2019).

Exercise is important in the post-natal period to return the mother to her pre-pregnancy condition. The first consideration in the post-natal period is that the mother's focus is now likely to be on meeting the needs of their baby and adjusting to their changes in circumstance. For some women this can take up all of their energy and may make exercise less of a priority. However, athletic females are often keen to return to training as quickly as possible and while this has benefits it also has risks.

The benefits of post-natal exercise include increased weight loss, improved aerobic fitness, better energy levels and reductions in post-natal mood disturbances (Temme, 2015). The Chief Medical Officer (2019) for the UK presents guidance for women after childbirth saying they should aim for 150 minutes of moderate intensity activity every week. Activities should start gently and can include walking, running, cycling, and stretching. Pelvic floor exercises should be started as soon as possible and activity while breastfeeding is fine.

Whereas previously a more conservative approach was taken to post-natal exercise now post-natal women are encouraged to start exercise as soon as they feel able to after birth. UK Sport (2021) recommends that athletes should wait until they have been discharged by their NHS post-natal maternity team to return to training. This usually occurs between weeks 6 and 8 but is dependent upon whether there were any complications during childbirth.

However, there are caveats regarding any return to exercise, such as physical activity should reflect pre-pregnancy activity levels and any commencement or return to exercise should start gradually, and in particular vigorous activity is not recommended for previously inactive women. The Royal College of Obstetricians and Gynaecologists (2019) recommends that more intense activities can gradually resume, building up intensity from moderate to vigorous over a period of three months, after the 6–8 week post-natal check. The amount and intensity of exercise is always dependent on how the woman feels and they should listen to their body.

According to the NHS (2023), starting postnatal exercise will depend on the type of pregnancy and delivery the woman had, and the doctor should be consulted before starting any fitness program. Although it is possible to start exercising as soon as a week after giving birth, the optimal time to return to exercise depends upon several factors such as:

- What type of delivery – abdominal birth or vaginal birth
- Were there any complications during the birth
- Condition of abdominals and pelvic floor muscles

If there is concern about the safety of post-natal exercise it may be preferable to wait until after the week 6 post-natal check up with a doctor, particularly before any high-impact exercise.

Once exercise is resumed it is advised to stay active for periods of 30 minutes a day and choose low-impact aerobic activities like walking, swimming, or yoga, to avoid excessive loading of the pelvic floor and abdominal muscles. If the birth has been without complications then it is important to start working to regain tone and strength in the abdominal muscles, starting with gentle tightening and relaxing exercises. It is also vital at this time that the breasts are well supported, and there is concern that a sports bra may compress the breasts and cause discomfort (Temme, 2015). It is advisable to wear a sports bra that supports rather than compresses the breasts (McGhee et al., 2013) as this may be more comfortable.

Diastasis recti

One major concern in the post-natal period is stretching and weakening of the abdominal muscles and in particular a condition called diastasis recti that can occur during pregnancy. Diastasis recti is characterised by a widening of the linea alba, which is a fibrous structure connecting the two sides of the rectus abdominis muscle (Mommers et al., 2017). It results in a splitting or widening of the rectus abdominus, as shown in Figure 10.4, and can cause a bulge in the midline when there is an increase in intra-abdominal pressure.

While diastasis recti can occur during the pregnancy when the contents of the enlarged abdomen press on the abdominal wall, it only becomes a consideration in the post-natal period. Owing to this weakening of these core muscles it can increase instability and cause poor posture and back pain. Initially the separation of the abdominal muscles will reduce over the first eight weeks but then it needs to be strengthened through a progressive programme of core training. Training should start with graded abdominal strengthening starting with breathing exercises and pelvic tilts (Royal University Hospital Bath, 2023).

For women who have particularly weak abdominal muscles after birth a set of breathing and exercises, called hypopressives, can be beneficial and a good starting point. These exercises involve breathing in fully and then sucking in the stomach after a full exhalation. The stomach is sucked in for around 10–20 seconds. These exercises also help to strengthen the pelvic floor that may have become weakened.

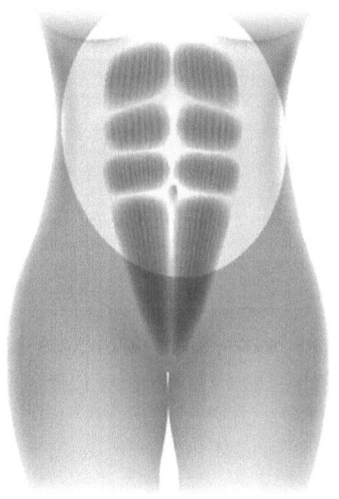
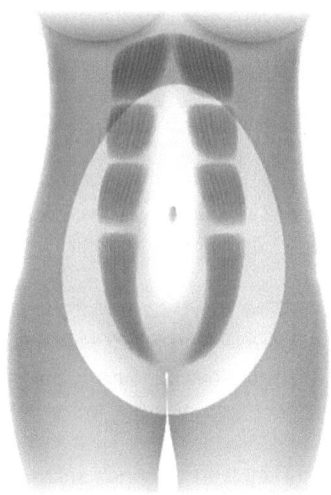

NORMAL ABDOMEN

DIASTASIS RECTI

FIGURE 10.4 Comparison of abdominal muscles showing diastasis recti and normal abdominal muscles
Source: Shutterstock

BOX 10.4 SPOTLIGHT ON RETURN TO SPORT POST-PREGNANCY

UK Sport (2021) recommends that all athletes should only return to their training programme once they have been discharged by their NHS doctor and midwife and also their sport's governing body and doctors are satisfied that they are ready. There is no set time frame to this, as UK Sport (2021) acknowledges that each case needs to be considered individually. They recommend a multidisciplinary approach to develop an effective strength and conditioning programme, including their main coach, strength and conditioning coach, physiotherapist and a physiotherapist specialising in pelvic health.

Considerations of exercise in the post-natal period

The following physiological changes need to be addressed during any return to sport training programme:

- Joint laxity owing to relaxin still being present, particularly if breast feeding
- Weakened pelvic floor muscles
- Weak abdominal muscles, particularly after a C-Section
- Possible symphysis pubis dysfunction, owing to uneven movement of the pelvis
- Muscle imbalances created during pregnancy
- Larger breasts as a result of lactation (if breast feeding)
- Amount and quality of sleep

Return to sport will be different for each athlete and dependent upon the specific demands of their sport. In particular athletes will need to consider:

- Is it high impact?
- How much twisting and turning is involved?
- What is the exercise intensity level?
- Is there risk of injury from external objects?

Many sports have high impact elements whether it is running or landing from jumps. High-impact activity is associated with a sudden increase in intra-abdominal pressure (Leitner et al., 2016) and this puts stress on the pelvic floor and also the looser joints. Athletes in the post-natal period need both adequate time to heal and train the pelvic floor to avoid dysfunction.

Athletes in sports such as netball and football need to be aware that the raised levels of relaxin in their body may cause joint laxity and, although it is not proven, may increase the risk of joint injury. Although it is not fully understood breast feeding alters the hormonal environment and results in relaxin staying in the body for longer.

This spotlight has focused on physiological changes in the postnatal period; however, there will be psychological changes as well and in particular the mother/athlete may experience changes to their identity. This is explored in Chapter 11 Motherhood and elite performance.

BOX 10.5 REAL-WORLD APPLICATION

As a female athlete, you should:

- Be familiar with exercise guidelines and be able to adapt training and performance to ensure they are safe during pregnancy.
- Be aware of the physiological changes that occur to the cardiovascular, respiratory, musculoskeletal systems, owing to the changing hormonal environment and how they impact on training and performance.
- Know the risks of injury owing to changes in hormone levels and the extra stress on the abdominal and pelvic floor muscles.
- Be able to identify warning signs of when to stop exercising and any contraindications to exercise.

As a coach, you should:

- Understand how pregnancy may affect the female body and athletic performance.
- adapt training schedules across the three trimesters in accordance with the physiological and hormonal changes that occur.
- adapt exercises to account for the bump, postural changes, and to avoid any potential harm to the foetus.
- adapt the training environment to limit any risk factors for foetal hypoxia or foetal hyperthermia.

Summary

Exercise in pregnancy and the post-natal period are both essential in ensuring the wellbeing and health of the mother and baby. Exercising correctly at these times will prepare the mother for the birth and ensure that they can return to normal everyday activities and functions after the birth. This is particularly important for female athletes who wish to return to competition as quickly as possible. However, all too often women reduce their activity levels during pregnancy as they do not know what to do and are worried that exercise will have a detrimental on their baby. This is referred to as 'benign neglect' of women and it can have undesirable, long term effects on both mother and baby (Segal and Chu, 2015). Understanding the changes to the body during pregnancy and how training needs to be adapted is vital for pregnant female athletes and those working with them.

The key messages to take away from this chapter are:

1. Exercise during pregnancy brings many benefits for both pregnant women and their babies, including less risk of high blood pressure, pre-eclampsia, and gestational diabetes.
2. Hormone levels in the body will increase to support pregnancy leading to a potential increase joint laxity and reduction in body stability.
3. The cardiovascular and respiratory systems adapt during pregnancy to increase blood volume and minute volume.
4. uring pregnancy the pelvic floor muscles can become stretched and weakened, owing to increased loading from the abdomen and this can cause stress incontinence.
5. UK Chief Medical Officer (2019) guidelines for women with uncomplicated pregnancies show that they should aim for 30 minutes of moderate intensity exercise a day and should include strength training twice a week.
6. Exercise in the post-natal period should start as soon as the woman feels ready, and they should aim for 30 minutes of moderate intensity exercise a day and should include strength training twice a week.
7. Post-natal exercise should focus on returning muscle strength and tone to the abdominal and pelvic floor muscles.

End-of-Chapter Quiz

Answers can be found after the References

1. Identify of the following hormones is responsible for vasodilation of the blood vessels during pregnancy:

   a   Oestrogen
   b   Relaxin
   c   Testosterone
   d   Progesterone

2. Identify what is meant by the term 'pre-eclampsia':

   a   Pregnancy related joint laxity
   b   Pelvic floor dysfunction
   c   Pregnancy related hypertension
   d   Gestational type 2 diabetes

3. Identify which of the following should not be performed from the second trimester onwards:

   a   Exercise at a high intensity
   b   Strength training exercises
   c   Exercise lying on the back
   d   Exercising every day

4. Identify which of the following is a post-natal guideline for exercise after birth:

   a   Women should exercise immediately after the birth
   b   Women should exercise when they feel ready
   c   Women should exercise after their week 6 check up
   d   Women should exercise once their abdominals have strengthened

5. Identify what is meant by 'diastasis recti':

   a   Splitting of the connection between abdominal muscles
   b   Stretched pelvic floor muscles resulting from pregnancy
   c   Post-pregnancy lower back pain from carrying a baby
   d   Pelvic pain resulting from the birth of the baby

References

American College of Obstetricians and Gynecologists (2020) ACOG Committee Opinion Number 804 'Physical Activity and Exercise During Pregnancy and the Postpartum period. *Obstetrics and Gynecology*, 135(4), 178–188.

Ahrens, K.A., Vladitiu, C.J., Mumford, S.L., Schliep, K.C., Perkins, N.J., Wactawski-Wende, J. and Schisterman, E.F. (2014) The effect of physical activity across the menstrual cycle on reproductive function. *Annals of Epidemiology*, 24(2), 127–134.

Barakat, R., Lucia, A. and Ruiz, J. (2015) Exercise and pregnancy. In M. Mountjoy (Ed.), *The Female Athlete*. New Jersey: Wiley.

Berghella, V. and Saccone, G. (2017) Exercise in pregnancy. *American Journal of Obstetrics and Gynecology*, 216, 335–337.

Bø, K., Artal, R., Barakat, R., Brown, W.J., Davies, G.A.L., Evenson, K.R., Haakstad, L.A.H, Kayser, B., Kinnunen, T.I, Larsen, K., Mottola, M.F, Nygaard, I., van Poppel, M., Stuge, B. and Khan, K.M. (2018) Exercise and pregnancy in recreational and elite athletes: 2016/2017 evidence summary from the IOC expert group meeting, Lausanne. Part 5 – Recommendations for health professionals and active women. *British Journal of Sports Medicine*, 52(17), 1080–1085.

Charkoudian, N. and Stachenfeld, N. (2016) Sex hormone effects on autonomic mechanisms of thermoregulation in humans. *Autonomic Neuroscience*, 196, 75–80.

Davenport, M.H., Kathol, A.J., Mottola, M.F., Skow, R.J., Meah, V.L., Poitras, V.J., Garcia, A.J., Gray, C.E., Barrowman, N., Riske, L., Sobierajska, F., James, M., Nagpal, T., Marchand, A., Slater, L.G., Adamo, K.B., Davies, G.A., Barakat, R. and Ruchat, S.M. (2019). Prenatal exercise is not associated with fetal mortality: A systematic review and meta-analysis. *British Journal of Sports Medicine*, 53(2), 108–115.

Draca, S. (2006) Estriol and progesterone: a new role for sex hormones. *International Journal of Biomedical Science*, 2(4), 305–307.

Dehghan, F., Haerian, B.S., Muniandy, S., Yusuf, A., Dragoo, J.L. and Salleh, N. (2014) The effect of relaxin on the musculoskeletal system. *Scandinavian Journal of Sports Science*, 24(4), 220–229.

Dunn, A.B., Jordan, S., Baker, B.J. and Carlson, N.S. (2017) The Maternal Infant Microbiome: Considerations for Labor and Birth. *American Journal of Maternity and Child Nursing*, 42(6), 318–325.

Fiat, F., Merghes, P.E., Scurta, A.D., Guta, B.A., Dehelean, C.A., Varan, N. and Bernad, E. (2022) The Main Changes in Pregnancy – The Therapeutic Approach to Musculoskeletal Pain. *Medicina (Kaunas)*, 58(8), 1115.

Goom, T., Donnelly, G. and Brockwell, E. (2019) Returning to running postnatal – guidelines for medical, health and fitness professionals managing this population. *Physiotherapy*, 107(1). doi:10.1016/j.physio.2020.03.276.

Gregg, V.H. and Ferguson, J.E. II (2017) Exercise in Pregnancy. *Clinical Sports Medicine*, 36, 741–752.

Kuhrt, K., Hezelgrove, N.L. and Shennan, A.H. (2015) Exercise in Pregancy. *The Obsterician and Gyaecologist*, 17, 281–287.

Leitner, M., Moser, H., Eichelberger, P., Kuhn, A. and Radlinger, L. (2016) Evaluation of pelvic floor muscle activity during running in continence and incontinence women: An exploratory study. *Neurourology and Urodynamics*, 36(6), 1570–1576.

McGhee, D.E., Steele, J.R., Zealey, W.J. and Takacs, G.J. (2013) Bra-breast forces generated in women with large breasts while standing and during treadmill running: implications for sports bra design. *Applied Ergonomics*, 44(1), 112–118.

Mommers, E.H.H., Ponten, J.E., Omar, A.K.A., Reilingh, T.S. de V., Bouvy, N.D. and Nienhuijs, S.W. (2017) The general surgeon's perspective of rectus diastasis> A systematic review of treatment options. *Surgical endoscopy*, 31(12), 4934–4949.

NHS (2023) Keeping fit and healthy with a baby. Available online at: www.nhs.uk/conditions/baby/support-and-services/keeping-fit-and-healthy-with-a-baby (Accessed 12 October 2023).

Pitchers, G., Elliott-Sale, K.J., DeVivo, M., Donelon, T., Mills, H., Brockwell, E. and Donnelly, G. (2020) Pregnancy in the Female Athlete – Part 1: Antenatal. *Professional Strength & Conditioning*, 58, 15–22.

Reese, M.E. & Casey, E. (2015) Hormonal influence on the neuromusculoskeletal system in pregnancy. In C.M. Fitzgerald & N.A. Segal (Eds), *Musculoskeletal Health in Pregnancy and Postpartum: An Evidence- Based Guide for Clinicians*, pp. 19–39. Cham: Springer International Publishing.

Roberts, C. and Kenatta, G. (2018) *Motherhood as an athletic transition*. Women in Sport and Physical Activity Conference, Stoke-on-Trent, Staffordshire.

Roberts, J.M., Pearson, G.D., Cutler, J.A. and Lindheimer, M.D. (2003) Summary of NHLBI Working Group on Research on Hypertension during Pregnancy. *Hypertension in Pregnancy*, 22, 143–146.

Royal University Hospitals Bath (2023) Diastasis Rectus Abdominis. Available online at: DRA (ruh.nhs.uk) (Accessed 12 November 2023).

Segal, N.A. and Chu, S.R. (2015) Musculoskeletal Anatomic, Gait, and Balance Changes in Pregnancy and Risk for Falls. In C.M. Fitzgerald & N.A. Segal (Eds), *Musculoskeletal Health in Pregnancy and Postpartum: An Evidence- Based Guide for Clinicians*, pp. 19–39. Cham: Springer International Publishing.

Soma-Pillay, P., Catherine, N., Tolpannen, H. and Mebazaa, A. (2016) Physiological changes in pregnancy. *Cardiovascular Journal of Africa*, 27(2), 89–94.

Temme, K.E. (2015) Exercise in pregnancy and Postpartum. In C.M. Fitzgerald and N.A. Segal (Eds), *Musculoskeletal Health in Pregnancy and Postpartum: An Evidence-Based Guide for Clinicians*. New York: Springer.

Tillet, E., DeVito, M., Mills, H. and Johnson, B. (2019) Royal College of Nursing Physical Activity Factsheet 11 – Physical Activity and Pregnancy.

UK Chief Medical Officer (2019) UK Chief Medical Officer's Physical Activity Guidelines. Available at: https://assets.publishing.service.gov.uk/media/5d839543ed915d52428dc134/uk-chief-medical-officers-physical-activity-guidelines.pdf (Accessed 17 October 2023).

UK Sport (2021) Pregnancy Guidance and Support for UK Funded Athletes. Available at: www.uksport.gov.uk/resources/pregnancy-guidance(Accessed 12 November 2023).

Verdière, S., Guinhouya, B.C., Salerno, D. and Deruelle, P. (2017) Should physical activity be contraindicated during pregnancy in relation to its potentially related risks? . *Gynecology Obstetrics Fertility and Senology*, 45(2), 104–111.

Westcott, W.L. and Faigenbaum, A.D. (2021) Clients who are preadolescent, older or pregnant. In B.J. Schoenfeld and R.L. Snarr (Eds), *NSCA's Essentials of Personal Training*. Champaign: Human Kinetics.

Wylie, L. (2005) *Essential anatomy and physiology in maternity care* (2nd ed.). London: Elsevier.

Answers

1. d
2. c
3. c
4. b
5. a

11

NAVIGATING MOTHERHOOD AND ATHLETIC PERFORMANCE

Candice Lingam-Willgoss and Jess Pinchbeck

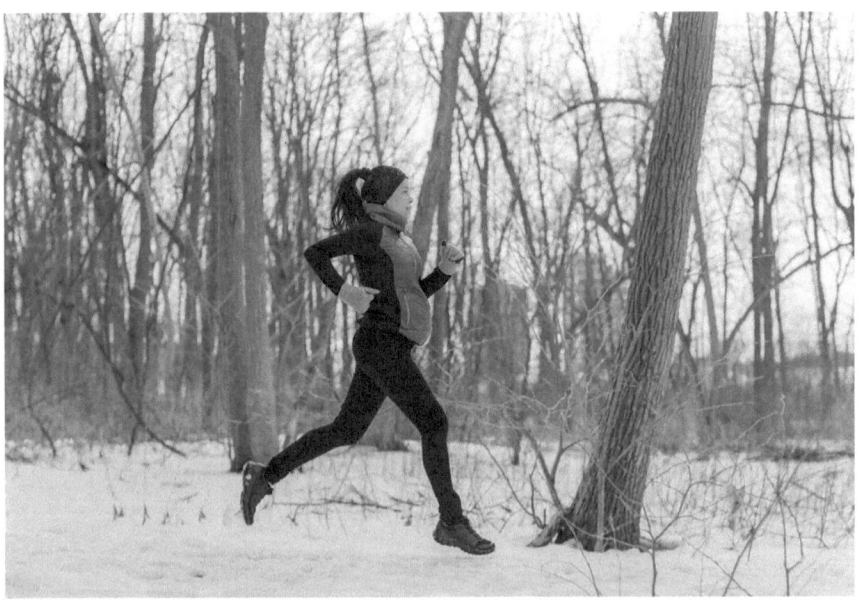

Introduction

The growth in female sport participation, has created a demand to develop the level of knowledge and understanding of specific factors related to elite female athletes (Castanier et al., 2021). One area that has generated research interest in recent years relates to the experiences of the mother athlete.

Becoming a parent has been recognised as one of the most significant events that can occur in a woman's life, and this transition can be all the

DOI: 10.4324/9781003330110-11

more meaningful for active females, because of both the physical implications and societal challenges related to gender ideology. Yet despite its importance, there is limited understanding of the impact of motherhood on participation and performance at both recreational and elite level. Traditionally women performing at elite level have been expected to coincide their retirement with starting a family due the expectation that they will be unable to resume the same standard of performance, owing to the physiological impact of childbirth as well as taking on childcare. While some female athletes do decide to wait until retirement to start a family it is becoming increasingly common for elite athletes to pursue their athletic career alongside motherhood and strive for both career and maternal success.

Several high-profile elite athletes have raised the visibility of athletic mothers. For example, Paula Radcliffe won the 2007 New York marathon 10 months after giving birth to her daughter. Likewise, ten months after giving birth to her second child, five-time Olympian Jo Pavey became the oldest female in European champion history to win the 10,000m gold at the 2014 European Championships. Following in their footsteps, more athletes, such as Laura Kenny (cycling) and Serena Williams (tennis) both successfully returned to elite sport after becoming mothers, although both have now retired, whereas Jessica Ennis-Hill struggled to return to elite sport once becoming a mother. Their stories highlight the need to further understand this transition with the aim of supporting more female athletes to compete following motherhood.

You have already been introduced to several of the physical challenges associate with pregnancy in Chapter 10, but it is important to contextualise the impact that the reduction in training during pregnancy has on an athlete's return to sport. Research by Tekavc et al. (2020) showed that the physical impact of pregnancy (both during and after) is also important, such as a decline in physical capabilities related to endurance, strength and balance. Furthermore, there have been many cases of elite athletes citing increases in injuries such as stress fractures which have been attributed to the limited post-partum advice available to them (Sundgot-Borgen et al., 2019).

For athletes, and those working alongside female athletes, it is important to recognise that the impact of motherhood is wider than just the physical impact. The return to sport may also involve conflict as women strive to manage both the demands of their sport and those of a mother. For example, both the emotional and psychological impact of motherhood, such as guilt and a loss of athletic identity, can present a challenge. This chapter will explore the various challenges of motherhood and sport illustrated below in Figure 11.1, and the impact of motherhood on the return to sport and athletic performance, for both elite and recreational athletes.

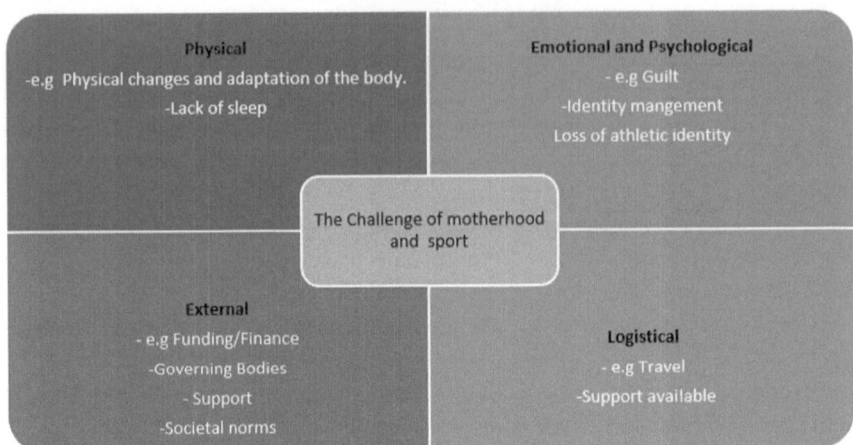

FIGURE 11.1 Factors to consider when balancing motherhood and sport
Source: adapted from Lingam-Willgoss and Heaney (2021)

Before we start to examine this topic more fully read the case study below in Box 11.1 where you are introduced to Yvonne, an elite runner who decided to have a baby in the middle of her career and return to competition.

BOX 11.1 YVONNE (RUNNER)

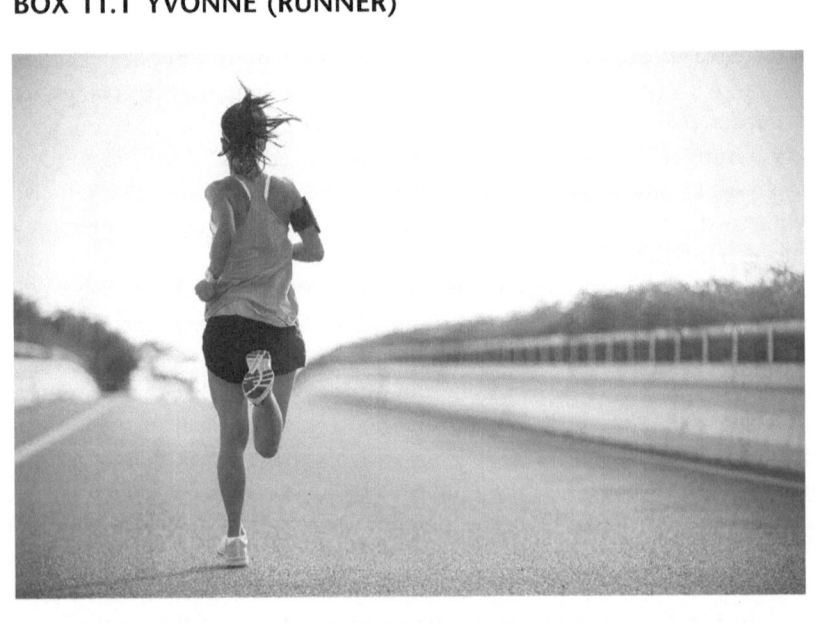

Yvonne is a 30-year-old runner and has represented Great Britain and has competed at Olympic level in the marathon. Following her last Olympics, she took a break from running to focus on having a baby as both her and her husband didn't want to wait any longer to start a family.

Yvonne had some concerns about getting pregnant as her sport meant she had relatively low body weight and her periods were at times irregular; however, she fell pregnant immediately. She managed to continue to run during her pregnancy although she carefully monitored her heart rate to ensure she wasn't stressing her body. She continued to run up until five days before giving birth to her daughter. Yvonne always planned to return to running and had thought maintaining running during her pregnancy would make her return easier.

She had a very challenging labour resulting in an emergency caesarean section. She spent several weeks unable to walk which impacted her mental health as she struggled to accept the changes to her body. Yvonne felt very lost and while her husband tried to support her she missed running as it was so much part of who she was. As her body began to recover, a visit from a new midwife marked a turning point for Yvonne. The midwife listened to her and shifted the focus away from being a mother and back to her, identifying the need to get her back doing what she loved.

Yvonne slowly started to return to running, and even if she went out and felt too tired to run, she used the time to walk and feel like herself again. While this was a slow return, 14 months after giving birth Yvonne represented Great Britain again at the European Championships. She recognised how her return was directly down to the support she received both from professionals (midwife), her husband and her coach who all provided tangible help in the form of advice and childcare.

Yvonne recognised how her career was different as a mother, as her priorities had shifted somewhat, while she loved to run and be an athlete, her identity as a mother was more important. She aimed to train in a way that minimised impact on her daughter and family to avoid feeling guilty and acknowledged how support was essential. She also noted how she felt less pressure once she had a child as even when things weren't going well she put that in the broader perspective of her life and was able to rationalise things better.

Yvonne's experience of pregnancy and motherhood are in no way unique but illustrate how there are several factors to consider for athletes as they negotiate their return to sport. The shift from athlete to mother athlete carries with it some significant adaptations to identity which can be a challenge to navigate. A key point noted in the case study is that getting the right support at the right time is key, if athletes are to make a return to training and competition.

Athletic identity and motherhood

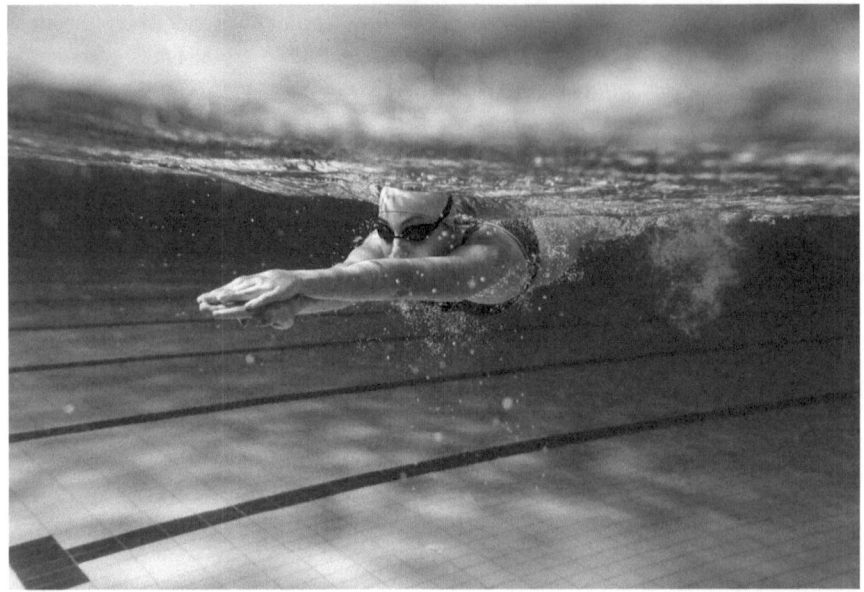

Before looking at athletic identity and motherhood in more depth it is key to consider the concept of identity more broadly. Erikson (1968) described identity as a largely unconscious and constantly evolving perception of who someone is, both as an individual and in terms of where they fit in broader society. For example, among other things you may be a student fitting into a college or university culture, thus reinforcing one aspect of your identity as 'the student'. In the context of this chapter 'athletic identity' is most relevant. A term conceptualised by Brewer et al. (1993, p. 237) as the 'degree to which an individual identifies with the athlete role'.

Athletic identity is shaped by three key factors: a) the strength of the individual's identification with the athlete role; b) the individual's response to setback or failures in this the athlete role (such as an injury); and c) whether they have any other roles (how exclusive is their athlete role). Athletic identity is particularly significant at elite level because athletes can develop a uni-dimensional identity where they only identify with the athletic side of themselves. Subsequently, when their athletic identity is threatened or disrupted athletes can experience several difficulties. Pregnancy and motherhood may cause a disruption to identity as this period will normally represent a time away from typical training and competition. This can result in the athlete feeling less connection with their athletic self as they are unable to fulfil their athlete role.

Research by Tekavc et al. (2020) showed that athletes attempting to combine motherhood with elite sports experienced a direct impact on their athletic identity. The women in their study felt since the birth of their child that their physical capabilities diminished, meaning they were less likely to feel like an athlete. Feelings such as these can carry with them several emotional and psychological challenges that are important for athletes and coaches to be prepared for and aware of.

Women can often struggle to balance their identity as a mother as well as an athlete. Palmer and Leberman (2009) found that elite females from a range of sports, who had all become mothers and continued to compete, did so successfully by finding ways to manage their two different roles. The women discussed how they put energy into negotiating guilt, because their athletic identity was so integral to who they were as people, it was essential that multiple identities were managed appropriately, something they termed 'identity management'. For example, the women would ensure they had fulfilled their role as a mother first so that they didn't feel guilty when they went to train.

These findings share similarities with those of Bean and Wimbs (2021), who examined the experiences of recreational runners. The women in their study strove to maintain their runner identity as well as their mother identity. This point raises an interesting learning for coaches who may perceive that the athlete mother is less committed to their sport, when in fact they are likely to have stronger commitment shown through their desire and ability to manage the two roles.

While the period of pregnancy can be a challenge where athletes have to adapt and sometimes refrain from training the return to sport post pregnancy can present different challenges. The strength of the mother identity has frequently been cited as superseding that of athlete, with athletes reporting that it can lead to a shift in priorities often knocking sport off the number one spot (Lingam-Willgoss, 2023). This was mentioned by our case study athlete Yvonne who noticed that running was no longer her top priority following the birth of her daughter.

Different sports and motherhood

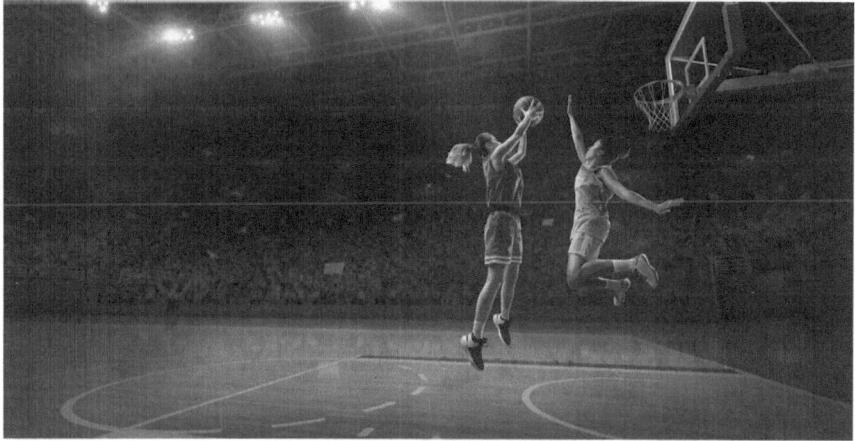

Research examining physical activity during pregnancy suggests that being physically active is beneficial to both mother and foetus, however, not all forms of physical activity or sport will be appropriate (Barakat et al., 2015). It is recommended that higher risk sports such as those with risk of trauma (e.g. hockey), physiological risk (e.g. scuba diving) and collision (e.g. downhill skiing) should be avoided (Barakat et al., 2015). In contrast, research exploring low risk sports has indicated that it is possible for competitive athletes to maintain strenuous regimes during their pregnancy and train at high volume (Kardel, 2005). This can result in a quicker return to high intensity training postpartum and a more rapid return to competition (Erdener and Budgett, 2016).

As well as the training implications of different sports both during pregnancy and when returning to sport, logistical differences between sports need to be considered. One such comparison is between team and individual sports. Team sport athletes have little control over their schedules with training and competition times and locations dictated by others. These constraints could prove problematic for a returning mother although research shows that team sport athletes with appropriate social support are able to overcome such logistical barriers (Pinchbeck, 2021). In contrast, a runner like Yvonne, faces fewer constraints as she can fit training around her life and child. A run can be completed at any suitable time straight from her home, and even indoors on a treadmill, her training is not dictated by external schedules.

Furthermore, while there are complexities attached to team sports environments there are some sports that carry even more logistical challenges. This was explored by McGannon and Schinke (2013), who looked at the varying experiences of athletes from different types of sport specifically those that require specialist settings and significant travel for competition and training. Both of these factors can take a mother away from her family making a return to training and competition even more problematic. For example, research with female winter sports athletes recognised childcare as the biggest challenge when travelling, and that their successful return to sport was only possible by family members travelling with them (Lingam-Willgoss, 2023). However, it is important to recognise that alongside these more obvious challenges athletic mothers also face less tangible unpredictable factors related to the emotional and psychological shifts that motherhood entails.

Motherhood, sport and guilt

For those athletes where participation is logistically and physically possible during motherhood, some women still face psychological barriers. Most studies that look at the balancing of motherhood with a career in elite sport identify the concept of mother guilt. For example, Sutherland (2010) concluded that mother guilt it is often viewed as an inherent part of motherhood by society and linked closely to fear of negative self-evaluation. Yet, this is not limited to elite athletes and mother guilt is frequently highlighted in the broader relationship between physical activity and parenthood (McGannon et al., 2012). Women accept, when they have children, they will feel guilty about anything they do for themselves (McGannon and Schinke, 2013)

This concept that guilt becomes part of all mother's lives can be heightened in the case of elite athletes, as identity is challenged as athletes seek to fulfil two roles (sometimes viewed as incompatible) and manage the associated guilt. Culture and society can also impact on the way in which athletes experience motherhood at both recreational and elite level, fuelled by the media. In a study of ten elite athletic mothers McGannon et al. (2015), reported the athlete and mother as conflicting identities which illustrated the polarised nature of these two roles. Media portrayals of the elite mothers were that they were in distress and felt guilt as a result of taking time away from their children for their sporting careers. Furthermore, the implication was that pursuing a career in sport could lead to them being inadequate mothers something that served to reinforce the guilt.

Later research by Darroch and Hillsbury (2017) on the postpartum return to training and international competition of elite distance runners revealed a predominant theme of the guilt associated with motherhood. Running required them to be selfish and motherhood demanded selflessness, presenting a tension between their athletic career and motherhood. Throughout their narratives, it was evident that these tensions stemmed from mothers constantly having to compromise, as if they reduce their training it impacts on their athletic performance and if they train more it increases their guilt. This resonates with findings by McGannon et al. (2015) whereby one participant was more 'at peace' with her training if she felt she had done what was required of her as a mother.

While the focus of this chapter so far has been on elite level athletes, many of the complexities of combining sport and motherhood are also seen at recreational level. Box 11.2 provides a brief summary of the challenges facing recreational athletes.

BOX 11.2 SPOTLIGHT ON: RECREATIONAL ATHLETES

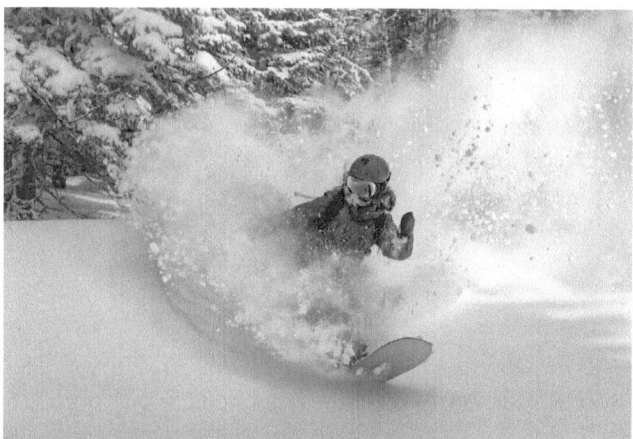

While elite athletic mothers may face tensions when combining these two roles many women who engage in recreational sport face similar challenges. Often, where women are engaged in the dual roles of both paid and domestic labour they face an impact on not only their time to engage in sport and physical activity but also their energies to do so (Scraton and Flintoff, 2013).

Women participating in recreational sport have to overcome challenges such as work demands including shift work and stress, competing hobbies, spending time with partners, childcare arrangements, children's own activities, as well as managing issues around cost, injury, and pregnancy (Pinchbeck, 2021).

For recreational athletes the pressure and the guilt experienced may even be greater than elite athletes as they are not leaving their child for work but for pleasure. In a study of snowboarding mothers Spowart et al. (2008) found that guilt was experienced when leaving their children to go snowboarding for the day or weekend. Yet, this was related to how the women felt they were being perceived, as a bad mother, with one mother saying she didn't admit to having a child when asked. This suggests that societal norms still underpin women's feelings about returning to sport as a mother, and that this can influence their feelings and lives at a subconscious level.

Research by Bean and Wimbs (2021) focused on the experiences of recreational marathon runners. Two clear themes generated from their findings were related to identity, conflict and management strategies, similar to studies on elite athletes. The decision to combine these two roles led to considerable internal conflict as all the mothers still prioritised their running, owing to the importance of their runner identity. Although this proved problematic with the women still feeling as though their runner identity was threatened. For example, one runner discussed how the shift from being defined as a runner who did adventure and long distance running to one who only managed 5km was hard on her ego. While all participants recognised that they shouldn't feel guilty they all still felt guilty about trying to balance multiple identities and not prioritising their mother identity, choosing running over other family related tasks. Their findings illustrate how even at recreational level the same challenges emerge that elite athletes have to contend with.

In addition to full time elite athletes and recreational athletes there are also those who perform at elite level but as a result of the nature of their sport have to remain in employment, meaning they have three conflicted roles linked to identity conflict and feelings of guilt.

The positive side to combining motherhood and sport

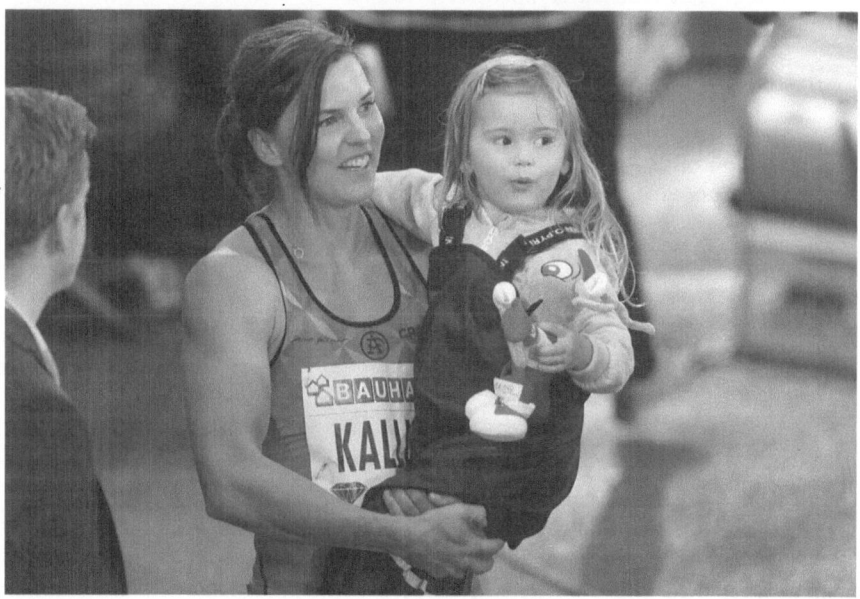

While there are challenges connected with motherhood and sport, there are also several positive outcomes. Within the case study Yvonne talked about how becoming a mother shifted her perspective and, in many ways, made her a better athlete as she was more able to cope with stressful events. This shift in perspective was also discussed by Darroch and Hillsbury (2017) who found that all the runners in their study linked motherhood to a changing of priorities and that this underpinned their change in perspective.

While this balancing act can result in some tension, research suggests that it can lead to positive outcomes. McGannon et al. (2012) examined this though a qualitative study that explored the development of multiple identities through textual analysis, specifically they examined the impact of the media on the construction of Paula Radcliffe's identity as both mother and athlete. They concluded that to successfully manage identity it could be that the two roles of mother and athlete are viewed as a 'newly melded identity' something which allowed Radcliffe to achieve both career and maternal success and negated conflict between identities. This new identity positions both roles as of equal importance that become intertwined suggesting that women can do both successfully. Furthermore, their findings suggest becoming a mother can give the athlete a different perspective on their sport allowing them to become a better athlete, which allows them to feel fulfilled in both areas of their life.

These findings are similar to earlier research of Appleby and Fisher (2009) that focused on runners. All of the women studied felt that the integration of their two identities of mother and athlete enriched their overall identity and signalled a form of self-enlightenment which allowed them to see motherhood as a strategy that reduced competitive pressure.

BOX 11.3 BEING A MUM MADE ME A BETTER ATHLETE

It's not a secret that I have my sights on 25 (Grand Slams), and actually, I think having a baby might help. When I'm too anxious I lose matches, and I feel like a lot of that anxiety disappeared when Olympia was born.

Serena Williams, tennis player, 2018, cited in Haskell, 2018

Before I became a mother, I would have been uptight and anxious about reaching my training targets, measuring my progress, worrying a session could have gone better; but [as a mother] I didn't have the time to dwell on it.

Jo Pavey, athlete, in Pavey, 2016

The positive side to combining a career in sport with motherhood was at the heart of research by McGannon et al. (2017) that focused on the comeback of tennis player Kim Clijsters who won three Grand Slam singles titles as a mother to add to the one she attained before motherhood. Their findings highlighted a shift in how sporting mothers were presented by the media. Her success was positioned in a positive way showing that it is possible to combine elite sport with motherhood. These findings contrast with more traditional narratives that a career (whether in sport or not) is incompatible with motherhood.

Findings such as these suggest that while motherhood does present challenges at the psychological and sociological level, there are ways to manage these and still pursue a (successful) elite career. Furthermore, the juggling of multiple roles may in fact make them better as parents allowing them time to themselves (McGannon et al., 2018). The concept that managing these two identities and allowing mothers time for themselves links to our case study athlete, Yvonne, who recognised a need to return to running to find herself again and the realisation that she felt she was a better mother when she had this time to herself. These findings are similar to those seen in recreational athletes where sport provides an opportunity to relieve the stresses of everyday life, including work and family, to provide a balance in women's lives and some 'time out' from life to maintain their mental wellbeing (Pinchbeck, 2021).

How to successfully combine motherhood and sport

So far within this chapter the complexities of the mother athlete dyad have been examined, however, a key theme in both the narratives of elite and recreational athletes is *how* sport and motherhood were managed and what strategies best support a successful return. Figure 11.2 illustrates how two key factors can facilitate the management of the athlete and mother role.

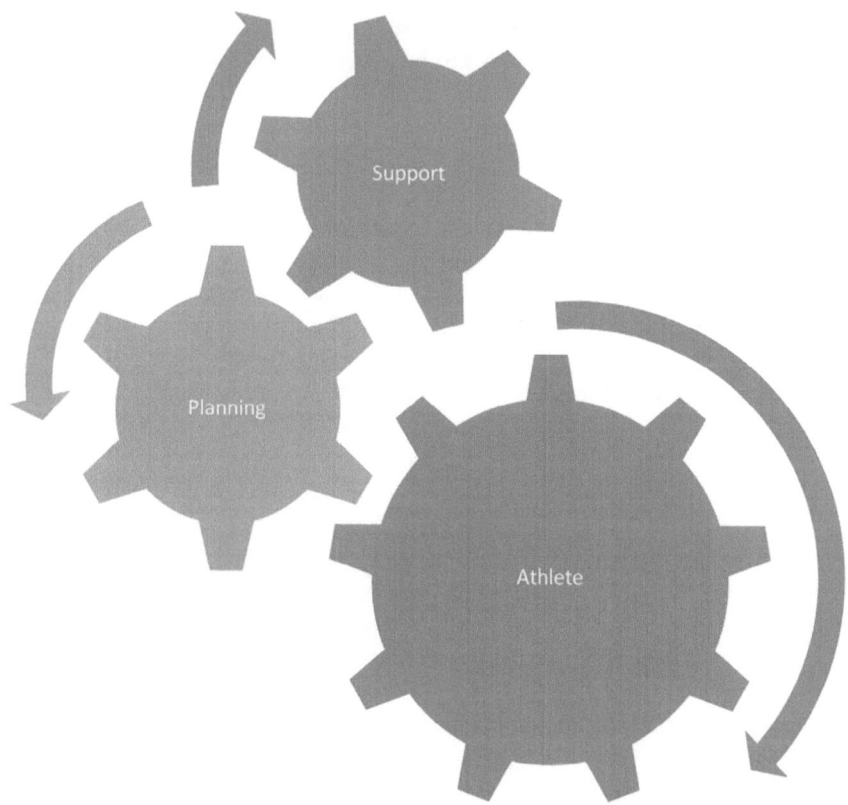

FIGURE 11.2 The key factors that allow athletes to return to sport

Support

The importance of support was considered by Bean and Wimbs (2021) from two perspectives. First, support was fundamental both in terms of whether a return was an option, and second, it proved essential when the athlete made the commitment to return. Specifically spousal support that was provided was both tangible in the form of childcare as well as emotional providing encouragement and motivation. The importance of spousal support was also discussed by Pinchbeck (2021) who reported that having children did not impact upon the participation of recreational netballers, however, being a mother did add an additional layer of negotiation to navigate, either involving childcare or the children's own activities. Support from partners, as well as parents, was vital in facilitating the women's netball participation. However, it is important to note that support is multifaced, it is provided by various sources and in different formats depending upon the specific needs of the athlete.

As well as the importance of emotional support, financial support is also a key consideration for the returning mother. Appleby and Fisher (2009) discussed how a lack of financial support could actually present a barrier to returning to sport. The importance of financial support was also discussed by Darroch et al. (2019) who explored the support from governing bodies and sponsors given to elite distance runners during pregnancy and the postpartum period. Athletes from five countries (Australia, Canada, Ireland, the UK, and the USA) reported a lack of support from corporate sponsors and governing bodies during pregnancy and the postpartum period. The athletes all discussed how there was an assumption that pregnancy marked the end of their career and as such financial support was removed including their sponsorship deals which carried significant financial implications for continuing their participation in sport.

A further point raised within Darroch et al's. (2019) study related to the lack of support in terms of policy for pregnant and returning athletes. The lack of clear policy saw pregnancy being treated in the same way as an injury or viewed as a clear sign that the athlete was retiring and did not warrant support. To mitigate for this the runners tried to manage and plan their pregnancies around competitions to reduce the financial impact and ensure they had adequate spousal support in cases where they had lost support from their governing body. While complex, the findings illustrate how female athletes may face considerable stress and uncertainty at this point in their career highlighting how some practices within elite sport environments may significantly disadvantage female athletes.

Planning

The notion of planning pregnancy to reduce impact on the athlete's career is not unique with research indicating that the timing of both the decision to have a baby and getting pregnant coincided in many cases with the four-year Olympic cycle (Tekavc et al. 2020). By timing their pregnancy, the athletes were able to minimise the impact of their time out of sport and reduce the number of major competitions missed. This was strengthened by maintaining a relatively high training volume during pregnancy, which allowed athletes the chance to return to high-intensity training postpartum, resulting in a more rapid return to competition (Kardel, 2005; Erdener and Budgett, 2016).

The maintenance of regular exercise was also discussed by Tekavc et al. (2020) who reported that athletes strived to maintain basic fitness to facilitate a quicker and more successful return to sport, although, athletes reduced training load during pregnancy and their level of athletic participation. However, as discussed this can partly relate to type of sport they play, as this can determine how long and what type of training an athlete can continue with. However, it is important to recognise that, while athletes tend to manage to maintain a level of training, there will nevertheless be a decline in fitness and physical capabilities which, like injury, can take time to regain (McGannon et al., 2012).

Recommendations for supporting athletic mothers

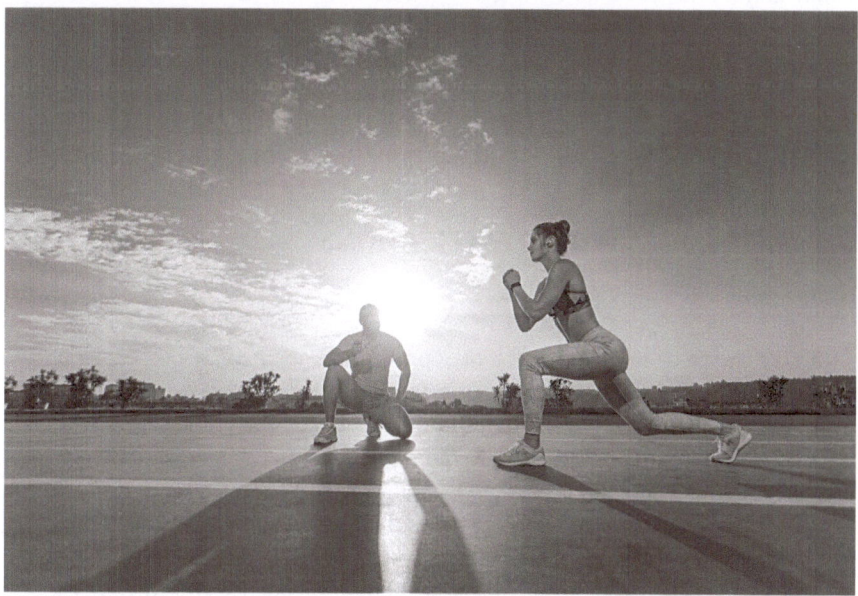

While some research has looked at the experiences of the returning mother there is still limited guidance on how to return to exercise after childbirth most notably when the return is to elite-level competition (Deering and Christopher, 2020). Of the limited research within this area, Sundgot-Borgen et al. (2019) concluded that most elite and non-elite athletes made a return to sport or exercise six weeks postpartum, however, during this time elite athletes reported stress fractures and concerns with body image, as well as feeling dissatisfied with the advice they were given. Chapter 10 provides further detail of the anatomical and physiological impact of birth and the postpartum issues. However, research indicates that there is still a lack of understanding, knowledge, and support during this potentially vulnerable period, suggesting that more needs to be done during this phase of the athlete journey to facilitate the returning athlete both in terms of knowledge and broader support.

While further studies are needed to fully appreciate how to support athletic mothers, research to date suggests that more work is needed from within sport to improve this experience for women. Greater education and awareness is needed of the psychological and physiological impact of pregnancy and motherhood on women. Specifically, those working with female athletes need to understand more about the impact on physical identity so that they are able to support women as they negotiate the changes to their physical as well as psychological self. Some fitness trainers and coaches specialise in pre- and postnatal training to support athletes; however, the elite athlete may need additional support beyond that of the coach.

More broadly, governing bodies and sponsors need to recognise that pregnancy and motherhood do not signal the end of an athlete's career and financial support should be maintained to allow their return to be managed in the most supportive manner. Finally, the lack of clear maternity policy in several sports leads to a lack of clarity about how to manage and support returning mothers. More work needs to be considered within this specific area to avoid inadequate or risky protocols being applied during the return to sport phase.

BOX 11.4 REAL-WORLD APPLICATIONS

As a female athlete, you should:

- Be aware of the importance of support throughout both pregnancy and motherhood. Support may come from family and friends but also from other sources such as the sporting organisation.
- Accept that motherhood will require a redefinition of self from athlete to mother athlete, often involving learning to accept some form of guilt.
- Be flexible in your approach to training both during pregnancy and during your return to sport as everyone's experience is different.
- Consider the demands of your sport both in pregnancy and when making a return.
- Talk to other mother athletes who have made a successful return to sport.

As a coach, you should:

- Ensure you understand the training implications both during pregnancy and when an athlete is returning to sport.
- Do not set targets for athletes until they are ready to do so.
- Have no set time frame for the return to training and competition.
- Appreciate the additional physiological, psychological and sociological demands on the athlete when they return as a mother.
- Ensure athletes have access to specialist advice when making their return to training.

Summary

Throughout this chapter you will have developed a more comprehensive understanding of both the challenges and experiences of combining motherhood with elite sport, as well as factors that are also applicable to recreational athletes. Key factors such as the impact on athletic identity and guilt have illustrated how this period can present several challenges to the elite athlete. However, in contrast to more established narratives the combining of an elite sports career with motherhood is achievable and can result in longer term success and a more fulfilled athlete. The chapter concludes by identifying some of the key points that athletes and coaches need to consider when either experiencing or working with an athletic mother.

The key messages to take away from this chapter are:

1. Combining an elite sports career with motherhood is achievable and does not have to impact on future success.
2. Athletes need to be well supported during their return to training and an element of flexibility is needed to accommodate the uncertainty related to the physical recovery post-partum.
3. Social support is essential for female athletes to return to sport following the birth of a child.
4. Motherhood sees an athlete have to manage two very strong identities and this may present a challenge.

End-of-Chapter Quiz

Answers can be found after the References

1. Identify the accurate definition of athletic identity:

    a   How much training an athlete does
    b   When an athlete competes at elite level
    c   degree to which an individual views themselves as an athlete
    d   how an athlete becomes more of an athlete the longer they have competed

2. Identify which of the following is NOT something athletes note a significant decline in during pregnancy and in the postpartum period:

    a   Decreased aerobic endurance
    b   Decreased muscular strength
    c   Decreased strategic awareness
    d   Decreased sense of balance

3. Which of the following two are benefits of being a sporting mother:

    a   You can present a positive role-model for your child
    b   Reduced sleep can enhance performance
    c   A shift in priorities which led to a reduction in anxiety.
    d   Having time away from your child to rest

4. What is the most important factor when it comes to elite athletic mothers managing their return to training and competition?

    a   A very strict and ridged training plan
    b   Ensuring a strong social support group

    c   Try and take their children with them to training

    d   Be motivated to re-gain lost funding

5.   As a coach, which of the following points is most important when supporting a returning female athlete?

    a   Ensure they are treated the same as all members of the team with no special treatment

    b   Ensuring you have a clear understanding of the training implications for the returning athlete post-partum

    c   Give them rigid time frames to return to training and competition

    d   Have competitive goals from the outset

References

Appleby, K.M. & Fisher, L.A. (2009). "Running in and out of motherhood": elite distance runners' experiences of returning to competition after pregnancy. *Women in Sport and Physical Activity Journal*, 18(1), 3–17.

Barakat, R., Perales, M., Garatachea, N., Ruiz, J.R. and Lucia, A. (2015) Exercise during pregnancy. A narrative review asking: what do we know? *British journal of sports medicine*, 49(21), 1377–1381.

Bean, C. and Wimbs, R.L. (2021) Running from (with) Mom Guilt: Exploring Experiences of Being a Mother and Training for and Running Marathons. *Leisure/Loisir*, pp. 1–23.

Brewer, B, Van Raalte, J. and Linder, D. (1993) Athletic identity: Hercules' muscles or Achilles heel? *International Journal of Sport Psychology*, 24(2), 237–254.

Castanier, C., Bougault, V., Teulier, C., Jaffré, C., Schiano-Lomoriello, S., Vibarel-Rebot, N., Villemain, A., Rieth, N., Le-Scanff, C., Buisson, C. and Collomp, K. (2021). The Specificities of Elite Female Athletes: A Multidisciplinary Approach. *Life*, 11(7), 622.

Darroch, F and Hillsbury, H. (2017) Keeping pace: Mother versus athlete identity among elite long distance runners. *Women's Studies International Forum*, 62, 61–68.

Darroch, F.E., Giles, A.R., Hillsburg, H. and McGettigan-Dumas, R. (2019) Running from responsibility: athletic governing bodies, corporate sponsors, and the failure to support pregnant and postpartum elite female distance runners. *Sport in Society*.

Deering, R.E., Christopher, S.M. and Heiderscheit, B.C., 2020. From Childbirth to the Starting Blocks: Are We Providing the Best Care to Our Postpartum Athletes? *Journal of orthopaedic & sports physical therapy*, 50(6), 281–284.

Erdener, U. and Budgett, R. (2016) Exercise and pregnancy: focus on advice for the competitive and elite athlete. *British Journal of Sports Medicine*, 50(10), 567.

Erikson, E.H. (1968) *Identity: Youth and crisis* (No. 7). WW Norton & Company.

Haskell, R. (2018) Serena Williams on motherhood, marriage, and making her comeback. *Vogue*, 10 January. Available at: www.vogue.com/ article/ serena-williams-vogue-cover-interview-february-2018 (Accessed: 12 November 2019).

Kardel, K.R. (2005) Effects of intense training during and after pregnancy in top-level athletes. *Scandinavian journal of medicine & science in sports*, 15(2), 79–86.

Lingam-Willgoss, C. (2023) Retirement From Sport: The Final Transition. In *Athletic Development*, pp. 54–69. Routledge.

Lingam-Willgoss, C. and Heaney, C. (2020) Session 6: Sportlight – parenthood and sport. Badged Open Course: The Athlete's Journey – Transitions Through Sport.

available at https://www.open.edu/openlearn/mod/oucontent/view.php?id=105610. Accessed 2nd March 2024

McGannon, K.R., Curtin, K., Schinke, R.J. and Schweinbenz, A. (2012) (De) Constructing Paula Radcliffe: Exploring media representation of elite running, pregnancy and motherhood through cultural sport psychology. *Psychology of Sport and Exercise*, Vol. 13, pp. 820–829.

McGannon, K.R., Gonsalves, C.A., Schinke, R.J. and Busanich, R. (2015) Negotiating motherhood and athletic identity: A qualitative analysis of Olympic athlete mother representations in media narratives. *Psychology of Sport and Exercise*, 20, 51–59.

McGannon, K.R., McMahon, J. & Gonsalves, C.A. (2018) Juggling motherhood and sport: A qualitative study of the negotiation of competitive recreational athlete mother identities. *Psychology of Sport and Exercise*, 36, 41–49.

McGannon, K.R., McMahon, J., Schinke, R.J. and Gonsalves, C.A. (2017) Understanding athlete mother transition in cultural context: A media analysis of Kim Clijsters' tennis comeback and self-identity implications. *Sport, Exercise, and Performance Psychology*, 6(1), 20.

McGannon, K.R. and Schinke, R.J. (2013) "My first choice is to work out at work; then i don't feel bad about my kids": A discursive psychological analysis of motherhood and physical activity participation. *Psychology of sport and exercise*, 14(2), 179–188.

Palmer, F., R. & Leberman, S., I. (2009) Elite athletes as mothers: Managing multiple identities. *Sport Management Review*, vol. 12, 241–254.

Pavey, J. (2016) *This mum runs*. London: Yellow Jersey Press.

Pinchbeck, J. (2021) *"It's more than just playing a sport"*. A socio-cultural analysis of participation in netball across the lifespan. (Doctoral Dissertation) Open University, UK.

Scraton, S. and Flintoff, A. (2013) Gender, feminist theory, and sport. In *A Companion to Sport*, pp. 96–111.

Spowart, L., Hughson, J. & Shaw, S. (2008) Snowboarding mums carve out fresh tracks: resisting traditional motherhood discourse? *Annals of Leisure Research*, 11(1–2), 187–204.

Sundgot-Borgen, J., Sundgot-Borgen, C., Myklebust, G., Sølvberg, N. and Torstveit, M. K. (2019) Elite athletes get pregnant, have healthy babies and return to sport early postpartum. *BMJ open sport & exercise medicine*, 5(1), e000652.

Sutherland, J.A. (2010) Mothering, guilt and shame. *Sociology Compass*, 4(5), 310–321.

Tekavc, J., Wylleman, P. and Cecić Erpič, S. (2020) Becoming a mother-athlete: female athletes' transition to motherhood in Slovenia. *Sport in Society*, 23(4), 734–750.

Answers

1. c
2. c
3. a and c
4. b
5. b

12

THE ROLE OF THE FAMILY IN SUPPORTING FEMALE ATHLETIC PERFORMANCE

Jess Pinchbeck and Candice Lingam-Willgoss

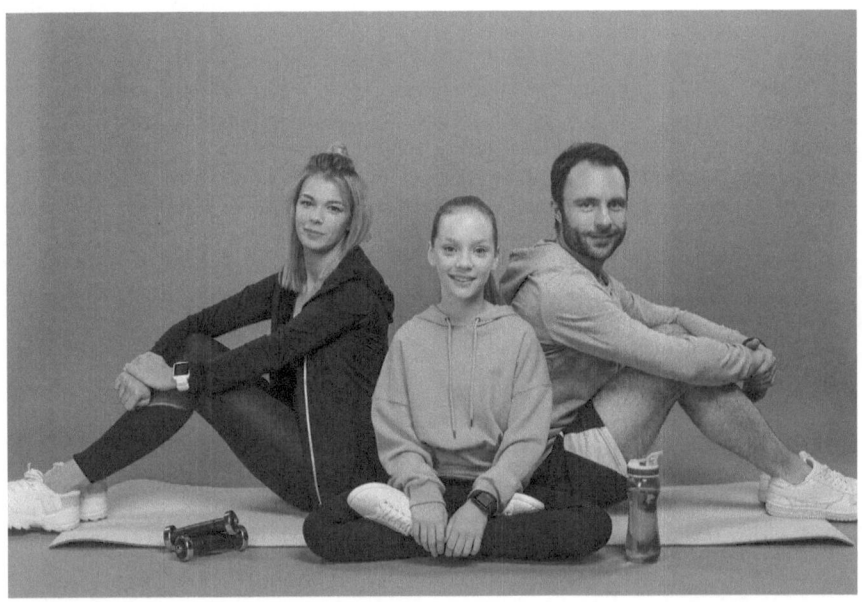

Introduction

The family unit is one of the most influential social constructions (Bourdieu, 1996) and the family environment a child grows up in, can shape their sports participation during childhood and even into adulthood. There are a variety of factors that can influence a child's sports participation, including the resources available to the family, the opportunities families are able to provide their children, and the way in which families support their children during sports

DOI: 10.4324/9781003330110-12

participation. Research shows that sport participation and experiences during childhood contribute to a person's mindset and approach towards sport into adulthood (e.g. Birchwood, Roberts and Pollock, 2008; Haycock and Smith, 2014). Therefore, it is important for those involved in youth sport to understand the socio-cultural influences of the family and how they can work together to create a positive environment for young girls that will be carried on throughout the lifespan.

Families form an integral part of the athletic journey for many athletes and the support offered throughout an athlete's career is invaluable to their success. Research suggests that in some instances parental support may be influenced by gender and this chapter explores this further, specifically focussing on parental opportunities and support provided for girls during childhood and adolescence. The nature of parental support an athlete requires throughout their sporting journey is also discussed. The case study, in Box 12.1, introduces you to 18-year-old Molly, a talented young golfer, and her family.

BOX 12.1 MOLLY (GOLFER)

Molly is an 18-year-old golfer who plays regional level golf. Molly attends monthly regional practice sessions as well as weekly strength and conditioning sessions, lab analysis sessions and normal training and competitions. Molly has two siblings; a younger brother, aged 14 and a younger sister aged 11. Her brother, Jonah, also plays golf but prefers playing cricket and has just been selected for the county U15s. Her sister, Abbie, enjoys team sports and plays in the school football and hockey teams.

Molly first experienced golf aged ten. Her primary school sent out leaflets from the local golf club advertising a week's golf camp over the summer holidays. Molly's mum decided to sign Molly up, mainly because it covered a week of childcare at a reasonable price, plus Molly's parents didn't think she was active enough. Both parents played sport in their youth and felt being active was important for their children. Molly hadn't wanted to go as she didn't know anyone there and she thought golf looked a bit boring! However, after the first couple of hours Molly was hooked, she realised she could be good if she practiced and loved the feeling of hitting the golf ball. She also made friends with two girls her own age. The coach suggested that Molly attend the weekly junior classes. Molly's parents discussed the cost and felt it was affordable as she could borrow some clubs to start with, and that they could manage to get her there.

Throughout secondary school Molly enjoyed PE, but her main sport remained golf. Aged 13, Molly entered her first season competing in national tournaments. Having posted some notable achievements across the season Molly was invited to apply for the regional squad. Following selection, the regional programme included weekly sessions, about an hours' drive away and her dad negotiated to finish work early on a Wednesday to get her there in time. Weekends were also taken up with squad golf sessions over the winter and competitions around the country during the playing season, sometimes involving an overnight stay. Typically, one parent accompanied Molly while the other stayed at home with Jonah and Abbie. This ensured that there was no resentment from her younger siblings, and they were genuinely pleased to see Molly do well. Likewise, Molly enjoyed watching her brother play cricket and taking him to the driving range with her. He enjoyed being at the club with Molly as everyone knew who she was and treated him well because of it. Molly didn't spend as much time with her sister, owing to the age gap, but Molly knew she looked up to her and wanted to be seen as sporty too.

At tournaments Molly was always grateful she had the parents she did. They were proud when she won or played well but they never shouted or got cross if she didn't, unlike some of the other parents. Even in the car to and from tournaments they often just chatted about school and friends and listened to music and only talked about golf if Molly started the conversation. She knew golf had cost her parents quite a bit of money over the years, but she never felt any pressure because of it, and now she was getting tiny bits of sponsorship here and there she felt very proud. They didn't even talk about golf that much at home, she was just Molly.

Now Molly is 18 and has passed her driving test she is becoming more independent and often drives herself to training and competitions. This allows her parents to spend more time with her younger brother and sister and their own activities, creating the family resources for her sister to join a local football team.

What the case study illustrates is some of the issues that families may face when children participate in sport and physical activity, and particularly as one child becomes identified as talented. As we move through this chapter, we will refer to Molly's case study to highlight some of the practical steps that can be taken by her family to support her to continue playing and improving, as well as how the coach can support the family in doing do. But first we will consider the nature of the family unit and the impact on female participation and performance.

The Importance of Creating a Sporting Habitus

Research has demonstrated important connections between sports participation as an adult and experiences of sport as a child (e.g. Birchwood, Roberts and Pollock, 2008; Haycock and Smith, 2014; O'Reilly, Brunette and Bradish, 2018; Scheerder et al., 2006; Tammelin et al., 2005). One way to explain how the culture of a family impacts the initial attraction and continued participation of children in sport is via the application of Bourdieu's theory of 'habitus' (Strandbu, Bakken and Stefansen, 2020).

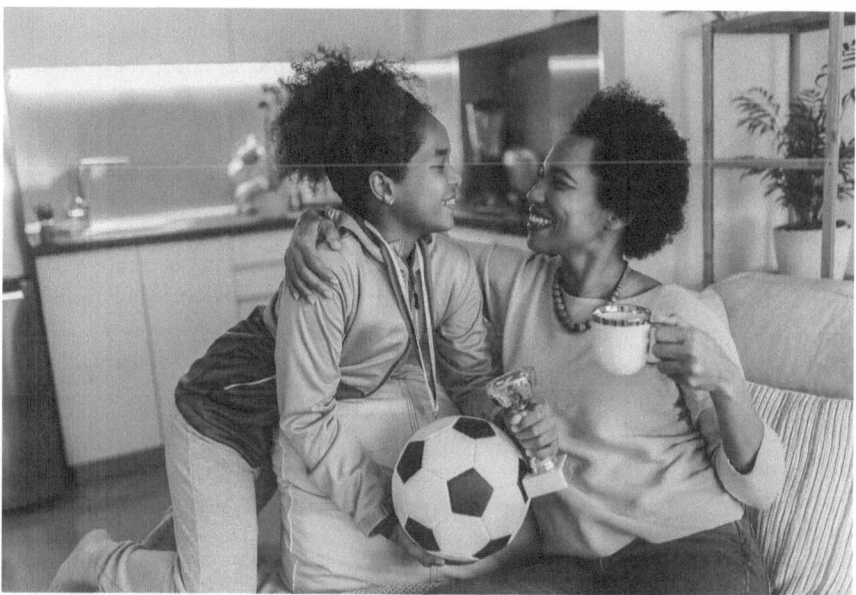

Bourdieu, a French sociologist, proposed that a person's behaviour, thoughts and emotions in every situation is controlled by their habitus (Stuij, 2015). The habitus is a set of dispositions that develop over time as a result of previous experiences, and it determines how an individual thinks and acts in a variety of situations. The structure of an individual's habitus is influenced by environments such as family upbringing and school experiences. For many people their early socialisation typically occurs within the family culture, and this socialisation forms the basis of all subsequent experiences. For example, a study by Birchwood, Roberts and Pollock (2008) suggested that, by the age of 16, an individual has already developed a disposition to participate in sport from their family, and that this habitus towards sports participation would endure into adulthood. Research by Wheeler (2012), supported the theory of a habitus with sporting cultures (beliefs and behaviours relating to sport) passed on through the family. More specifically, Wheeler found that parents own sport experiences shaped the goals and approaches they adopted for their children's sport participation. This was either wanting their child to experience something they had not, or by wanting their child to have similar experiences to their own. This would suggest that both sporty and non-sporty parents can create a habitus for sports participation for their daughter.

Socialisation into sport

Socialisation into sport typically occurs during childhood and the family a girl grows up in influences her physical activity levels as well as her attitudes and behaviours towards being active (Strandbu, Bakken and Stefansen, 2020). It is a combination of both nature and nurture that contribute to a child's sport participation. Inherited genes may be a factor in possessing certain natural abilities, however, it is the family that encourage and develop these abilities (Tucker and Collins, 2012). Organised sport is typically started at some point during young childhood (Coakley, 2011) and although a child may show a desire to start a certain sport, the final decision is usually one made by her parents. Such a decision is often informed by whether the activity is viewed to be worthwhile, affordable, and logistically possible and there are several factors that will influence this decision including the resources, structure, and values of the family. For example, Molly entered into the sport of golf purely because her mum thought that the summer sports camp was good value for money and cheap childcare over the summer holidays.

The following quotes in Box 12.2 are from female athletes who demonstrate links between their family and sport participation.

BOX 12.2 WHAT DO THE ATHLETES SAY?

Sometimes it takes a family. When you don't have a family, a family can be replaced with friends and people that believe in you. It's important to have a system like that. We couldn't have done it without ours.

Serena Williams, tennis player (cited in Ashtakoula, 2021)

My parents are the greatest. They would sacrifice anything and they would take the shirts off their backs for us. We wouldn't be here without them.

Nelly Korda, Golfer (cited in Murray, 2021)

Family resources

The amount and type of physical activity a child participates in is significantly influenced by the cultural, physical and economic resources a family possess (Dagkas and Stathi, 2007). For example, middle-class parents, typically have the resources to support their daughter's sport as well as valuing sport as an activity (Wheeler and Green, 2014). This has been attributed to the social perception that providing opportunities for sport and parental support is seen in middle-class social networks as 'good' parenting (Wheeler and Green, 2019) and therefore parents seek out sport opportunities for their daughters. For those parents who do not have the resources to support their daughter in organised sport then sports participation becomes more difficult, even if they value sport as an activity.

Families of low socioeconomic status (SES) often do not have the funds to pay for the initial costs associated with organised sports participation, and as a result families with lower SES are associated with lower levels of participation (Grima et al., 2017). As well as greater participation those from higher social classes have also been shown to engage in a wider range of family activities such as kayaking or skiing, and this diversity can have a positive impact on a child's athletic development (Lundy et al., 2019). Though it is worth noting that higher financial investment into a child's sport has also been linked to greater perceptions of parent pressure, accompanied by lesser enjoyment of and commitment to the sport by the child (Dunn et al., 2016). Therefore, the allocation of resources and the participation of young female athletes in sport is not a straightforward one.

There also appear to be connections between socioeconomic status during childhood and adult participation with research suggesting that greater parental socioeconomic position in childhood leads to a greater amount of time spent doing physical activity in adulthood (Elhakeem et al., 2017). Therefore, to encourage greater female participation that also continues into adulthood it is important to consider the intricate connections between family resources and taking part in organised sport, as well as the various pathways that young athletes may take (McMillan, McIsaac and Jannssen, 2016). Clubs and organisations should seek to provide opportunities for girls from a wide variety of families with varying resources.

Family structure

The composition of the family may also impact upon a girl's sport participation with children living in both single-parent and reconstituted families (comprising a step-parent), experiencing a reduction in organised sport participation (McMillan, McIsaac and Jannssen, 2016). However, the financial situation of the family has been shown to act as a mediator to sports participation.

The number of siblings within a family may also have relevance to a child's initial and continued participation. A family environment with more siblings is typically associated with more time spent playing sport or being physically active, as a result of more children playing together (Blazo and Smith, 2018). However, once again financial resources are likely to play a part as more children within the family unit can reduce the resources available to each child. For example, Molly and her brother both take part in sport outside of school, yet the youngest sibling only just started playing football once Molly became more independent and freed up some of the family resources.

Some research has also shown a gender difference in the influence of siblings. For example, Trent and Spitze (2011), reported that male children with no siblings took part in more sport compared to those who grew up with siblings whereas, female children with no siblings had lower sport participation levels. Gender effects were also found by Osai and Whiteman (2017) whereby only siblings of the same gender influenced one another regarding sport participation. However, Lundy et al. (2019) observed that younger siblings profited, regardless of gender, from the exposure to their older sibling's sport experiences. For example, Molly's younger brother who enjoys going to the golf club with her.

Overall, research shows that the presence of siblings throughout childhood does appear to have some influence over a child's sport and physical activity participation, yet the relationship appears complex and diverse, and more investigation is required, particularly around gender influences. Owing to females' participation in sport constantly evolving and changing, it is likely that the influence of female siblings will also evolve, permitting more female sibling role models and gender-related sibling influences.

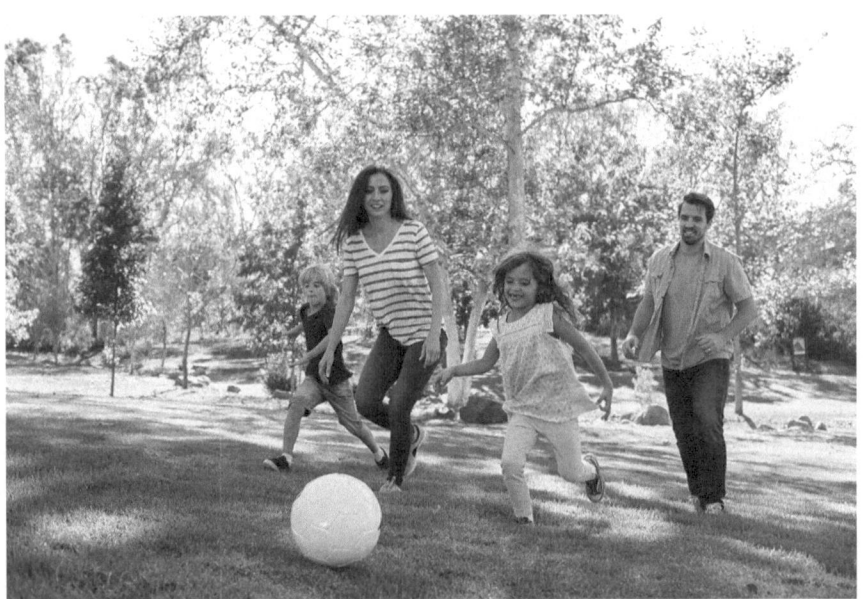

Family culture

Parents are commonly seen as key role models for their daughters, and children often observe and copy their parents' behaviours. Studies typically show a positive relationship between parent and child physical activity with more active parents having more active children (Petersen et al., 2020). Yet, parents can still be role models even if they do not actively participate in sport themselves, such as by coaching sport (Fredricks and Eccles, 2004) or through taking pleasure in sport (Dixon, Warner and Bruening, 2008). For example, Dixon, Warner and Bruening (2008) found that mothers who did not have the opportunity to participate in sport when they were younger wanted to ensure that their daughters did and so they actively conveyed the message that sports participation was positive. This appeared to have a strong and lasting effect on their daughters' sports involvement and demonstrates how parental attitudes towards sport can be just as powerful as

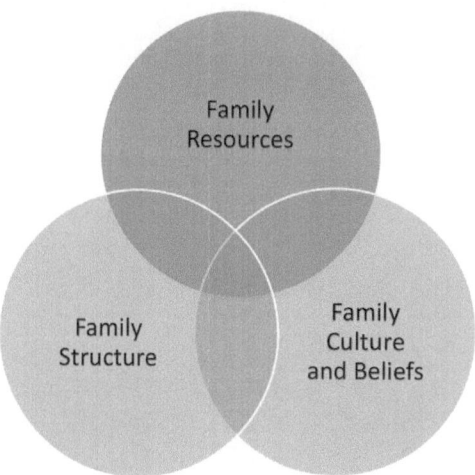

FIGURE 12.1 Family factors that influence socialisation into sport

parental participation. This is reflected by Molly's parents wanting her to be outside and more active as they felt this was beneficial for her as a child.

The theories and concepts of Bourdieu are a useful lens through which to view how parents make decisions to provide opportunities for their daughter's sport participation. Bourdieu used the term 'capital' to refer to "a form of power, the capacity individuals and groups might have to impact upon, change or control situations" (Tomlinson, 2004, p. 168). As this section has discussed parents hold the power to impact their daughter's participation through the distribution of the family resources or capital. Parents typically make decisions on how they will allocate any economic, social and cultural resources for their daughter (Wheeler and Green, 2014), and such decisions are shaped by the parent's own values and attitudes towards sport. In summary, girls are more likely to take part in sport if they grow up in a family culture where sport is valued. Parental distribution of capital can also be influenced by the role of gender and the type of activities that they encourage their daughter to participate in.

Gender and sports socialisation

The family unit, as well as the wider social environment, also plays a key role in shaping a child's beliefs around gender (Boiché et al., 2014). The way that boys and girls view, and value sport is extremely powerful and often become apparent at a very young age. These attitudes typically occur through the process of socialisation rather than any gender differences in 'natural' abilities (Eccles and Harold, 1991).

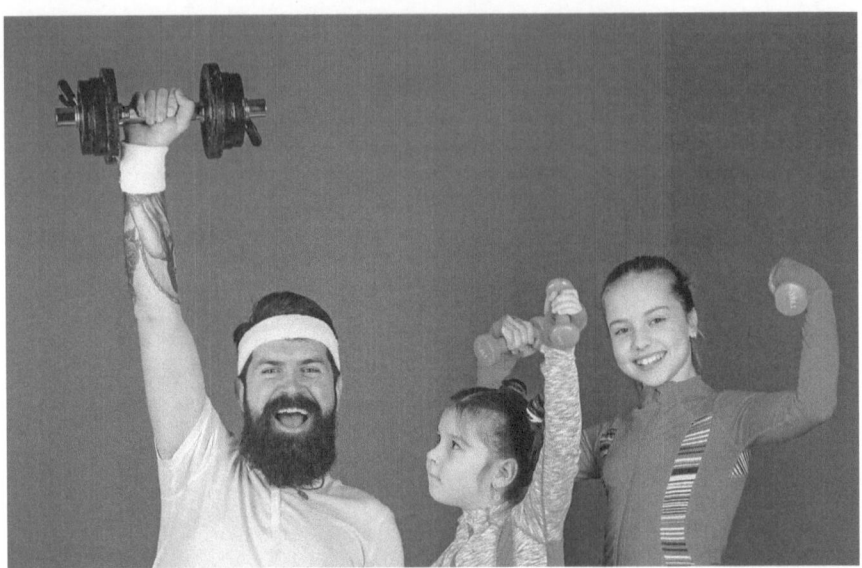

Research evidence suggests that boys take part in more physical activity and are in receipt of greater parental support than girls, indicating a powerful gender difference in physical activity levels (Gustafson and Rhodes, 2006). Parents place a greater value on sport for sons, than for daughters, both ideologically and financially, and gender role beliefs about their daughters' participation in sport, shape their daughter's participation and the type of sports they take part in (Heinze et al., 2017). In a report by The Women's Sport Foundation (2020), 32.2 per cent of parents held the belief that boys were more competent than girls at sport. In a society where girls typically meet greater challenges to their participation than boys (such as those evidenced in Chapter 9) the role of the family in supporting their daughter's sports participation is crucial, demonstrated by Molly's parents encouraging her to be active.

As previously mentioned the family are often the most influential role models in a child's life and even though male family members can be good role models, Daniels (2016) has argued that active females within the family are extremely powerful role models for girls' involvement in sports, especially mothers. Although both mothers and fathers influence female sports participation, mothers are usually more involved in their daughter's participation and have less influence over their son's involvement (e.g. Bauer et al., 2008; Milošević and Vesković, 2013; Sukys et al., 2014). It is not only the physical activity of parents that is associated with a daughter's sport participation, but also parental attitudes to provide opportunities and support. More recent studies showed a shift towards equal support provided by parents to both boys and girls to be physically active, although with differing levels of impact, and perhaps encouragement towards different types of activities (Pinchbeck, 2021).

How do families influence activity choice?

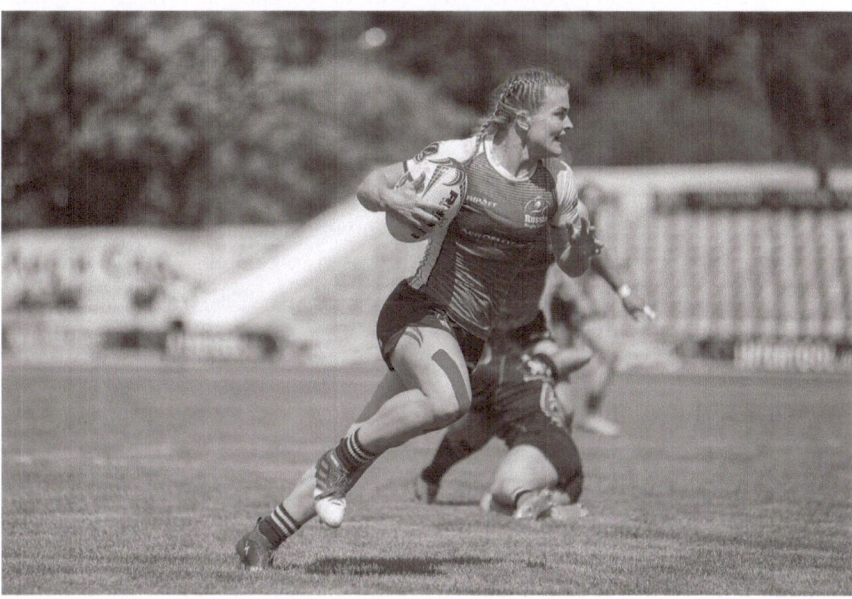

In certain societies some sports activities may be viewed as masculine, feminine, or neutral and it is typically during childhood where the gender roles associated with certain sports are formed (Chalabaev et al., 2013). Although society is constantly changing, especially in terms of what is considered to be masculine and feminine, some sports continue to be viewed as gender-specific. Sports that emphasise appearance and attractiveness, such as tennis and gymnastics, are considered to be feminine, whereas sports with an element of danger and risk, like rugby and boxing, are identified as masculine (Koivula, 2001). Some studies suggest that women will avoid sports that are viewed as masculine territories (e.g. Hanlon, Morris and Nabbs, 2010) although Roster (2007) argued that society no longer allocates activities as only being for men or for women but instead provides women with greater choices for sports participation. Yet, women who take part in a sport viewed as a masculine domain often find that they have their femininity and their sexuality questioned (McGannon, McMahon and Gonsalves, 2018; Scheadler and Wagstaff, 2018).

It is within social contexts where children learn what are considered to be masculine and feminine characteristics (Paechter, 2007), typically reflective of the culture and demonstrated by the sports activities that they participate in. For example, Wheeler (2012) found evidence of stereotyped activity participation, with boys choosing football, taekwondo and water sports, with dancing and ice skating more popular choices for girls. Gender influence was also evident in a study by Carlin, Murphy and Gallagher (2015), whereby 11–13-year-old British males preferred structured sport, which was more intense and competitive, and females favoured activities like dance. Such gender stereotypes conveyed within sport have been linked to dropout in female adolescents (Boiché et al., 2014) and therefore as coaches and parents it is important to recognise this and try to combat such stereotypes. For girls that do take part in traditionally masculine sports Bevan et al. (2021) found that social connectedness, mentors and same-sex role models are all factors that help the girls to navigate their sports participation.

The research presented illustrates how, although sport has developed to permit wider sport provision for females, gender stereotypes in society persist as a negative factor in female sports participation. With activities often still labelled as masculine or feminine such stereotypes influence the type of activity girls opt to take part in. In addition (as discussed in Chapter 9) adolescent girls often feel conflicted over developing their bodies for athletic prowess and the ideal physique associated with traditional notions of femininity.

Parental behaviour at sports events

There is growing evidence to suggest that, if the early experiences of girls include participating in a variety of sports that are fun and enjoyable, they are likely to have greater positive experiences and increased developmental outcomes. The family environment that appears to be most effective in encouraging participation in sport is one which is caring and supportive and where sport is not taken too seriously (Allender, Cowburn and Foster, 2006). As well as creating opportunities for participation, parents can also influence their daughter's sporting experience.

Enjoyment of the activity is often determined by the quality of the experience and both can influence whether children choose to continue (Bailey, Cope and Parnell, 2015). When girls are involved in organised sport the level of parental involvement varies greatly and the nature of this involvement can significantly impact the quality of a girl's sporting experience in a multitude of ways. Key findings from the Women's Sport Foundation Report, 'Keeping Girls in the Game' showed the multiple roles that parents played in either helping or hindering their daughter's sports participation, and that working with parents to improve the engagement and support can lower girls' rates of sport dropout (Zarrett, Veliz and Sabo, 2020).

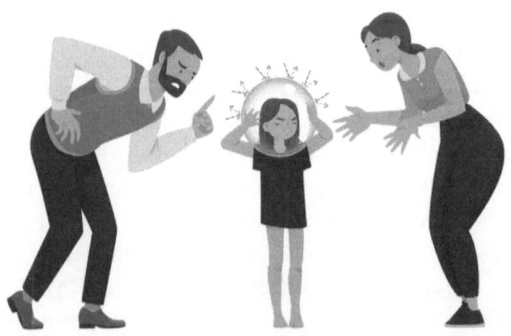

BOX 12.3 SPOTLIGHT ON: FAMILY PRESSURES AND DROPOUT

It is only natural that not all girls will be able to maintain consistently high levels of performance, or that they will want to continue on a performance pathway. Girls drop out of sport at various stages of their athletic development for a variety of reasons. This can be due to academic pressures, injuries, other interests or in some cases an inability to cope with the demands placed on them causing chronic stress, known as burnout. Burnout is typically defined as a psychological, physical, and emotional withdrawal from an activity that was previously enjoyable and motivating caused by persistent or chronic stress (Smith, 1986). Excessive parental pressure can sometimes contribute to young female athletes experiencing burnout and withdrawing from sport completely.

In a study on predominantly adolescent female swimmers (15 female and five male) Fraser-Thomas, Côté and Deakin (2008) reported certain parental characteristics present in the parents of children that dropped out of swimming. These included providing coaching tips when watching practices and competitions, providing incentives for good performances, and placing significant pressure on their child to continue swimming when the child was contemplating withdrawing from the sport. The dropout athletes within this study also discussed two contrasting factors contributing to parent pressure that occurred during adolescence. Parents either pressurised children to stay involved in swimming because they themselves had not been afforded such opportunities in their youth or parents applied pressure to swim and perform well because they had been high-level athletes.

The influence of family members, particularly parents, on youth sport participation and performance has been well established in the sporting literature, predominantly by Knight and colleagues (e.g. Harwood and Knight, 2015; Knight, Boden and Holt, 2010; Knight and Holt, 2014). To help identify what types of parental behaviours young tennis players preferred during competitions Knight, Boden and Holt (2010) conducted a study of 42 male and female 12–15-year-old tennis players. Results showed that players wanted their parents to be supportive without placing unnecessary pressure upon them. More specifically players felt that parents should not give technical and tactical advice, but that they should comment on effort and attitude, offer practical advice, follow tennis etiquette, and match nonverbal behaviours with supportive comments. Though, it is likely that the nature of the sport (i.e. individual or team), as well as gender of the athletes, could also lead to different preferences. The study of adolescent female athletes is underrepresented in sports literature however there are some studies to draw upon. For example, Knight, Neely and Holt (2011) conducted a study with early adolescent female athletes' (aged 12–15 years) at team sport competitions and found that prior to competition athletes wanted parents to help them physically and mentally prepare. During competition the preferences were slightly more complex with four behaviours that athletes would like parents to display; encouraging the entire team, focusing on effort rather than outcome, interacting positively with athletes throughout the game, maintaining control of their emotions, and three behaviours that athletes would prefer parents not to display; drawing attention to themselves or their daughter, coaching, and arguing with officials. After competition the participants had clear preferences that they wanted their parents to provide positive and realistic post game feedback. Knight, Neely and Holt (2011) concluded that athlete preferences of parental behaviour is not only about parents displaying the desired behaviour but a need to display the right behaviour at the right time.

Bringing together the wealth of research in this area via a position statement on parenting expertise in youth sport Harwood and Knight (2015) compiled six key postulates, or recommendations, of parenting expertise. For the purposes of this chapter the postulates have been adapted and applied to female youth sports participation (see Figure 12.2), yet there is still the need to conduct specific research with adolescent female athletes because, as demonstrated in Chapter 9, they face different issues than young male athletes. One such study by Pynn, Dunn and Holt (2019) with adolescent females showed support for all six postulates though they concluded further investigation was required to determine how parental support and the level of involvement changes over time.

A coach and parent partnership

It is not just parents that hold power over girls' sports experiences but coaches play a key role as well (Eliasson, 2015). The female athletes, coaches and parents, all form part of the socialisation process within youth sport and the relationship between these three parties is often referred to as 'the sporting triangle' (Byrne, 1993). The athletic development of girls will be impacted by the interaction and social system within the sporting triangle (Lisinskienė and Šukys, 2014), which in turn is likely to have an effect on their continued participation.

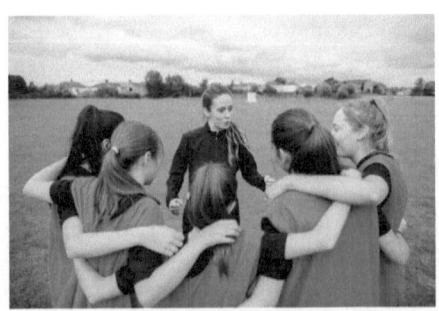

Postulate no. 1: parents select the appropriate sporting opportunities for their daughter and provide necessary types of social support	• parents provide opportunities for their child to participate in a range of fun and enjoyable sporting activities with limited emphasis on competition and a focus on learning through play • parents and children have shared and communicated goals about what children want to achieve and parents provide the appropriate opportunities • parents provide appropriate tangible, emotional and informational support relevant to the child's needs
Postulate no. 2: parents understand and apply an authoritative or autonomy-supportive parenting style	• parents create create a healthy emotional climate for their daughter, through their application of specific parenting styles • parent's work separately or together in applying an authoritative or autonomy-supportive style with their daughter
Postulate no. 3: parents manage the emotional demands of competition and serve as emotionally intelligent role models for their daughter	• parents effectively manage the various emotional demands of competition • parents understand their daughter's emotional needs, appreciate values such as effort, sportpersonship, independence, honesty, composure, and constructive feedback, and behave in a manner that role models these values to their daughter
Postulate no. 4: parents foster and maintain healthy relationships with significant others in the youth sport environment	• parents support the coach with relevant input but they allow the coach to drive the pace of learning and development without interference • parents take responsibility for the behavior of their daughter, and support the coach on reinforcing appropriate attitudes and behaviors in training and competition • parents foster and maintain healthy parent-parent relationships
Postulate no. 5: parents manage the organisational and developmental demands placed on them as stakeholders in youtg sport	• parents cope with demands by means of a variety of intrapersonal, interpersonal and organizational skills and strategies • parents ability to manage a range of stressors and cope with the demands they encounter in youth sport will influence the extent to which parents offer appropriate support to their daughter
Postulate no. 6: expert parents adapt their involvement and support to different stages of their daughter's athletic development and progressions	• as girls initiate and progress through sport, parents' roles, experiences, demands, and responsibilities change • parents are able to positively adapt their involvement in tandem with their daughter's sporting progressions and developmental needs • to recognize and successfully negotiate shifting roles as girls transition through the stages of athletic development

FIGURE 12.2 Postulates of good parenting
Source: Adapted from Harwood and Knight (2015)

Extensive research has been conducted to improve the understanding of coaching expertise in youth sport (Harwood and Knight, 2015). To facilitate positive development in youth sport literature indicates that the quality of relationships and communication between coaches, young athletes and parents are the two most important factors (Lisinskienė and Šukys, 2014). In interviews with adolescent competitive swimmers, Fraser-Thomas and Côté (2009) reported that each participant identified both positive and negative experiences. Most athletes discussed the special relationships they had with coaches, though coaches' intimidating demeanour, their preference for favourites, and their inappropriate behaviours were also mentioned by many. The conduct of sports coaches is a prominent topic, particularly owing to cases of abuse being reported in the media in gymnastics and cycling (Scott, 2020). The coach is central to a young female athlete's development and participation and Navin (2016) recommended that coaches reduce the focus on winning and instead aim to develop the individual holistically, supported through frequent and transparent communication with parents.

Taking into consideration the research in this area and the six postulates, Box 12.4 provides recommendations on how parents can support their daughter's sports participation.

BOX 12.4 REAL-WORLD APPLICATION

As a parent of a female athlete, you should:

1. Provide as many opportunities as possible for your daughter to participate in a range of sports.
2. Provide an environment whereby your daughter can choose her own sporting activities.
3. Discuss improvement and enjoyment with your daughter rather than winning and competition.
4. Ask your daughter what type of support they would like before, during and after competition.
5. Form an effective relationship with the coach through regular communication and where you can both be honest and open with each other.

Coaches of female athletes can also play an important role in supporting families to encourage the continued participation of their young female athletes. Box 12.5 presents some ideas around how a coach can support their athletes.

BOX 12.5 TIPS FOR COACHES TO SUPPORT FAMILIES OF FEMALE ATHLETES

1. Take the lead to provide regular communication and ensure effective working relationships with parents.
2. Use education to make families aware of the type of support they should provide and behaviour expectations at training and competition.
3. Take steps to involve parents in decision making about their daughter's sporting journey.

4. Be aware of any family circumstances that may impact the young female athlete's sporting experience and provide the appropriate support.
5. Work together with parents to overcome any issues around physical and emotional development that may impact on the young female athlete.

Summary

Having completed this chapter, you will now have developed a more detailed understanding of the complex issues faced by the families of female athletes. In particular you will appreciate how participation during childhood and adolescence can often depend upon the values that parents place on playing sport and being physically active and the resources they have available to support this. It is most important to understand the societal pressures that face female athletes and how gender can impact the type of support families provide and the types of activities that are encouraged. You will also have explored the importance of parental behaviour and attitudes during competition and training and the value of a good working relationship between the coach, athlete, and family.

The key messages to take away from this chapter are:

1. Family resources, structure and culture influence the sporting opportunities a family can provide for their daughter.
2. Gender influences can play a role in the level of support provided by the family and the type of sporting activity they feel is suitable.
3. Families should aim to provide a variety of fun sporting experiences for their daughter during childhood and adolescence.
4. Both mothers and fathers can influence their daughter's sporting journey.
5. Parents should talk to their daughter about the type of support they would like before, during and following competition.
6. The relationship between parents, coaches and athletes is key to effective female athletic development and continued participation.

End-of-Chapter Quiz

Answers can be found after the References

1. Identify why it is important for girls to participate in sport from a young age:

    a To create a sporting habitus for life
    b To accrue as many hours practice as possible
    c To increase their chances of becoming a professional sports person
    d To develop a work ethic

2. Identify which three family factors below most influence a child's socialisation into sport:

   a Sporty parents, having a brother, being the oldest sibling
   b Family resources, family structure and family culture
   c Having grandparents, owning a car, money
   d Having more than two siblings, a sporty mum, living near a park

3. Identify which statement is true in regard to influence over their daughter's physical activity and sport participation:

   a Only the mother influences their daughter's sport participation
   b Only the father influences their daughter's sport participation
   c Neither mother nor father have any influence over their daughter's sort participation
   d Both mother and father influence their daughter's sport participation

4. Identify which three behaviours female adolescent team sport athletes do not want their parents to display:

   a drawing attention to themselves or their child, coaching, arguing with officials
   b shouting, clapping and talking to other parents
   c smiling, shaking the coach's hand, thanking the officials
   d talking to their teammates, shouting praise, filming on their phone

5. How many postulates of parenting expertise did Knight and Holt develop:

   a Ten
   b Five
   c Six
   d Eight

References

Allender, S., Cowburn, G. and Foster, C. (2006) 'Understanding participation in sport and physical activity among children and adults: a review of qualitative studies', *Health education research*, 21(6), 826–835.

Ashtakoula, S. (2021) *"Couldn't Have Done It": Serena Williams Credits Family for the Success of Venus and Herself*. Essentially Sports: the fans perspective. Available at: https://www.essentiallysports.com/wta-tennis-news-couldnt-have-done-it-serena-williams-credits-family-for-the-success-of-venus-and-herself/ (Accessed: 19th December 2022).

Bailey, R., Cope, E. and Parnell, D. (2015) 'Realising the benefits of sports and physical activity: the human capital model', *Retos*, 28, 147–154.

Bauer, K.W., Nelson, M.C., Boutelle, K.N. and Neumark-Sztainer, D. (2008) 'Parental influences on adolescents' physical activity and sedentary behavior: longitudinal findings from Project EAT-II', *International Journal of Behavioral Nutrition and Physical Activity*, 5(1), 1–7.

Bevan, N., Drummond, C., Abery, L., Elliott, S., Pennesi, J.-L., Prichard, I., Lewis, L.K. and Drummond, M. (2021) 'More opportunities, same challenges: adolescent girls in sports that are traditionally constructed as masculine', *Sport, Education and Society*, 26(6), 592–605.

Birchwood, D., Roberts, K. and Pollock, G. (2008) 'Explaining differences in sport participation rates among young adults: Evidence from the South Caucasus', *European Physical Education Review*, 14(3), 283–298.

Blazo, J.A. and Smith, A.L. (2018) 'A systematic review of siblings and physical activity experiences', *International Review of Sport and Exercise Psychology*, 11(1), 122–159.

Boiché, J., Plaza, M., Chalabaev, A., Guillet-Descas, E. and Sarrazin, P. (2014) 'Social antecedents and consequences of gender-sport stereotypes during adolescence', *Psychology of Women Quarterly*, 38(2), 259–274.

Bourdieu, P. (1996) 'On the family as a realized category', *Theory, culture & society*, 13 (3), 19–26.

Byrne, T. (1993) 'Coaching children in sport: principles and practice', in M. Lee (Ed.), *Coaching children in sport*, pp. 39–47. London: E & FN Spon.

Carlin, A., Murphy, M.H. and Gallagher, A.M. (2015) 'Current influences and approaches to promote future physical activity in 11–13 year olds: a focus group study', *BMC Public Health*, 15(1), 1–12.

Chalabaev, A., Sarrazin, P., Fontayne, P., Boiché, J. and Clément-Guillotin, C. (2013) 'The influence of sex stereotypes and gender roles on participation and performance in sport and exercise: Review and future directions', *Psychology of Sport and Exercise*, 14(2), 136–144.

Coakley, J. (2011) 'Youth Sports: What Counts as "Positive Development?"', *Journal of Sport & Social Issues*, 35(3), 306–324.

Dagkas, S. and Stathi, A. (2007) 'Exploring social and environmental factors affecting adolescents' participation in physical activity', *European Physical Education Review*, 13(3), 369–384.

Daniels, D. (2016) 'Introduction: Becoming a Female Athlete', in E. Staurowsky (Ed.), *Women and Sport: Continuing a Journey of Liberation and Celebration*, pp. xv–xxvii. Human Kinetics.

Dixon, M.A., Warner, S. M. and Bruening, J.E. (2008) 'More Than Just Letting Them Play: Parental Influence on Women's Lifetime Sport Involvement', *Sociology of Sport Journal*, 25(4), 538–559.

Dunn, C.R., Dorsch, T.E., King, M.Q. and Rothlisberger, K.J. (2016) 'The impact of family financial investment on perceived parent pressure and child enjoyment and commitment in organized youth sport', *Family Relations*, 65(2), 287–299.

Eccles, J.S. and Harold, R.D. (1991) 'Gender differences in sport involvement: Applying the Eccles' expectancy-value model', *Journal of Applied Sport Psychology*, 3(1), 7–35.

Elhakeem, A., Hardy, R., Bann, D., Caleyachetty, R., Cosco, T.D., Hayhoe, R.P., Muthuri, S. G., Wilson, R. and Cooper, R. (2017) 'Intergenerational social mobility and leisure-time physical activity in adulthood: a systematic review', *Journal of Epidemiology and Community Health*, 71(7), 673–680.

Eliasson, I. (2015) '"In different sports worlds": Socialisation among children, coaches, and parents in girls' and boys' football teams', *European Journal for Sport and Society*, 12(2), 187–214.

Fraser-Thomas, J. and Côté, J. (2009) 'Understanding Adolescents' Positive and Negative Developmental Experiences in Sport', *Sport Psychologist*, 23(1), 3–23.

Fraser-Thomas, J., Côté, J. and Deakin, J. (2008) 'Understanding dropout and prolonged engagement in adolescent competitive sport', *Psychology of Sport and Exercise*, 9(5), 645–662.

Fredricks, J.A. and Eccles, J.S. (2004) 'Parental influences on youth involvement in sports', in M.R. Weiss (Ed.), *Developmental sport and exercise psychology: A lifespan perspective*, pp. 145–164. Michigan: Fitness Information Technology.

Grima, S., Grima, A., Thalassinos, E., Seychell, S. and Spiteri, J.V. (2017) 'Theoretical Models for Sport Participation: Literature Review', *International Journal of Economics & Business Administration*, 5(3), 94–116.

Gustafson, S.L. and Rhodes, R.E. (2006) 'Parental correlates of physical activity in children and early adolescents', *Sports Medicine*, 36(1), 79–97.

Hanlon, C., Morris, T. and Nabbs, S. (2010) 'Establishing a successful physical activity program to recruit and retain women', *Sport Management Review*, 13(3), 269–282.

Harwood, C.G. and Knight, C.J. (2015) 'Parenting in youth sport: A position paper on parenting expertise'. *Psychology of Sport and Exercise*, 16(1), 24–35.

Haycock, D. and Smith, A. (2014) 'A family affair? Exploring the influence of childhood sport socialisation on young adults' leisure-sport careers in north-west England', *Leisure Studies*, 33(3), 285–304.

Heinze, J.E., Heinze, K.L., Davis, M.M., Butchart, A.T., Singer, D.C. and Clark, S.J. (2017) 'Gender role beliefs and parents' support for athletic participation', *Youth & Society*, 49(5), 634–657.

Knight, C.J., Boden, C.M. and Holt, N.L. (2010) 'Junior tennis players' preferences for parental behaviors', *Journal of Applied Sport Psychology*, 22(4), 377–391.

Knight, C.J. and Holt, N.L. (2014) 'Parenting in youth tennis: Understanding and enhancing children's experiences'. *Psychology of Sport and Exercise*, 15(2), 155–164.

Knight, C.J., Neely, K.C. and Holt, N.L. (2011) 'Parental Behaviors in Team Sports: How do Female Athletes Want Parents to Behave?', *Journal of Applied Sport Psychology*, 23(1), 76–92.

Koivula, N. (2001) 'Perceives Characteristics of Sports Categorized as Gender-Neutral, Feminine and Masculine', *Journal of Sport Behavior*, 24(4), 377–393.

Lisinskienė, A. and Šukys, S. (2014) 'The athlete triangle: Coach, athlete and parents as an educational system', *Global Journal of Sociology*, 4(2), 46–51.

Lundy, G.I., Allan, V., Cowburn, I. and Cote, J. (2019) 'Parental Support, Sibling Influences and Family Dynamics across the Development of Canadian Inter-university Student-Athletes', *Journal of Athlete Development and Experience*, 1(2), 87–97.

McGannon, K.R., McMahon, J. and Gonsalves, C.A. (2018) 'Juggling motherhood and sport: A qualitative study of the negotiation of competitive recreational athlete mother identities', *Psychology of Sport and Exercise*, 36, 41–49.

McMillan, R., McIsaac, M. and Janssen, I. (2016) 'Family structure as a correlate of organized sport participation among youth', *PloS one*, 11(2). Available at: https://doi.org/10.1371/journal.pone.0147403 (Accessed: 5 January 2023).

Milošević, V. & Vesković, A. (2013) 'Family as an agent for sport socialization of youth', *Serbian Journal of Sports Sciences*, 7(3), 143–149.

Murray, E. (2021) 'Nelly Korda's PGA Championship win elevates remarkable family dynasty'. *The Guardian*, 28 June. Available at: https://www.theguardian.com/sport/2021/jun/28/golf-tennis-nelly-korda-pga-championship-family-dynasty-seb-korda-wimbledon (Accessed: 8 June 2023).

Navin, A. (2016) 'Introduction to coaching youth participants', in A. Navin (Ed.), *Coaching Youth Netball: An Essential Guide for Coaches, Parents and Teachers*, pp. 10–25. London: The Crowwood Press.

O'Reilly, N., Brunette, M. and Bradish, C. (2018) 'Lifelong Female Engagement in Sport: A Framework for Advancing Girls' and Women's Participation', *Journal of Applied Sport Management*, 10(3), 15–30.

Osai, K.V. and Whiteman, S.D. (2017) 'Family Relationships and Youth Sport: Influence of Siblings and Parents on Youth's Participation, Interests, and Skills', *Journal of Amateur Sport*, 3(3), 86–105.

Paechter, C. (2007) *Being boys; being girls: Learning masculinities and femininities: Learning masculinities and femininities.* Maidenhead: McGraw-Hill Education (UK).

Petersen, T.L., Møller, L.B., Brønd, J.C., Jepsen, R. and Grøntved, A. (2020) 'Association between parent and child physical activity: a systematic review', *International Journal of Behavioral Nutrition and Physical Activity*, 17(67), 1–16.

Pinchbeck, J. (2021) *"It's more than just playing a sport". A sociocultural analysis of netball participation across the lifespan.* PhD thesis. The Open University. Available at: https://oro.open.ac.uk/79807 (Accessed: 14 August 2023).

Pynn, S.R., Dunn, J.G. and Holt, N.L. (2019) 'A qualitative study of exemplary parenting in competitive female youth team sport', *Sport, Exercise, and Performance Psychology*, 8(2), 163.

Roster, C.A. (2007) '"Girl power" and participation in macho recreation: The case of female Harley riders', *Leisure Sciences*, 29(5), 443–461.

Scheadler, T. and Wagstaff, A. (2018) 'Exposure to women's sports: Changing attitudes toward female athletes', *The Sport Journal*, 19, 1–17.

Scheerder, J., Thomis, M., Vanreusel, B., Lefevre, J., Renson, R., Vanden Eynde, B. and Beunen, G.P. (2006) 'Sports participation among females from adolescence to adulthood: A longitudinal study', *International Review for the Sociology of Sport*, 41(3–4), 413–430.

Scott, L. (2020) *UK Sport notified of 19 allegations of emotional abuse or neglect of athletes since 2017.* Available at: www.bbc.co.uk/sport/53837137 (Accessed: 19 April 2022).

Smith, R. E. (1986) 'Toward a cognitive-affective model of athletic burnout', *Journal of Sport Psychology*, 8(1), 36–50.

Strandbu, Å., Bakken, A. and Stefansen, K. (2020) 'The continued importance of family sport culture for sport participation during the teenage years'. *Sport, Education and Society*, 25(8), 931–945.

Stuij, M. (2015) 'Habitus and social class: a case study on socialisation into sports and exercise', *Sport, Education & Society*, 20(6), 780–798.

Sukys, S., Majauskienė, D., Cesnaitiene, V.J. and Karanauskiene, D. (2014) 'Do Parents' Exercise Habits Predict 13–18-Year-Old Adolescents' Involvement in Sport?', *Journal of Sports Science & Medicine*, 13(3), 522–528.

Tammelin, T., Näyhä, S., Hills, A.P. and Järvelin, M.-R. (2005) 'Adolescent participation in sports and adult physical activity', *American Journal of Preventive Medicine*, 24(1), 22–28. doi:10.1016/S0749-3797(02)00575-00575.

Tomlinson, A. (2004) 'Pierre Bourdieu and the sociological study of sport: Habitus, capital and field', in R. Giulianotti (Ed.), *Sport and Modern Social Theorists*, pp. 161–172. Hampshire: Palgrave Macmillan.

Trent, K. and Spitze, G. (2011) 'Growing up without siblings and adult sociability behaviors', *Journal of Family Issues*, 32(9), 1178–1204.

Tucker, R. and Collins, M. (2012. 'What makes champions? A review of the relative contribution of genes and training to sporting success', *British Journal of Sports Medicine*, 46(8), 555–561.

Wheeler, S. (2012) 'The significance of family culture for sports participation', *International Review for the Sociology of Sport*, 47(3), 235–252.

Wheeler, S. and Green, K. (2014) 'Parenting in relation to children's sports participation: generational changes and potential implications', *Leisure Studies*, 33(3), 267–284.

Wheeler, S. and Green, K. (2019) '"The helping, the fixtures, the kits, the gear, the gum shields, the food, the snacks, the waiting, the rain, the car rides…": social class, parenting and children's organised activities'. *Sport, Education and Society*, 24(8), 788–800.

Zarrett, N., Veliz, P. and Sabo, D. (2020) Keeping Girls in the Game: Factors That Influence Sport Participation. *Women's Sports Foundation*. Available at: https://files.eric.ed.gov/fulltext/ED603915.pdf (Accessed: 5 January 2023).

Answers

1. a
2. b
3. d
4. a
5. c

13

THE EFFECT OF PERIMENOPAUSE AND MENOPAUSE ON THE ATHLETIC FEMALE

Simon Rea

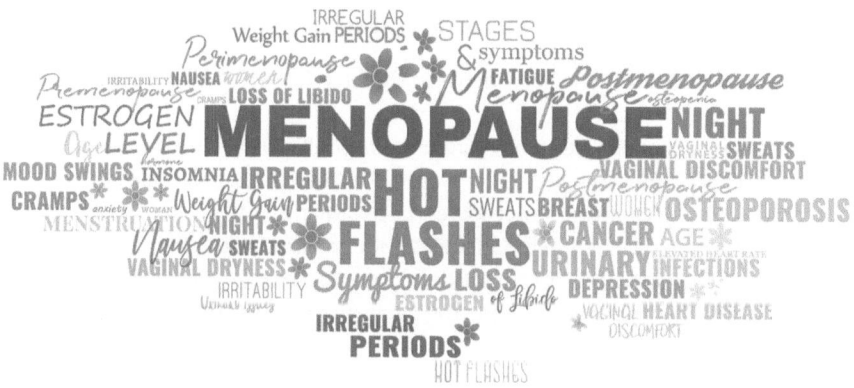

The menopause is the stage in a female's life where their periods stop, owing to lower hormones levels. The menopause is when a female has not had a period for one year (Newson, 2019). The word 'menopause' comes from Greek terms with 'menos' meaning the menstrual cycle and 'pause' meaning stop, referring to the last menstrual period. It usually occurs between the ages of 45–55, with 51 being the average age at menopause (NHS Choices, 2022). However, about 1 per cent of females will experience a premature menopause that occurs before the age of 40 (British Menopause Society, 2015). The menopause is not exclusive to females as it may affect transgender men as well. There is a period before the menopause, called perimenopause, where reducing levels of hormones can lead to some menopausal symptoms being experienced.

You may think that because the menopause occurs in later life, and after the athletic peak of most females, that it may not be something you need to consider. However, some female athletes may experience an early

DOI: 10.4324/9781003330110-13

menopause, in their 30s or 40s, and many females athletes continue competing in masters' events well into their 40s and 50s. In addition to these master athletes, many females will continue to exercise once their competitive careers have finished. Also, as exercise is recommended as a means of managing menopausal symptoms it is important for coaches and fitness professionals to know the symptoms of the menopause and the effect of the anatomical, physiological, and psychological changes that may occur. Understanding these profound changes that occur will enable professionals involved in strength and conditioning to support the physical activity of individuals during this stage of the lifecycle.

In this chapter we will develop a detailed knowledge of the menopause and its accompanying symptoms, how it is caused by changes in hormone levels, and assess the impact of these changes on athletic performance. Then we will explore how exercise and training can help manage the condition and what other measures can be taken. Box 13.1 presents the definitions of the stages of the menopause that will be used throughout this chapter.

BOX 13.1 STAGES OF THE MENOPAUSE

Premenopause: The time span between puberty (onset of menstrual periods) and perimenopause.

Premature menopause (premature ovarian insufficiency): A menopause that occurs at or before the age of 40, which may be the result of genetics, autoimmune disorders, medical procedures, or treatments.

Perimenopause: The time that begins with changes to the frequency, duration or flow during the menstrual cycle, and the start of menopause-related symptoms. It extends through menopause and up to one year after menopause.

Menopause: The natural end of the menstrual cycle, which can be confirmed after 12 consecutive months without a period. This time marks the permanent end of menstruation and fertility. It is a normal, natural event associated with reduced functioning of the ovaries, resulting in lower levels of ovarian hormones.

Post-menopause: The span of time after menopause.

Adapted from North American Menopause Society, 2022

The terms 'menopause' and 'post-menopause' are often used interchangeably, although they are technically slightly different. The menopause is the point where a woman has not had a period for 12 consecutive months, and after this point a woman is post-menopausal.

Before we examine the menopause read the case study in Box 13.2 where you will meet Mia who is a tennis player.

BOX 13.2 MIA (TENNIS PLAYER)

Mia is a tennis player who started playing as a teenager and represented her county. When she became a senior player at the age of 35 she started playing in the Senior's County Cup. However, by her mid-40s she found herself struggling with some difficult symptoms that were affecting her performance.

Here Mia tells her story:

Up until my mid-40s I had regular periods and although I did experience some symptoms during my period they never significantly affected my performance. Each period was regular and was fairly similar in its flow. However, in my mid-40s my periods started to change slightly as sometimes they started earlier and sometimes they started later, sometimes they were heavy and sometimes they were light. Around this time I was finding it harder to concentrate and was becoming irritable at home for no particular reason. I had started to have interrupted sleep as I was getting up around 4 am, then not being able to get back to sleep as I was having really anxious thoughts about all the bad things that could happen.

This was making finding the energy and enthusiasm for training harder. This may sound stupid but sometimes when I was playing tennis I started to lose track of the match score and even forgot the name of my opponent on a couple of occasions.

I just felt a bit off and was aware that something was happening to me. I was aware of the menopause but reassured myself I was too young for that, and these feelings would soon pass.

I did finally go to the doctor, and they informed me that I was experiencing symptoms of the perimenopause. The mention of the word 'menopause' scared me as I thought I was too young for that. These symptoms worsened and when I got to age 51 my periods stopped completely.

By this point I was having bad night sweats, as I would wake up in the small hours of the night covered in sweat with my bed sheets soaking as well. It got to the stage where I had to change my pyjamas every night and sometimes even the bed sheets. Also I was experiencing a lot of pain as my joints were becoming stiff and swollen and I had to reduce the amount of tennis I was playing.

Also at this time I was feeling extreme fatigue and frequently anxiety to the point where I was expecting the worse things to happen to my family. This was affecting my mood and my motivation to be active. I was ready to stop playing tennis altogether. When I shared this with my doctor they suggested I see a menopause specialist. This menopause specialist encouraged me to try hormone replacement therapy (HRT) and keep exercising as it would help me with my symptoms. Within a few weeks the symptoms lessened, and I have been able to keep playing tennis and start enjoying it again. In hindsight I wish I had started taking HRT sooner.

As you move through this chapter you will discover that initially Mia is experiencing perimenopausal symptoms until they worsen at the time around her menopause.

What happens at the menopause?

A person will be in the menopause when they have not had a period for 12 consecutive months. This is an indication that their body has stopped ovulating and the levels of their hormones have fallen to the point where they can no longer conceive. In particular oestrogen, progesterone and testosterone levels fall and this not only results in the loss of the menstrual cycle, but it has an effect on other organs and systems of the body.

Oestrogen, along with progesterone, are the driving forces of the menstrual cycle. Oestrogen is produced predominantly in the ovaries but there is also some produced in the liver, adrenal glands, and fat cells. While its predominate role is in ovulation there are oestrogen receptors all over the body, including in the brain, bones, joints and in the heart. At the brain oestrogen plays a role in cognitive health and it helps to maintain memory and cognition functions as well as regulating mood (Newson, 2019). Oestrogen helps to regulate serotonin that is referred to as the 'feel good' hormone and is also involved in the control of body temperature. In the heart oestrogen protects the arteries, while it is also central to the process of bone growth (Newson, 2019).

As oestrogen levels drop across the lifespan its reduction, as in Figure 13.1, is associated with low mood, increased anxiety, brain fog, rapid variations in body temperature, loss of bone density (osteoporosis and osteopenia) and an increased risk of heart disease. The impact of the reduction of oestrogen on the brain, skeleton, cardiovascular system, and the reproductive system can be

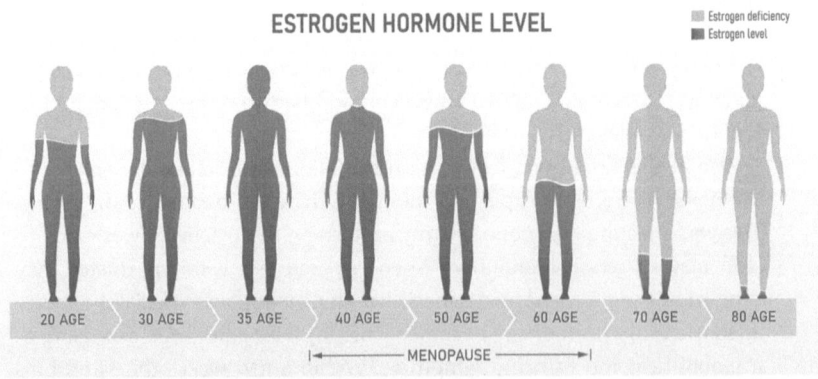

FIGURE 13.1 How oestrogen levels decline throughout the lifespan
Source: Shutterstock

minimised through hormone replacement therapy (HRT), and this is examined in Box 13.3 later in the chapter.

Progesterone is another hormone that helps to maintain the menstrual cycle along with oestrogen. It provides a balance with oestrogen by preparing the lining of the uterus for the fertilised egg to lie in. Its levels start to reduce before oestrogen levels meaning that oestrogen dominates during the perimenopausal stage, causing symptoms such as increased anxiety, sleeping difficulties and breast tenderness (Mansberg, 2020).

Testosterone is produced by the adrenal glands and is often mistakenly regarded as an exclusively male hormone. It is also present in females and its reduction leads to a lowering of sex drive, lower moods, and poorer concentration as well as a reduced ability to build bone and develop muscle (Newson, 2019).

Perimenopause: the change before the change

The perimenopause, or menstrual transition, is an undefined time span that starts with menstrual irregularity and ends when there has been 12-months without a period (Santoro, 2016). On average the perimenopausal stage starts at 47.5 years of age and last for around four years (Rayner and Fitzgerald (2016), although there are differing figures on this. There are two stages to the perimenopause: the early transition where cycles are mostly regular but there are a few changes; and the late transitions where periods may be up to 60 days apart.

It is worth saying that everyone who goes through the perimenopausal, and menopausal stages will have their own experiences of the stages. Their symptoms will differ, and they will respond differently to any treatments they undertake. The next section examines the menopause and the looks at some of the 31 associated physical and cognitive symptoms identified by Newson (2019).

Good menopause, bad menopause?

As stated previously 51 is the average age when the menopause begins. However, this age is dependent upon a range of genetic, lifestyle, and environmental factors (Hillyard et al., 2017). Genetics is a significant factor, and it is likely that a female will start their menopause a similar age to when their mother started theirs (Henpicked, 2020). This is particularly the case for women who experience an early menopause, as although it is not hereditary, many females who have an early menopause find out that other family members also had an early menopause (Newson, 2019). Lifestyle factors, such as smoking and stress, can lead to an earlier menopause as can surgical history (hysterectomy) and medical treatments such as chemotherapy (Henpicked, 2020).

While there is some variability in the age when the menopause starts there is also variation in the types and severity of symptoms that females will experience. There are some females who will not experience any symptoms. Of those females who do experience symptoms 25 per cent will have mild symptoms, 50 per cent will have moderate symptoms that affect their daily life, and 25 per cent will have severe symptoms that seriously impact on their wellbeing (The Well HQ, 2022).

There's more to it than hot flushes: symptoms of the menopause

The symptoms of the menopause are caused predominantly by the changes in hormone levels and the balance between the hormones. As virtually every cell in the body has receptors for oestrogen any changes will be felt widespread across the body. Figure 13.2 presents symptoms of the menopause, although there many, many others.

Authors have identified up to 62 symptoms of the menopause, including restless legs, dizziness/fainting, and tinnitus (Potter, 2022). We will now explore some of the most common and debilitating symptoms females may experience.

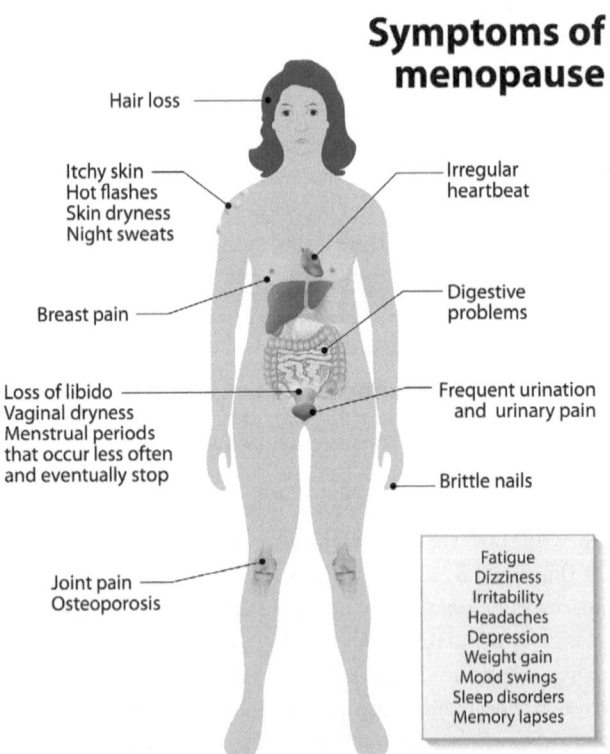

FIGURE 13.2 Symptoms of the menopause
Source: Shutterstock

Hot flushes and night sweats

Hot flushes are the symptoms most commonly associated with the menopause, and they are experienced by up to three out of four menopausal women (Women's Health Concern, 2022. Hot flushes and night sweats are characterised by a rapid surge in cutaneous vasodilation (opening up of blood vessels in the skin), an increase in heart rate, an increase in sweat rate and sometimes feelings of faint (Bailey et al., 2016). A hot flush has been described as an intense heat that comes on suddenly and spreads through the face, neck, chest, and body (Newson, 2021). Most hot flushes last between 5 seconds up to 5 minutes and they can happen a few times a day or even more regularly. Night sweats are similar to hot flushes, but they are characterised by an intense sweating that happens at night, and they often contribute to insomnia (Kaye, 2020).

It is not totally clear what causes hot flushes, but they may be related to the reduction of oestrogen causing a malfunction of the thermoregulatory control centre in the hypothalamus (Binkley et al., 2021). Thurston et al., (2009) identified that women with a high body mass index reported worse hot flushes, particularly in the perimenopausal phase. Smoking, anxiety, low mood have also been identified as contributory factors (Santoro, 2016). There is evidence to suggest that exercise can have an impact on reducing hot flushes and night sweats, as it can enhance blood flow to the thermoregulatory control centre and the skin, as well as decreasing resting body temperature, and the earlier onset of sweating to regulate body temperature (Bailey et al., 2016).

Mood changes

As well as the physical symptoms, many psychological symptoms are experienced as well. In particular the sudden changes of mood, such as being angry one minute and tearful the next. Mood changes are common during the perimenopause and menopause stages, and the following are some of the other psychological symptoms identified:

- Anger
- Frustration
- Irritability
- Lack of joy
- Reduced self-esteem

(Potter, 2022)

These changes may be related to reductions in oestrogen, as oestrogen promotes the production of serotonin. Serotonin is a neurotransmitter than is seen as a 'feel good chemical' as it has a positive effect in mood, energy levels, and sleep (Newson, 2019). The reduction in serotonin can negatively impact mood, and in conjunction with disturbed sleep and other symptoms, the psychological impact can be significant.

Anxiety and depression

Women are twice as likely to experience anxiety and depression than men at any age, but the prevalence of depression increases during the menopausal transition (Sassarini, 2016). Women who had previously had no symptoms of depression or anxiety become more likely to develop symptoms of depression during the perimenopause and anxiety during the menopause than before (Mulhall et al., 2017). Worryingly, the highest rate for suicides in females is in the 45–64 age group (Office for National Statistics, 2021) which includes the age bracket of the typical age of females going through the menopause.

Sleep disturbances

Insomnia and disturbed sleep patterns are experienced by 40–60 per cent of women going through the menopause with around 50 per cent of menopausal women getting fewer than 6 hours sleep a night (Baker et al., 2015). Rising anxiety levels during the menopause can make falling asleep more difficult while insomnia is related to depression in perimenopause, menopause and post-menopause stages (Terauchi et al., 2018).

There are many other causes that contribute to insomnia in menopause. For example, falling levels of oestrogen leading to hot flushes and night sweats. There may be urinary issues causing frequent bathroom trips as well as anxiety and depression. Levels of progesterone, which promotes rest and relaxation, and is beneficial to sleep quality are also falling (Newson, 2019). As sleep quality is impaired feelings of fatigue will be experienced during the day including morning grogginess and afternoon slumps in energy.

Brain fog

In Box 13.2, Mia, the case study, said that she would find it difficult to recall the score of the tennis game and indeed her opponent's name. These examples of brain fog, or menopausal fog, are typical and as the menopause is characterised by difficulty in focusing or concentrating and even this short term memory loss. Again, this is due to the effect that reduced oestrogen levels have on hormone receptors in the brain (Newson, 2019).

Musculoskeletal and cardiovascular considerations for menopausal and perimenopausal female athletes

The changes in the levels of hormones that occur in women from around their mid-40s impact on the muscular, skeletal, cardiovascular, and endocrine systems. All of the systems are vital in the production of optimal athletic performance. As a result, an awareness of these changes is vital when planning and designing training programmes. Some of these changes can be minimised, delayed, or even reversed. Before we look at training we will investigate the significant changes that occur to the body during the perimenopausal and menopausal stages.

1 Loss of muscle mass

Sarcopenia is the term used to describe the loss of skeletal muscle mass, muscular strength, and the accompanying loss of function as a result (Santilli et al., 2014). The reduction in muscle mass is due to a decrease in the size of type II (fast twitch) muscle fibres in particular, as well as a reduction in the number of type II motor units (Khalidar, 2019). This reduction in the number of type II muscle fibres and their cross sectional area will result in decreased muscular power and slower reaction times (Rothschild, 2022).

This loss of muscle is a natural effect of ageing as much as the result of the reduction in levels of the anabolic hormone testosterone. Women and men will both achieve peak muscle mass and muscular strength between the ages of 20 and 30 when the muscles' cross-sectional areas achieve maximum size (McArdle, Katch and Katch, 2022). Muscular strength declines progressively every decade, and by the age of 70 it will have decreased by 30 per cent. This loss of muscle, that also reduces basal metabolic rate, is accompanied by an increase in body fat of around 3 per cent each decade, even in individuals who train continuously (McArdle, Katch and Katch, 2022).

The menopause has a negative effect on body composition (ratio of lean body mass to fat body mass) with increased intra-abdominal (within the abdomen) and gluteo-femoral (hip, thigh, and legs) fat deposits (Seidelin et al., 2017). Unfortunately, this accumulation of intra-abdominal fat along with a reduction in lean body mass leads to potential insulin resistance and an increased risk of type 2 diabetes mellitus as well (Kalyani et al., 2014).

While some studies say that even individuals who train regularly will gain body fat each decade, there are other studies that say that remaining physically active can prevent the age-related loss of muscle and reduce the typical accumulation of body fat (McArdle, Katch and Katch, 2022). While muscular strength and power reduce in line with the reduction of type II muscle fibres it has been observed that in masters athletes the number of type I (slow twitch) muscle fibres is maintained or even increased (Rothschild, 2022). This means that in older athletes there is an increased reliance on type I muscle fibres during exercise and this can account for the reduction in power and speed in older age but maintenance of aerobic fitness. An early study by Powell (2005) concluded that changes in training routine that occur with age were more likely causing the change in the distribution of muscle fibres and body composition than ageing, and thus an appropriate training programme could reverse the changes in muscle fibre distribution to levels similar to younger athletes.

2 Reduction in bone density

The reduction in oestrogen in the perimenopausal and menopausal stage can have devasting effects on bone mass as oestrogen is central to the bone building process. Peak bone mass is reached in a female's third decade after which bone loss starts (Chadha et al., 2022). Accelerated bone loss starts during the menopause transition stage of the perimenopause and continues up to 10 years after with a total bone loss of between 10–15 per cent (Greendale et al., 2012). This can lead to fractures, disability, pain, and the diagnosis of diseases, such as osteoporosis and osteopenia. Osteoporosis is a condition where bones lose mineral density and strength meaning that it is more likely that they will fracture (Royal Osteoporosis Society, 2022), while osteopenia is the precursor to osteoporosis. Osteoporotic fractures generally occur at the spine, hip, and wrist. While these fractures may seem reversible the lack of activity resulting from fractures can have serious consequences. For example, there is a mortality rate of 10–24 per cent within one year of a hip fracture for females (Teng et al., 2008).

Low bone mass can also increase the risk of stress fractures. Female long distance runners are particularly prone to stress fractures to the femur and tibia, as a result of the repetitive loading on bones with low mineral density (Loudon, 2016). Athletes who have previously experienced relative energy deficiency in sport (RED-S) or have had previous menstrual disruption are more at risk of osteoporosis as this may have caused bone density loss previously (Rothschild and Schellhase, 2022).

Weight-bearing exercise, where forces pass through bones, helps prevent the damaging effects of osteoporosis associated with ageing and the perimenopause and menopause stages (McArdle, Katch and Katch, 2022). This is because exercise will promote bone building and development. However, exercise needs to be relative to age, and weight bearing activities such as walking, running and resistance training will be more beneficial than activities such as swimming, where the body is supported by buoyancy and limited force passes through bones. That said, any activity is preferable to inactivity when preventing or treating osteoporosis.

3 Declining pelvic floor health

As explored in Chapter 7, pelvic floor health is vital in sports and activities that involve high impact movements, such as running and gymnastics. These activities rely on the pelvic floor being able to withstand the forces placed on them, or else the result is leakage of urine, or urinary incontinence (UI). Oestrogen plays a key role in maintaining the pelvic floor and this is affected by the reduction in its levels. Also this reduction of oestrogen can lead to the thinning of the lining of the bladder and the urethra (the tube that carries urine from the bladder) (Newson, 2019). These factors can contribute to leaking from the bladder when the pelvic floor muscles are put under pressure from coughing, sneezing or sudden loading movements, such as when landing during running or jumping. The pelvic floor muscles may have already been weakened through vaginal child birth or obesity. Pelvic floor exercises should be performed daily and as part of a strength and conditioning programme to maintain pelvic floor function and avoid any leakage.

4 Increased risk of cardiovascular conditions

Cardiovascular performance reduces as part of the ageing process, with age-related decreases in maximum heart rate (HRmax) and maximal oxygen consumption (Vo_2max), but the menopause may have an impact on cardiovascular health as well. The link between the menopause and risk of cardiovascular disease in unclear, but it has been identified that an early menopause can lead to an increased risk of heart failure and atrial fibrillation while a later menopause is linked to reduced risk (Shin et al., 2022).

The reduction in oestrogen and progesterone seem to affect the autonomic control of the heart rate and blood pressure. The autonomic nervous system is responsible for inducing the force of contraction of the heart and heart rate. It also controls peripheral resistance of blood vessels, and these are impacted by the changes in hormones.

Changes in blood pressure may also be related to the changes in the lipid profiles in the blood at menopause. The changes include an increase in total cholesterol, triglycerides, low density lipoproteins (LDLs) while there is a decrease in high density lipoproteins (HDLs) that protect against heart disease. It is this increase in the ratio between total cholesterol and HDLs that leads to a higher risk of cardiovascular disease (Stefanska et al., 2015). The decrease in oestrogen at the menopause may cause the lipid profile to alter (Bade et al., 2014).

BOX 13.3 SPOTLIGHT ON: HORMONE REPLACEMENT THERAPY (HRT)

What is it?

Hormone replacements therapy (HRT) is a treatment where the hormones that have become deficient during the perimenopause and menopause are replaced. HRT always contains oestrogen, and it often contains progesterone as well. Some women are also prescribed testosterone. HRT works to reduce the symptoms of the menopause, such as the hot flushes, mood changes and urinary issues.

Oestrogen and progesterone are available as a patch, gel or spray and they are derived from the yam plant which is a root vegetable. It is described as being 'body identical' as it has the same molecular structure as oestrogen produced by the body.

Testosterone is prescribed for women who are experiencing symptoms of fatigue, brain fog and low sex drive

What effect will it have?

Many women find that while it may take a couple of months their symptoms do improve. In particular sleep quality, mood and concentration levels improve and the incidence of hot flushes and night sweats reduces. Often doses of hormones have to be altered to achieve the most benefits so it is important to have regular check-ups with your GP.

HRT also reduces the risks of health problems that derive from low hormone levels. The risk of osteoporosis is reduced as oestrogen protects the bones against reductions in bone mass and research shows that the risks of heart problems and strokes are reduced by 50 per cent. HRT can also protect against the development of other diseases such as Alzheimer's disease, type 2 diabetes, and osteoarthritis.

What are the risks?

In 2002 a study by the Women's Health Initiative identified that HRT may increase the risk of breast cancer and heart disease. However, an examination of the research study showed that the women in the study had an average age of 63, many were obese and had had heart attacks in the past. As well as having major risk factors for cancer and heart disease they were also using older forms of oestrogen and progesterone that are no longer prescribed.

Subsequent studies have shown that if women start taking HRT under the age of 60 and use the newer forms of HRT the benefits seriously outweigh any risks. The actual risk of developing cancer depends upon many factors including age, family history, lifestyle, and general health and overall 1 in 7 women will develop breast cancer in their lifetime (Breast Cancer Now, 2022).

Taking oestrogen only HRT is actually linked to a reduced risk of breast cancer while combined HRT (oestrogen and progesterone) containing older types of progesterone has a higher risk when compared to oestrogen and new micronized forms of progesterone. Research studies have shown that the risk of breast cancer with any type of HRT is either not present or very low and there is no increased risk in women under the age of 51.

(Adapted from Newson, 2021)

Training and exercise – the solution to managing the effects of the menopause?

Research strongly suggests that exercise is an effective treatment for people experiencing the psychological symptoms and physical changes that occur during the menopause. Exercise may even be as effective as medical treatments, such as hormone replacement therapy (HRT), with the combination of traditional treatments with exercise offering the best outcomes (Pederson and Saltin, 2015).

However, the thought of exercise for some people going through the menopause is not always appealing. Feeling depressed, anxious, fatigued, sleep deprived and experiencing low self-esteem may not produce the ideal psychological state for embarking on a training regime or new forms of exercise. We can see that in the case study of Mia in Box 13.2 she says how feelings of extreme fatigue and anxiety were affecting her mood and motivation to exercise. That said, the benefits of exercise will far outweigh the risks of not exercising for the majority of post-menopausal women. Therefore, coaches and trainers need to find opportunities to present the benefits of training for post-menopausal women, and training schedules need to be specific to protect against the negative effects of the menopause and ageing (Binkley et al., 2021).

The key goals of a training programme for perimenopausal and post-menopausal females are to protect the functioning of the cardiovascular system, maintain or develop muscle and bone mass, minimise weight gain through fat accumulation, and ensure against a reduction in insulin sensitivity contributing to the development of type 2 diabetes. The menopause is accompanied by the natural process of ageing that has additional effects, such as loss of balance, co-ordination, and flexibility and these need to be considered as well. A specific training programme for females in the perimenopausal and post-menopausal stages should include the following types of training.

Aerobic training

Aerobic training that increases the heart rate is vital during the perimenopause and the menopause. This is because reductions in the level of oestrogen can increase the risks of developing high blood pressure and coronary heart disease (Binkley et al., 2021). Aerobic training can protect against these by lowering blood pressure and increasing arterial circulation (Ward, 2022). However, the fitness level and exercise preferences of the individual need to be considered before developing a training programme. Walking has been identified as the preferred exercise type by menopausal women (Daley et al., 2011), however, jogging, running, cycling, rowing, and dancing may all be appropriate activities. Table 13.1 presents aerobic training recommendations for menopausal females of differing fitness levels

Resistance training

Resistance training has positive benefits on muscle size and strength, bone mass density, type 2 diabetes, fat accumulation, cardiovascular health and physical performance (Leite et al., 2010). In particular resistance training addresses the issues of osteoporosis and sarcopenia that impact on both performance and function in daily life. Resistance training can take many forms other than gym based training, and can include using resistance bands, body weight or water to provide resistance to work against.

TABLE 13.1 Aerobic training recommendations for menopausal women

Training level	Training recommendations
Novice (Beginner or presence of risk factors, osteoporosis, heart disease)	Frequency – 3–5 days a week Intensity – low to moderate (30–50 per cent of maximum heart rate) Time 10–30 minutes/day Progression – start with short bouts of exercise then increase time before increasing pace.
Intermediate (Some training history or moderate risk factors)	Frequency – 3–5 days a week Intensity – moderate to vigorous (50–70 per cent of maximum heart rate) Time 20–60 minutes/day Progression – increase time exercising and then gradually increase pace.
Advanced (Athlete, or recent training history with low risk factors)	Frequency – 3–5 days a week Intensity – moderate to vigorous (70–85 per cent of maximum heart rate) Time 30–75 minutes/day Progression – increase time exercising and then gradually increase pace.

Source: Adapted from Binkley et al. (2021)

Resistance training should focus on working the major muscle groups of the body – glutes, quadriceps, hamstrings, latissimus dorsi and pectorals. Once these muscles have been worked then the minor muscles – deltoids, trapezius, biceps, triceps, and calves. Resistance training should include exercises for the pelvic floor as well to decrease any issues with incontinence. Table 13.2 presents resistance training recommendations for menopausal females of differing fitness levels.

Impact training

Impact training, such as walking, dancing, and jumping, is vital in the prevention of osteoporosis to stimulate both growth and bone maintenance in post-menopausal women (Binkley et al., 2021). During impact exercise forces will be transmitted through bones from ground reaction forces when the feet make contact with the ground and when muscles exert forces on bones to produce movement and promote bone development.

The choice of impact, or weight bearing exercises, needs to take into account the individual's level of conditioning and their body mass. For less conditioned women walking, marching, lunging and step ups would be appropriate. For moderately well-conditioned women side step ups, single leg hopping, and squat jumps would be beneficial, while for well-conditioned women and athletes depth jumps, star jumps and backwards/forwards squat jumps would produce the overload required (Daly et al., 2019).

TABLE 13.2 Resistance training recommendations for menopausal women

Training level	Training recommendations
Novice (Beginner or presence of risk factors, osteoporosis, heart disease)	Frequency – 2–3 days a week Intensity – low (40–60 per cent of 1 rep max) Sets – 1–3 Repetitions – 8–12 Rest – 1–2 minutes between sets Progression – start with short bouts of exercise then increase time before increasing pace.
Intermediate (Some training history or moderate risk factors)	Frequency – 3–4 days a week Intensity – moderate (60–80 per cent of 1 rep max) Sets – 2–4 Repetitions – 8–12 Rest – 1–2 minutes between sets Progression – start with short bouts of exercise then increase time before increasing pace.
Advanced (Athlete, or recent training history with low risk factors)	Frequency – 4–6 days a week Intensity – high (80 per cent+ of 1 rep max) Sets – 3–6 Repetitions – 8–12 Rest – 1–2 minutes between sets Progression – start with short bouts of exercise then increase time before increasing pace.

Source: Adapted from Binkley et al. (2021)

Balance and co-ordination

Balance and co-ordination exercises can lead to improved balance and stability and can improve physical function (Dipietro et al., 2019). Improved balance can help to protect against osteoporotic fractures, particularly at the hip and wrist, that result from falls. Activities such as yoga, Tai Chi and Pilates are recommended with care being taken with females who have osteoporosis.

Flexibility

Flexibility training to include dynamic stretching in the warm-up and static stretching in the cool-down should be included to maintain or even increase the range of movement of joints (Binkley et al., 2021). Musculoskeletal connective tissue, such as tendons and ligaments become less pliable with age and more prone to injury (Loudon, 2016). This loss of pliability can increase joint stiffness and limit joint movement with estimates suggesting flexibility declines by 6 per cent every decade after the age of 50 years resulting in a negative impact on athletic performance (Ganse and Degens, 2021).

Dynamic stretching in a warm-up should mimic the movements that will be undertaken in the training or exercise session, while in the cool-down, static stretches should be applied to all muscles that have been contracting during the training or exercise session.

BOX 13.4 REAL-WORLD APPLICATION

As a female athlete, you should:

1. Be able to identify the physical and mental symptoms you might experience at the perimenopausal and menopausal stages of life and make preparations when the time comes.
2. Include resistance training in your training schedule at least twice a week to preserve muscle mass, maintain functional movements and protect bone density to reduce the risk of developing osteoporosis.
3. Address any lifestyle issues such as smoking, excess alcohol intake and stress that may predispose you to an early menopause, particularly if a close relative has had an early menopause.
4. Track your menstrual cycle and record any changes in timing, flow, and regularity.
5. Consult a doctor or menopause specialist when you start to experience menopausal symptoms.

As a coach, you should:

1. Develop a coaching environment and coach-athlete relationships where you are able to discuss issues around the menopause and how they may be affecting female athletes.
2. Be able to identify the signs and symptoms of perimenopause and menopause in your athletes.
3. Be able to advise on the types of exercise and activities that athletes should be undertaking to manage the symptoms and physiological changes that occur in perimenopausal and menopausal stages.
4. Develop a network of professionals around you and your athletes that you can trust and refer your athletes to if you identify any need for further help.

Summary

Having completed this chapter you will now have developed a more detailed understanding of the stages of the menopause, the challenges that female athletes may face and the physical and psychological symptoms that can be experienced. In particular you will understand the benefits of exercising during the stages of the menopause and the types of training that can protect against, or slow down, some of the anatomical and physiological changes that can occur during these stages. Resistance and impact training assume even more important during this life stage to protect the bones against the reduction in bone mineral density that occurs with lowered oestrogen levels.

The key messages to take away from this chapter are:

1. The menopause is the life stage when the menstrual cycle stops, and the female has not had a period in the least 12 months.
2. It is possible that a female may experience menopause type symptoms from their mid-40s during a stage called the perimenopause.
3. The menopause is characterised by reductions in the production of ovarian hormones, oestrogen and progesterone, and the symptoms and physical effects caused by this change.
4. The average age for the menopausal is 51 and its symptoms commonly include hot flushes, night sweats, mood swings, brain fog, anxiety, and depression.
5. There are several physical changes to the body that may impact on athletic performance, including a reduction in muscle mass, an increase in fat mass, reduction in bone density, weaking pelvic floor muscles and an increased risk of cardiovascular conditions.
6. Exercise is recommended to manage and reduce some menopausal symptoms.
7. Training is essential to protect against physical changes that occur, and a training schedule should include aerobic, resistance and impact training as well as balance and co-ordination exercises.

End-of-Chapter Quiz

Answers can be found after the References

1. Identify when a female is considered to be in the menopause stage:

   a   When they start to experience symptoms that affect wellbeing
   b   When oestrogen and progesterone levels start to reduce
   c   When periods become irregular in duration and frequency
   d   When they have not had a period for 12 consecutive months

2. Identify the average age at which the menopause starts:

   a   45
   b   47.5
   c   51
   d   54.5

3. Identify which of the following is not a recognised symptom of the menopause:

   a   Anxiety
   b   Osteoarthritis
   c   Incontinence
   d   Osteoporosis

4. The reduction in muscle size and strength is called:

   a   Osteopenia
   b   Ovarian insufficiency
   c   Sarcopenia
   d   Vasodilation

5. Identify why impact training is so important for menopausal females?

   a   It protects against loss of muscle mass
   b   It increases joint stability
   c   It improves maximal oxygen uptake
   d   It promotes bone development

References

Bade, G., Shah, S., Nahar, P. and Vaidya, S. (2014) Effect of menopause on lipid profile in relation to body mass index. *Chronicle of Young Scientists*, 5, 20–24.

Bailey, T.G., Cable, T.N., Aziz, N., Atkinson, G., Cuthbertson, D.J., Low, D.A. and Jones, H. (2016) Exercise training reduces the acute physiological severity of post-menopausal hot flushes. *Journal of Physiology*, 594, 657–667.

Baker, F.C., Willoughby, A.R., Sassoon, S.A., Colrain, I.M. and Zambotti, M. (2015) Insomnia in women approaching menopause: Beyond perception. *Psychoneuroendocrinology*, 60, 96–104.

Binkley, H.M., Phillips, K.L. and Wise, S.L. (2021) Menopausal Women: Recognition, Exercise, Benefits, Considerations and Programming Needs. *National Strength and Conditioning Association*, 43(4), 87–104.

Breast Cancer Now (2022) What is breast cancer?. Online at: *What is breast cancer?* (breastcancernow.org) (Accessed 11 October 2022).

British Menopause Society (2015) Premature ovarian insufficiency. Online at: *Premature ovarian insufficiency – British Menopause Society* (thebms.org.uk) (Accessed 4 October 2022).

Chadha, M., Chaddha, R., Divakar, H. and Kalyan, H.K. (2022) Osteoporosis: Epidemiology, Pathogenesis, Evaluation and Treatment. *Open Journal of Orthopedics*, 12 (4), 153–182.

Daley, A., Stokes-Lampard, H., Wilson, S., Rees, M., Roalfe, A. and McArthur, C. (2011) What women want? Exercise preferences of menopausal women. *Maturitas*. 68, 174–178.

Daly, R.M., Via, J.D., Duckham, R.L., Fraser, S.F. and Helge, E.W. (2019) Exercise for the prevention of osteoporosis in post-menopausal women: an evidence based guide to the optimal prescription. *Brazilian Journal of Physical Therapy*, 23, 170–180.

Dipietro, L., Campbell, W.W., Buchner, D.M., Erickson, K.I., Powell, K.E., Bloodgood, B., Hughes, T., Day, K.R., Piercy, K.L., Vaux-Bjerke, A. and Olson, R.D. (2019) Physical activity, injurious falls, and physical function in aging. *Medicine and Science in Sports and Exercise*, 51, 1303–1313.

Ganse, B. and Degens, H. (2021) Current insights in the age-related decline in sports performance of the older athlete. *International Journal of Sports Medicine*, 42, 879–888.

Greendale, G.A., Sowers, M.F., Han, W, Huang, M-H., Crandall, C., Lee, J.S. and Karlamangla, A. (2012) Bone mineral density loss in relation to the final menstrual period in a multiethnic cohort. *Journal of Bone and Mineral Research*, 27, 111–118.

Henpicked (2020) When will I start the menopause? Online at: *When will I start the menopause? | Menopause Hub – Expert information, useful resources, top tips and women's stories* (henpicked.net) (Accessed 4 October 2022).

Hillard, T., Abernethy, K., Hamoda, H., Shaw, I., Everett, M., Ayres, J. and Currie, H. (2017) *Management of the Menopause* (6th ed.). Marlow: British Menopause Society.

Kalyani, R.R., Corriere, M. and Ferucci, L. (2014) Age related and disease-related muscle mass: The effect of diabetes, obesity and other diseases. *The Lancet Diabetes and Endocrinology*, 2(10), 819–829.

Kaye, P. (2020) *The M Word: Everything You Need to Know About the Menopause*. London: Vie Books.

Khalidar, S.S. (2019) Musculoskeletal disorders and menopause. *Journal of Obstetrics and Gynaecology India*, 69, 99–103.

Leite, R.D., Prestes, J., Pereira, G.B., Shiguemoto, G.E. and Perez, S.E. (2010) Menopause: Highlighting the effects of resistance training. *Sports Medicine*, 31, 761–767.

Ley, S.H., Li, Y., Tobias, D.K., Manson, J.E., Rosner, B., Hu, F.B. and Rexrode, K.M. (2017) Duration of reproductive lifespan, age at menarche, and age at menopause are associated with risk of cardiovascular disease in women. *Journal of American Heart Association*, 6, 1–11.

Loudon, J.K. (2016) The master female athlete. *Physical Therapy in Sport*, 22, 123–128.

Mansberg, G. (2020) *The M Word: How to Thrive in Menopause*. London: Murdoch Books.

McArdle, W., Katch, F.I. and Katch, V.L. (2022) *Exercise Physiology: Nutrition, Energy and Human Performance* (9th ed.). Philadelphia: Wolters Kluwer.

Mulhall, S., Andel, R. and Anstey, K.J. (2017) Variations in symptoms of depression and anxiety in midlife women by menopausal status. *Maturitas*, 108, 7–12.

North American Menopause Society (2022) Menopause Glossary. Online at: *Menopause Glossary, Menopause Resources | The North American Menopause Society, NAMS* (Accessed 4 October 2022).

Newson, L. (2021) *Preparing for the menopause*. United Kingdom: Penguin Life.

Newson, L. (2019) *Menopause; all you need to know in one concise manual*. Yeovil: Haynes.

NHS Choices (2022) Menopause Overview. Online at: *Menopause – NHS* (www.nhs.uk) (Accessed 4 October 2022).

Office for National Statistics (2021) Suicides in England and Wales: 2021 registrations. Online at: *Suicides in England and Wales – Office for National Statistics* (ons.gov.uk) (Accessed 10 October 2022).

Peterson, B.K. and Saltin, B. (2015) Exercise as medicine – evidence for prescribing exercise as therapy in 26 different chronic diseases. *Scandinavian Journal of Sports Medicine*, 25(3), 1–72.

Potter, N. (2022) Menopause symptoms checklist. Online at: *Menopause Symptom Checklist – Menopause Care* (Accessed 6 October 2022).

Powell, A.P. (2005) Issues unique to the masters athlete. *Current Sports Medicine Reports*, 4, 335–340.

Rayner, S. and Fitzgerald, P. (2016) *Making Friends with the Menopause*. Sarah Rayner: Amazon Fulfilment.

Rothschild, C.E. and Schellhase, K.C. (2022) Considerations for the female adult endurance runner: A survey analysis. *Journal of Women's Physical Health Therapy*, 44, 3–8.

Royal Osteoporosis Society (2022) Information and Support. Online at: *Osteoporosis –
Low bone density | ROS* (theros.org.uk) (Accessed 7 October 2022).

Santilli, V., Bernetti, A., Mangone, M. and Paoloni, M. (2014) Clinical definition of
sarcopenia. *Clinical Cases of Mineral and Bone Metabolism*, 11, 177–180.

Santoro, N. (2016) Perimenopause: From Research to Practice. *Journal of Womens
Health*, 25(4), 332–9.

Sassarini, J. (2016) Depression in midlife women. *Maturitas*, 94, 161–175.

Seidelin, K., Nyberg, M., Piil, P., Jorgensen, N.R., Hellsten, Y. and Bangsbo, J. (2017)
Adaptations with intermittent exercise training in post- and premenopausal women.
Medicine and Science in Sports and Exercise, 49(1), 96–105.

Shin, J., Han, K., Jung, J.H., Park, H.J. and Kim, W. (2022) Age at menopause and risk
of heart failure and atrial fibrillation: a nationwide cohort study. *European Heart
Journal*. doi:10.1093/eurheartj/ehac364.

Stefanska, A., Bergmann, K. and Sypniewska, G. (2015) Metabolic syndrome and
menopause: Pathophysiology, clinical and diagnostic significance. *Advanced Clinical
Chemistry*, 72, 1–75.

Teng, G.G., Curtis, J.L. and Saag, K.G. (2008) Mortality and Osteoporotic Fractures: Is
the Link Causal and is it Modifiable? *Clinical and Experimental Rheumatology*, 26,
125–137.

Terauchi, M., Odai, T., Hirose, A., Akiyoshi, M., Masuda, M., Tsunoda, R., Fushiki,
H. and Miyasaki, N. (2018) Dizziness in peri- and postmenopausal women is associated with anxiety: a cross-sectional study. *BioPsychoSocial Medicine*, 12, 12–21.

Thurston, R.C., Sowers, M.R., Sternfield, B. and Gold, E.B. (2009) Gains in Body Fat and
Vasomotor Symptom Reporting Over the Menopausal Transition: The Study of
Women's Health Across the Nation. *American Journal of Epidemiology*, 170(6), 766–74.

Ward, T. (2022) Female athletic performance: managing the menopause. *Sports Injury
Bulletin*. Online at: *Female athletic performance: managing menopause* (sportsinjur
ybulletin.com) (Accessed 11 October 2022).

Women's Health Concern (2022) The Menopause. Available at: www.womens-hea
lth-concern.org/wp-content/uploads/2022/12/15-WHC-FACTSHEET-The-Menopause-
NOV2022-B.pdf (Accessed 2 April 2024).

The Well HQ (2022) @menopause FAQs. Online at: www.thewell-hq.com/menopause/m
enopause-faqs (Accessed 6 October 2022).

Answers

1. d
2. c
3. b
4. c
5. d

14

THE PSYCHOLOGY OF COACHING FEMALE ATHLETES

Candice Lingam-Willgoss

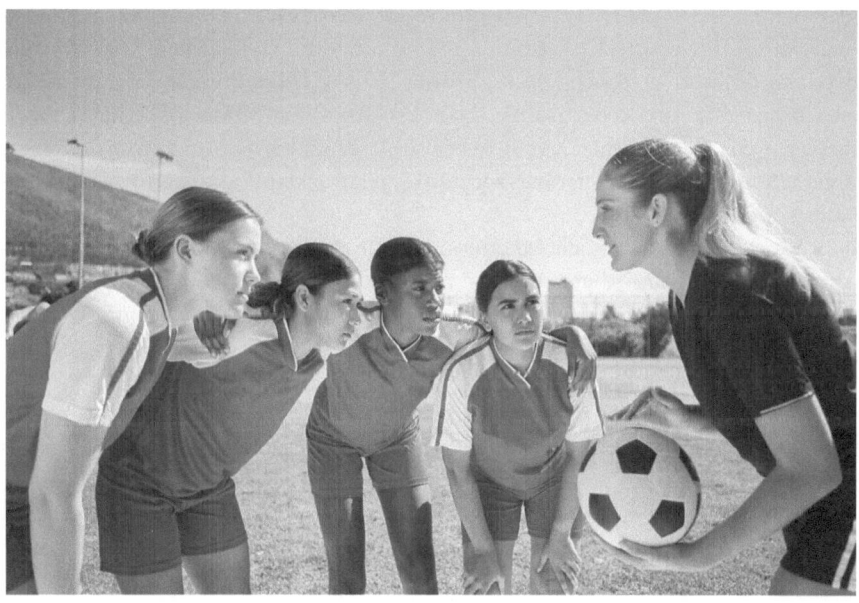

The current movement within research on female sports performance, and much of this book, tends to focus on the many biological differences between the sexes and the implication these differences may have on the support female athletes require. However, these are not the only differences between men and women, and it is important for those working with female athletes to also consider the variations in the psychology of men and women. For example, research suggests that there are several subtle differences when looking at the psychology of men and women including, goal orientation, cohesion, sources of

DOI: 10.4324/9781003330110-14

confidence and preferred coaching style (Pitchers and Elliott-Sale, 2019). While an appreciation of the right physical training an athlete needs is fundamental to performance improvement, without acknowledging the different psychological needs of women optimal performance is unlikely to be achieved.

One of the main distinctions between male and female athletes lies in what drives their participation and performance. Findings by Moradi et al. (2020), suggested that male athletes ranked situational factors, fun and teamwork as most important whereas female athletes ranked teamwork, fun and fitness. These differences link to previous findings that suggest men are more motivated by competition and females by friendship and health (e.g. Egli et al., 2011). Differences such as these illustrate the importance of coaches understanding the motivations of the female athletes they coach to ensure that they are considering their psychological needs. For example, if teamwork is more important to female athletes even within an individual setting, the importance of the team needs to be foregrounded within the training environment.

The preference of coaching styles has also received significant interest in the coaching literature with findings indicating that female athletes tend to prefer democratic styles (where they have some control of their training) in contrast to male athletes who tend to prefer a more autocratic style (where they are told what to do by their coach) (Wałach-Biśta, 2019). These differences in preferred coaching style are inextricably linked to communication, whether that is between coach and athlete or between athletes and it is imperative that these interactions remain positive if successful relationships and performance outcomes are to be created.

Regardless of how much expertise a coach may have when they are ineffective communicators it can present a significant barrier to the coach/athlete relationship in particular when that relationship is a male coaching working with female athletes. Research within this area suggests that it is key for coaches to align their coaching to the preferences of female athletes, who predominantly prefer strong relationships with their coach that are based on trust and when they feel that they can be involved with the decision-making process (Lau et al., 2020).

Preferences in coaching style and motivational factors are not the only psychological differences that coaches need to be aware of when working with female athletes. For example, men see interpersonal comparison and winning as sources of confidence, in contrast women thrive off personalised goals, performance or process related, with a more task-oriented approach to training and competition (Hays et al., 2007). Tailoring coaching approaches and support to align with female athlete preferences are likely to positively impact participation and performance.

As we move further through this final chapter we will start to examine in more detail the evidence base that looks at the psychology of coaching women as well as some of the challenges that can present themselves. Before we start to examine these areas you are introduced to Molly, a 25-year-old swimmer.

BOX 14.1 MOLLY (ELITE FREESTYLE SWIMMER)

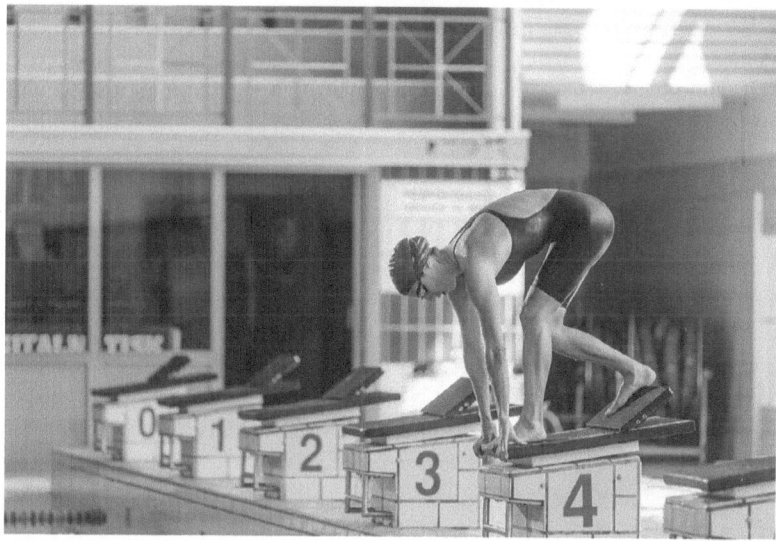

Molly has been swimming competitively since she was eight years old, now aged 21 years she has been selected for the England swim team. This has seen a change in the coaching setup around her as she is now training with the England squad and rarely gets to train with her regional team, as a result of a clash in training sessions.

Her previous coach Mark had worked with her since she entered the senior squad at 17 and he had built up a very positive relationship with her. His style of coaching was highly individualised, as he focused very much on what worked best for each individual rather than a one size fits all approach. Molly had always been very involved in setting her training plan and often questioned what she was being asked to do and sought out extra insights into her weekly schedule. Mark was always open to her insights but equally explained to Molly if her suggested changes weren't feasible or likely to be productive. This approach saw a very collaborative relationship between Mark and Molly where she contributed her thoughts on training plans and they were developed together.

Her new coach Ray is a very well-known and a highly successfully swim coach, renowned internationally for the improvements that are seen in the athletes he coaches. However, Molly is struggling with the change in coach, mainly because Ray is so different to Mark. Ray sets drills and training for the whole squad without little explanation of why and everyone just seems to get on with the session. At her second session Molly asked the purpose of the session as well as the plan for the rest of the week. Ray's response was that he knows what works and she should trust him. Being new, Molly has just got on with the training, but she isn't enjoying things as she just feels like just another athlete with no specific focus on her individual needs or specific feedback on her training. She knows that Ray has been successful but is struggling with the loss of input into her training and is contemplating leaving and going back to the regional squad.

What the case study illustrates is some of the issues that females face when being coached, in this instance two male coaches working with two contrasting approaches. As we move through this chapter, we will refer to Molly's case study to highlight some of the practical steps that can be taken to support her, and women in general, within the coaching environment, starting with communication styles and the potential issues that can impact the participation and performance of women.

Communication styles

When working with athletes it is key for coaches to understand how to best communicate with each and every individual and communication can be viewed as the key driver for developing and maintaining the relationships between coach and athlete. Research by Davis et al. (2019) highlighted that using the right communication style links to the positive enhancement of the quality of the coach/athlete relationship as well as the athlete's experience of sport satisfaction. Furthermore, their research showed it is important to consider how an individual's perception of another's communication is key as what one athlete perceives as helpful another may perceive as challenging. This raises a key point, which suggests coaches need to consider how their communication may be perceived differently by individual athletes. We saw in the case study how Molly is finding it difficult to adapt to a different type of coaching as Ray doesn't communicate with her in the same way as Mark, this is also starting to impact on her enjoyment and sport satisfaction. Her former coach Mark adopted a style known as an 'athlete-centred approach' which allowed him to take the athletes perspective into account and work collaboratively. This variation on the person-centre approach developed by psychologist Carl Rogers works off the principle that there are three pillars needed to create the right climate around the athlete which are illustrated in Figure 14.1 below.

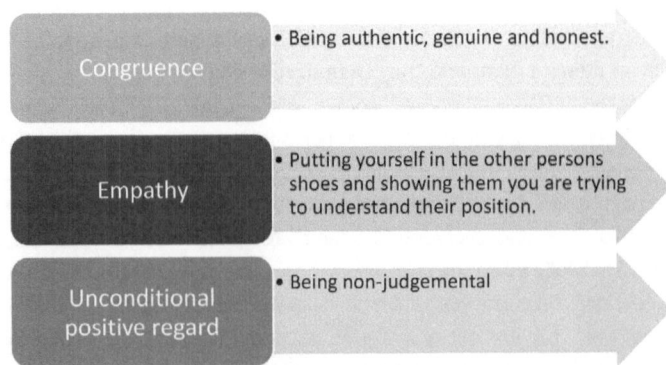

FIGURE 14.1 The three factors required to create an open coaching environment
Source: Adapted from Nelson et al. (2014)

It seems likely that the factors shown in Figure 14.1 are what led to Molly and Mark having such a positive coach/athlete relationship. Mark would always listen to Molly's suggestions and consider her point of view and remained genuine and honest with her, resulting in her feeling empowered and cared for. This aligns to the findings of Lau et al. (2020), who also concluded that trust was key to building a positive relationship between coach and athlete. Likewise, research into social support (e.g. Brown et al., 2018) found that it was of fundamental importance to athletes to feel cared for and that they could trust their coach. From the coach's perspective, they acknowledged how knowing the athlete so well allowed them to be more effective, as they knew how to get the best from them – in turn allowing them to coach the person, not the athlete.

The psychology of female athletes

The preferences of female athletes in terms of communication style illustrates one significant difference in the psychology of female athletes to male athletes. With the upward trajectory of female participation in both recreational and elite sport there has been a greater interest in these subtle psychological differences. In a review article by Herrero et al. (2021) they examined a number of psychological factors that were pertinent to elite female athletes, including those around mental health and wellbeing. For example, one of the studies within their review (Pluhar and McCracker, 2019), suggested that anxiety and depression rates tend to be higher among female athletes, especially for those within individual sports. This one factor is pertinent to coaches understanding of athletes as increased levels of anxiety have been shown to positively correlate with increased injury risk (Herrero et al., 2021). These findings echoed the earlier research of Correia and Rosado (2019) whose comparative study of male and female athletes from a range of team and individual sports also concluded that female and individual sports athletes revealed much higher levels of sport-related anxiety.

A further difference between male and female athletes was observed by Özdemir (2019) who concluded that male elite athletes reported much higher levels of psychological resilience than their female counterparts. Athletes' ability to perform under pressure is fundamental to their success in sport, as the high-performance sports environment requires athletes to adapt to and manage different demands on a daily basis (Fletcher, 2018). This high-pressure environment often sees athletes overcoming adversity, in turn facilitating the development of resilience which is a quality underpinning sustained success in sport (Fletcher, 2018). The importance of the development of resilience for female athletes, is also salient when placed in the context of research by Tekavc et al (2020) who concluded that female athletes often face more challenges in their career related to sport inequality, body image and mental distress, highlighting how this is an area of great significance for coaches to be aware of and to foster an environment that allows the development of resilience.

In addition to resilience, gender differences have also been documented within research exploring self-compassion (caring for yourself), which is a mediator of mindfulness and burnout. Amemiya and Sakairi (2020) reported that female athletes tended to score lower on mindfulness and self-compassion than male athletes, a finding that is similar to that of non-athletic females. Such findings point to a need for coaches to understand differences between male and female athletes which may see them manage situations in different ways.

The importance of the coach–athlete relationship

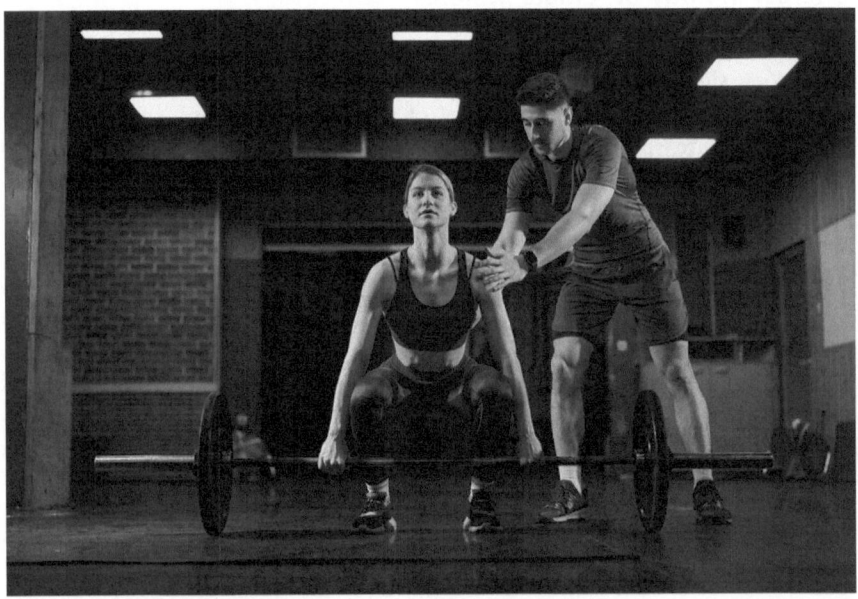

There has been extensive research looking at the importance of the coach/athlete relationship within the athletic development literature (Shipherd et al., 2019). Jowett and Poczwardowski (2007) have defined this relationship as one that sees the athlete and coach start to work as one with their cognitions, feelings and behaviours being somewhat interrelated with an interdependence between them. Jowett (2007) developed this aspect of interdependence to ascertain the extent of connection between the coach and athlete which can in turn shape the coaching interactions. What this explanation further highlights is the element of mutuality within the relationship and how both the coach and the athlete have responsibility for it. When managed correctly this can lead to highly effective interpersonal exchanges and in turn facilitative relationships. In contrast without a strong base of communication skills even with the right technical expertise it will be hard for a coach to successfully transfer their knowledge (Cherubini, 2019). We have seen this directly in the example of Molly, when she changed coaches whereby the positive coach/athlete relationship was lost which had a huge impact on her, resulting in Molly losing motivation and questioning her place within the team.

The importance of this relationship becomes even more relevant when you consider a number of the factors we have looked at throughout this book, for example the impact of the menstrual cycle on performance. Clarke et al. (2021) focused on what male coaches felt they needed to know about their female athletes around their menstrual cycle in a bid to better support them, of the five areas coaches felt the most important area they needed to understand more about was how to communicate with their athletes about this topic and when was best to do it. This paper shows some steps forward by male coaches to understand the needs of female athletes but also how there is a desire to learn more about how to communicate more effectively as well.

Gender, power imbalances, and communication

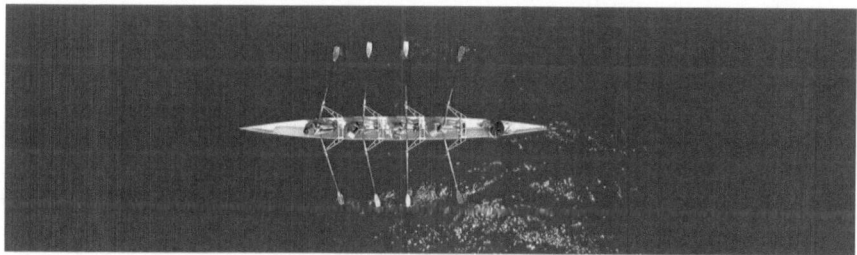

In earlier chapters we have talked about the gendered nature of sport and how this is often perpetuated by the power imbalances that remain within these environments. These imbalances can present female athletes with additional stressors within sport when they are faced with patronising attitudes, gender stereotypes and inequality in the way they are treated (Pitchers and Elliott- Sale, 2019). This power imbalance is similar to that seen between young athletes and coaches when acquiescence occurs with young athletes remaining silent, this lack of balanced dialogue sees the coach in control of the situation and the conversation (Groom et al., 2012). It is key to address this area as Norman and French (2013) discuss, coaches hold a very powerful position in the life of the elite female athlete and if their practices fail to be personalised and positive they will have a significant impact on all aspects of the athlete journey.

This difference in treatment of female vs male athletes was the focus of De Haan and Knoppers (2019) examination of elite level rowing and the behaviours of 12 elite-level coaches. They found that coaching behaviour was heavily influenced by their own experiences of coaching and while they perceived all athletes were treated equally their prominent discourses positioned the female athletes as inferior when compared to male norms. Findings such as these further emphasise the gendered nature of sport with men positioned as superior.

These findings link to work that has considered how unconscious bias is often at play within coaching settings and how when we meet new people it may influence how we then communicate. Unconscious bias is explained in Box 14.2.

BOX 14.2 WHAT IS UNCONSCIOUS BIAS?

Unconscious bias arises when we make initial judgements about people based on previous experiences, often termed learnt stereotypes, ingrained within our beliefs. From childhood we start to build up a series of unconscious pathways between cues we pick up from people we meet and how we judge them. Each time a judgement is unchallenged the pathway strengthens reinforcing the way we both automatically and subconsciously interact with new people we meet (Marino et al., 2021).

The impact of unconscious bias was seen in research looking at the range of factors that affect the coaching of elite female athletes. These findings suggested that coaches differentiate their practice based on gender influenced by both their perception of the value of sports participation by women as well as their own background (De Haan and Sotiriadou, 2019). Within sports environments people are frequently forming new relationships whether that is between coach and athlete or athlete and athlete and it is important for all those working within sport to recognise their own unconscious bias and how this might impact their communications (Levi et al., 2023). Furthermore, Levi et al. (2023) suggest it is key that coaches avoid stereotyping athletes and recognised the gendered world that female athletes find themselves within.

BOX 14.3 SPOTLIGHT ON: THE DARKER SIDE OF COACHING: ABUSE IN SPORT

While we have looked at some of the challenges that can be seen within the coach/athlete relationship when communication isn't managed in the most productive way, there is the potential for more dramatic failings within some coaching environments. For some athletes sport is not a positive space and can be an environment where abuse is present and allowed to continue as it is deemed the norm. Abuse in a coaching setting can range from bullying behaviour by coaches, over-prioritisation of performance outcomes, to the most severe of sexual abuse as was seen in the case of Larry Nassar (American gymnastics coach) (Hobson and Boren, 2018). What is most concerning is how some of the behaviours typical of emotional abuse in sport are viewed as normal or a necessary means of coaching (Kerr et al., 2020), with athletes also perceiving this as normal (Stafford et al., 2015).

The impact of this type of coaching has serious implications for the athlete. Kerr et al. (2020) examined the experiences of female Canadian athletes and the impact of emotionally abusive coaching practice. The impact affected all aspects of the athlete's life, including a range of negative psychological effects (depression, decreased confidence), a negative impact on their relationship with sport and finally implications on their life outside of sport with it having a serious bearing on their social lives. Longer term these experiences had implications for their life after sport such as difficulties forming new relationships or engaging in abusive relationships. The athletes in their study presented several reflections on their experiences with abusive coaches which are illustrated in Figure 14.2 below.

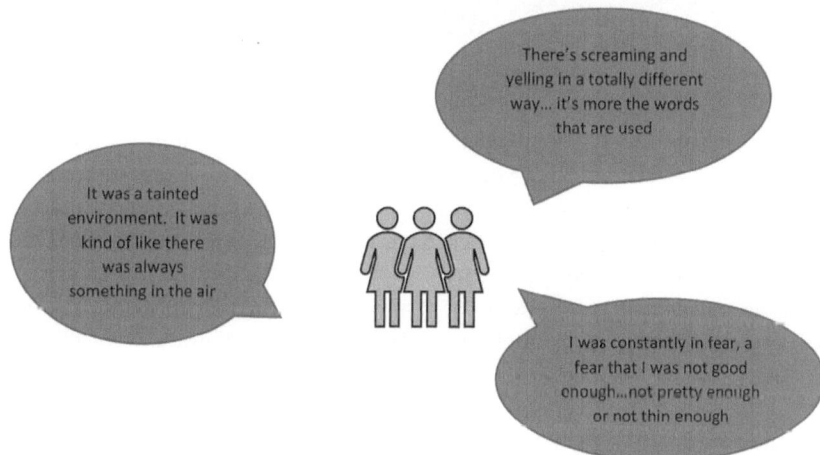

FIGURE 14.2 Athlete reflections of their experiences with abusive coaches
Source: Adapted from Kerr et al. (2020)

This small selection of quotations illustrate the way these emotionally abusive coaching environments made the athletes feel, from always feeling on edge to self-doubt and fear. Likewise, later research by Willson and Kerr (2022) explored body shaming as a form of emotional abuse, within female national level athletes from aesthetic sports. They concluded that coaches would use methods such as body shaming to control athletes' weight and in turn this was a form of abuse. Findings such as this indicate that some coaches seem unlikely to know the right way to communicate with athletes and rather than consider the process focus on the outcome of getting the athlete to lose weight.

Social media and female athletes

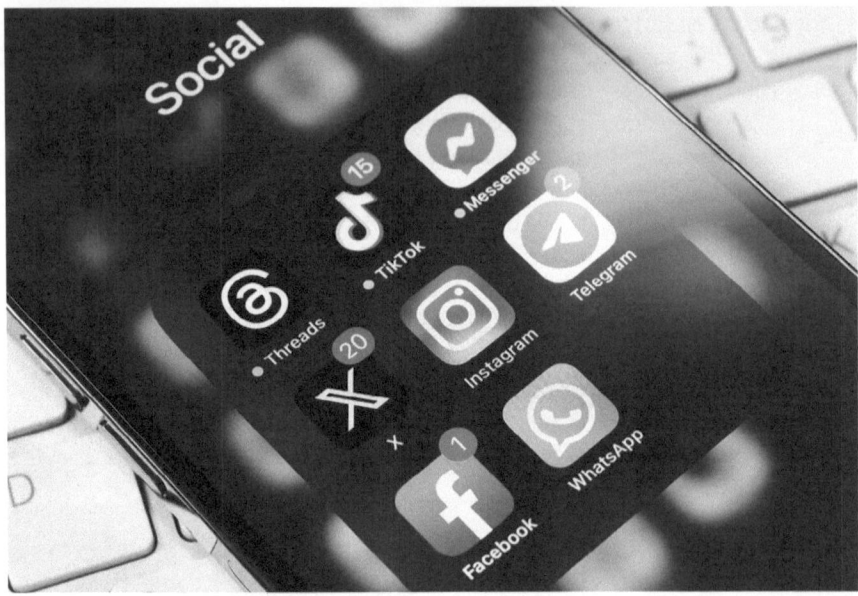

The era of social media has seen yet another communication method that must be considered when working with athletes. This medium of communication has allowed athletes to be directly connected to their fans and be in charge of the messages they send, however, they have no control over the response. While these channels have seen a different way for athletes to gain publicity they also illustrate another avenue that may result in negative psychological responses. To protect themselves from the potential negative responses, research within this area has found that female athletes are often less open than their male counterparts when engaging with media, owing to concerns over public scrutiny which can potentially have an impact on their confidence and self-image (Kovacs and Doczi, 2020). However, somewhat ironically the main motivations for their self presentation on social media are to both seek approval and avoid disapproval (Li et al., 2021).

The impact of messages on athletes was discussed by The Australian Olympic Committee who noted how both negative feedback from the public and online bullying can all result in negative emotions (Australian Olympic Committee, 2015). There is limited research addressing this with female athletes, however, the impact of this is seen in the 2018 study by Smith et al. which examined the impact of social media on male cricket captains and found that the 24-hour nature of social media can make it more of a stressor than traditional media channels and in turn intensify the level of scrutiny athletes felt they were under.

The impact of social media at major sport events was the focus of research by Hayes et al. (2020) and interviews with both male and female athletes on the athlete's perception of social media found the use of social media to be a distraction diverting athletes' attention from their sport. They also concluded that unwanted messages increased the likelihood of negative emotions, making the athletes feel as though they weren't good enough. A further point raised in their research was that athletes looked at their competitor's social media which served to increase anxiety and stress. The research drew some helpful conclusions for managers and coaches which are summarised below:

- Organisations need to better support athletes about when they should and should not engage with social media.
- Practitioners should consider strategies that allow the filtering of social media content.
- Athletes need support to develop appropriate coping strategies to help with the impact of social media responses.
- Social support is key to athletes coping with the social media pressures.
- Development of resilience is key to allow athletes to cope with pressure including those related to social media.

(Hayes et al., 2020)

As well as the more general negative comments that athletes may experience on social media Kavanagh et al. (2016) noted that of growing concern are the more universally recognised forms of abuse that may take place online. Geurin (2017) also examined this and noted how female athletes are often subject to direct sexist remarks either privately or on posts they have made which have negative implications and can make the athletes feel very uncomfortable. These negative impacts of social media are also seen throughout recreational sport with Prichard et al. (2020) examining women's interaction with Instagram finding that those exposed to images pertaining to 'fit-spiration' (a motivator to improve health and fitness) tended to have higher levels of body dissatisfaction and negative mood. Findings such at this present an area that coaches need to consider, owing to the potential impact on the athlete, including mood and general behaviour, and presents a further complexity to consider.

BOX 14.4 REAL-WORLD APPLICATIONS

As a female athlete, you should:

- Be open with your coach about your preferred means of communication and coaching and if things aren't working talk to them.
- Acknowledge that a strong coach/athlete relationship can take some time to develop as a coach needs to understand the athlete and vice versa.
- Recognise your relationship with social media and identify if it is helpful or a hindrance and consider how you interact with it moving forward.
- Understand that bullying or abusive behaviour by a coach is not normal and should not be tolerated.

As a coach, you should:

- Develop your understanding of each athlete's preferred coaching style and how involved they want to be in the decision-making process.
- Reflect on your own unconscious bias when coaching athletes.
- Focus on developing an open coaching environment in which you are authentic, genuine, honest empathetic and non-judgemental.
- Facilitate the development of a positive coach/athlete relationship by ensuring that your athletes feel cared for.
- Strive to develop a mutually respectful environment that sees the appropriate balance of power between athlete and coach.
- Call out any signs of abusive practice by other coaches to prevent it being normalised.

Summary

Throughout this chapter we have examined a number of factors related to the psychology of coaching women in sport. The differences in preferred coaching style and the importance of developing positive communication strategies illustrate how female athletes may need coaches to tailor their interactions and understand their individual needs. Furthermore, the importance of the coach/ athlete relationship highlights how this is most beneficial when there is mutuality and effective interpersonal exchanges. This relationship is perhaps of even more importance for male coaches working with female athletes, owing to the range of factors that are unique to women, for example preferred coaching style and the menstrual cycle. No chapter looking at coaching can avoid the fact that sport remains heavily gendered and as such is an arena where power imbalances are often apparent. These need to be acknowledged and addressed to avoid positions where coaches hold all of the power and athletes are acquiescent. Finally, the impact of social media on athletes' self-perception must be considered by coaches as this can impact on their emotional wellbeing.

The key messages to take away from this chapter are:

- Female athletes tend to prefer a more democratic style of coaching where they have some input and control of their training.
- Women will tend to adopt different motivational factors to men and it is important to consider this when coaching.
- A person-centred approach to coaching will allow a coach to tailor their practice to the athlete and meet their needs.
- There are a range of psychological differences between the sexes that need to be considered, such as those related to confidence and anxiety.

- The development of a positive coach/athlete relationship is key to positive athletic development through the successful transfer of knowledge.
- There remains gender imbalance within sport which can see female athletes experience ineffective coaching, inequality or emotional abuse.
- Social media is a factor to consider when coaching women as the public scrutiny can have an impact on self-image, confidence and in turn mental health.

End-of-Chapter Quiz

Answers can be found after the References

1. What coaching style do female athletes prefer?

   a   Mixed
   b   Autocratic
   c   Democratic
   d   No preference.

2. Which of the following factors is NOT key to creating an open coaching environment?

   a   Congruence
   b   Judgement
   c   Empathy
   d   Unconditional positive regard

3. Men tend to exhibit more anxiety than female athletes.

   a   True
   b   False

4. The coach/athlete relationship is a/an _____ relationship:

   a   Independent
   b   Challenging
   c   Interdependent
   d   Autonomous

5. Which of the following sentences best summarises how a coaching relationship should work?

   a   It is preferable that coaches hold the power in the coach/athlete relationship so that the best decisions are made.
   b   Athletes should do what the coach tells them and not question their methods as this can lead to time wasting.
   c   Coaches should work with athletes to identify the preferred coaching style and understand their needs.
   d   It is normal for coaches to get upset and shout at their athletes as a way to ensure they get results.

References

Amemiya, R. and Sakairi, Y. (2020) The role of self-compassion in athlete mindfulness and burnout: Examination of the effects of gender differences. *Personality and Individual Differences*, 166, 110167.

Australian Olympic Committee (2015) Athletes prepare for social media distraction. www.olympics.com.au.

Brown, C.J., Webb, T.L., Robinson, M.A. and Cotgreave, R. (2018) Athletes' experiences of social support during their transition out of elite sport: An interpretive phenomenological analysis. *Psychology of Sport and Exercise*, 36, 71–80.

Cherubini, J. (2019) Strategies and communication skills in sports coaching. In M.H. Anshel, T.A. Petrie, and J.A. Steinfeldt (Eds), *APA handbook of sport and exercise psychology*, Vol. 1. Sport psychology, pp. 451–467. American Psychological Association.

Clarke, A., Govus, A. and Donaldson, A. (2021) What male coaches want to know about the menstrual cycle in women's team sports: Performance, health, and communication. *International Journal of Sports Science & Coaching*, 16(3), 544–553.

Correia, M. and Rosado, A. (2019) Anxiety in athletes: Gender and type of sport differences. *International Journal of Psychological Research*, 12(1), 9–17.

Davis, L., Jowett, S. and Tafvelin, S. (2019) Communication strategies: The fuel for quality coach-athlete relationships and athlete satisfaction. *Frontiers in psychology*, 10, 2156.

De Haan, D. and Knoppers, A. (2020) Gendered discourses in coaching high-performance sport. *International Review for the Sociology of Sport*, 55(6), 631–646.

De Haan, D. and Sotiriadou, P. (2019) An analysis of the multi-level factors affecting the coaching of elite women athletes. *Managing Sport and Leisure*, 24(5), 307–320.

Egli, T., Bland, H.W., Melton, B.F. and Czech, D.R. (2011) Influence of age, sex, and race on college students' exercise motivation of physical activity. *Journal of American College Health*, 59(5), 399–406.

Fletcher, D. (2018) Psychological resilience and adversarial growth in sport and performance. In *Oxford Research Encyclopedia of Psychology*.

Geurin, A.N. (2017) Elite female athletes' perceptions of new media use relating to their careers: A qualitative analysis. *Journal of Sport Management*, 31(4), 345–359.

Groom, R., Cushion, C. and Nelson, L. (2012) Analysing coach–athlete "talk in interaction" within the delivery of video-based performance feedback in elite youth soccer. *Qualitative Research in Sport, Exercise and Health*, 4(3), 439–458.

Hayes, M., Filo, K., Geurin, A. and Riot, C. (2020) An exploration of the distractions inherent to social media use among athletes. *Sport Management Review*, 23(5), 852–868.

Hays, K, Maynard, I, Thomas, O. and Bawden, M. (2007) Sources and types of confidence identified by world class sports performers. *Journal of Applied Sport Psychology*, 19, 434–456.

Herrero, C.P., Jejurikar, N. and Carter, C.W. (2021) The psychology of the female athlete: how mental health and wellness mediate sports performance, injury and recovery. *Annals of Joint*, 6.

Hobson, W. and Boren, C. (2018) Michigan State settles with Larry Nassar victims for $500 million. *The Washington Post*.

Jowett, S. (2007) Interdependence Analysis and the 3+1Cs in the Coach-Athlete Relationship. In S. Jowette and D. Lavallee (Eds), *Social Psychology in Sport*, pp. 15–27. Human Kinetics.

Jowett, S., and Poczwardowski, A. (2007) Understanding the Coach-Athlete Relationship. In S. Jowette and D. Lavallee (Eds), *Social Psychology in Sport*, pp. 3–14. Human Kinetics.

Kavanagh, E., Jones, I. and Sheppard-Marks, L. (2016) Towards typologies of virtual maltreatment: Sport, digital cultures & dark leisure. *Leisure Studies*, 35(6), 783–796.

Kerr, G., Willson, E. and Stirling, A. (2020) "It was the worst time in my life": The effects of emotionally abusive coaching on female Canadian national team athletes. *Women in Sport and Physical Activity Journal*, 28(1), 81–89.

Kovacs, A. and Doczi, T. (2020) Elite athletes and media appearances: opportunity or obligation? *Sport in Society*, 23(7), 1136–1145.

Lau, E.S., Chung, H.J. and Hwa, M.C.Y. (2020) Voices of Singapore national beach volleyball female athletes: What is an ideal coach? *International Journal of Sports Science & Coaching*, 15(5–6), 642–652.

Levi, H., Wadey, R., Bunsell, T., Day, M., Hays, K. and Lampard, P. (2023) Women in a man's world: Coaching women in elite sport. *Journal of Applied Sport Psychology*, 35 (4), 571–597.

Li, B., Scott, O.K., Naraine, M.L. and Ruihley, B.J. (2021) Tell me a story: Exploring elite female athletes' self-presentation via an analysis of Instagram stories. *Journal of Interactive Advertising*, 21(2), 108–120.

Marino, K.R., Vishnubala, D., Ahmed, O.H., Zondi, P.C., Whittaker, J.L., Shafik, A., Le, C.Y., Chatterjee, D., Odulaja, A., Jones, N.E. and Thornton, J.S. (2021) Embrace your discomfort: leadership and unconscious bias in sport and exercise medicine. *British Journal of Sports Medicine*, 55(6), 303–304.

Moradi, J., Bahrami, A. and Amir, D. (2020) Motivation for participation in sports based on athletes in team and individual sports. *Physical Culture and Sport*, 85(1), 14–21.

Nelson, L., Cushion, C.J., Potrac, P. and Groom, R. (2014) Carl Rogers, learning and educational practice: Critical considerations and applications in sports coaching. *Sport, Education and Society*, 19(5), 513–531.

Norman, L. and French, J. (2013) Understanding how high performance women athletes experience the coach-athlete relationship. *International Journal of Coaching Science*, 7, 3–24.

Özdemir, N. (2019) The investigation of elite athletes' psychological resilience. *Journal of Education and Training Studies*, 7(10).

Pitchers, G. and Elliot-Sale, K. (2019) Considerations for coaches training female athletes. *Prof Strength Cond*, 55, 19–30.

Pluhar, E and McCracker, C. (2019) Team Sport Athletes May Be Less Likely To Suffer Anxiety or Depression than Individual Sport Athletes. *J Sports Sci Med*, 18, 490–496.

Prichard I., Kavanagh E., Mulgrew K.E., *et al.* (2020) The effect of Instagram #fitspiration images on young women's mood, body image, and exercise behaviour. *Body Image*, 33, 1–6.

Shipherd, A.M., Wakefield, J.C., Stokowski, S. and Filho, E. (2019) The influence of coach turnover on student-athletes' affective states and team dynamics: An exploratory study in collegiate sports. *International Journal of Sports Science & Coaching*, 14 (1), 97–106.

Smith, M.J., Arnold, R. and Thelwell, R.C. (2018) "There's no place to hide": exploring the stressors encountered by elite cricket captains. *Journal of Applied Sport Psychology*, 30(2), 150–170.

Stafford, A., Alexander, K. and Fry, D. (2015) "There was something that wasn't right because that was the only place I ever got treated like that": Children and young people's experiences of emotional harm in sport. *Childhood*, 22(1), 121–137.

Tekavc, J., Wylleman, P. and Cecić Erpič, S. (2020) Becoming a mother-athlete: female athletes' transition to motherhood in Slovenia. *Sport in Society*, 23(4), 734–750.

Wałach-Biśta, Z.M. (2019) What do we want and what do we get from the coach? Preferred and perceived leadership in male and female team sports. *Human movement*, 20 (3), 38–47.

Willson, E. and Kerr, G. (2022) Body shaming as a form of emotional abuse in sport. *International journal of sport and exercise psychology*, 20(5), 1452–1470.

Answers

1. c
2. b
3. b
4. c
5. c

INDEX

Note: *Italic* page numbers refer to *figures* and **bold** page numbers reference to **tables**.